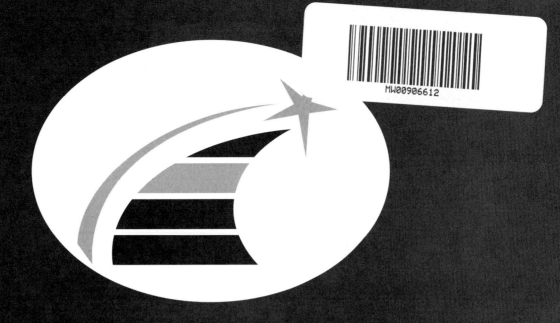

Step 3: Certify

"The average salary across the board is 17% higher for a certified coder."

— AAPC Salary Survey, 2007

Congratulations on reaching the certification step in your career! As you know, certified coders are in top demand in today's marketplace. That's why, as a lifelong coder and educator, I have dedicated myself to providing the most up-to-date, comprehensive, and user-friendly certification review books on the market. I update this book every year so you will have the best tool possible when studying for your certification exam. It's time to hit the books. ***You can do it! I know you can!***

— Carol J. Buck, MS, CPC-I, CPC, CPC-H, CCS-P

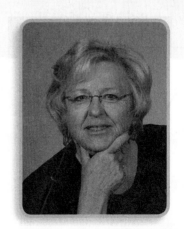

Track your progress!

See the checklist in the back of this book
to learn more about your next step toward coding success!

80265

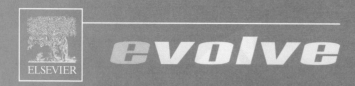

ELSEVIER

evolve

∴ *To access your Student Resources, visit:*

http://evolve.elsevier.com/Buck/ccs/

Evolve® Student Resources for *Buck: CCS Coding Exam Review 2009: The Certification Step* offer the following features:

Student Resources

- **Study Tips**
  Thoughts and advice from the author to help medical coding students.

- **Content Updates**
  The latest content updates from the author to keep you current with recent developments in this area.

- **WebLinks**
  Links to places of interest on the web specific to your needs.

- **HCPCS and ICD-9-CM Updates**
  The latest developments and rules for these coding sets.

CCS CODING EXAM REVIEW

The Certification Step

2009

CCS CODING EXAM REVIEW

The Certification Step

CAROL J. BUCK
MS, CPC-I, CPC, CPC-H, CCS-P
Program Director, Retired
Medical Secretary Programs
Northwest Technical College
East Grand Forks, Minnesota

Karla R. Lovaasen, RHIA, CCS, CCS-P
Coding and Consulting Services
Abingdon, Maryland

Debra Kroll, RHIT
Altru Health System
Grand Forks, North Dakota

Judith Neppel, RN, MS
Executive Director
Minnesota Rural Health Association
University of Minnesota, Crookston
Crookston, Minnesota

Marilyn Rasmussen, RHIA, CPC
Coding, Reimbursement, Compliance Specialist
Albert Lea, Minnesota

Cynthia Stahl, CPC, CCS-P, CPC-H
Reimbursement and Coding Specialist
Lebanon, Indiana

SAUNDERS

ELSEVIER

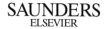

11830 Westline Industrial Drive
St. Louis, Missouri 63146

CCS CODING EXAM REVIEW 2009:　　　　　　　ISBN: 978-1-4160-3686-9
THE CERTIFICATION STEP

Notice

Neither the Publisher nor the Author assumes any responsibility for any loss or injury and/or damage to persons or property arising out of or related to any use of the material contained in this book. It is the responsibility of the treating practitioner, relying on independent expertise and knowledge of the patient, to determine the best treatment and method of application for the patient.

The Publisher

NOTE: *Current Procedural Terminology, 2009,* was used in updating this text.

Current Procedural Terminology (CPT) is copyright 2008 American Medical Association. All Rights Reserved. No fee schedules, basic units, relative values, or related listings are included in CPT. The AMA assumes no liability for the data contained herein. Applicable FARS/DFARS restrictions apply to government use.

Library of Congress Cataloging-in-Publication Data

CCS coding exam review 2009 : the certification step / Carol J. Buck . . . [et al.]. — 2009 ed.
　　p. ; cm.
　Includes index.
　ISBN 978-1-4160-3686-9 (pbk. : alk. paper)　1. Nosology—Code numbers—Examinations, questions, etc.　2. Diseases—Code numbers—Examinations, questions, etc.　3. Medical records—Management—Examinations, questions, etc.　I. Buck, Carol J.
　[DNLM:　1. Anatomy—classification—Examination Questions.　2. Disease—classification—Examination Questions.　3. Forms and Records Control—Examination Questions.　4. International Classification of Diseases—Examination Questions. 5. Terminology as Topic—Examination Questions.　WB 18.2 C386 2009]
　RB115.C38 2009
　616.001′2—dc22

　　　　　　　　　　　　　　　　　　　　　　　　　　2008036691

Publisher: Michael S. Ledbetter
Developmental Editor: Joshua S. Rapplean
Publishing Services Manager: Melissa Lastarria
Publishing Services Manager: Pat Joiner-Myers
Senior Designer: Renee Duenow
Senior Designer: Amy Buxton

Printed in Canada

Last digit is the print number:　9　8　7　6　5　4　3　2　1

Dedication

*To coding instructors,
who each day strive to enhance the lives
of their students and provide the next generation
of knowledgeable medical coders.
Karla Lovaasen, a dedicated educator
with superlative expertise in diagnosis coding,
who is always willing to share that knowledge.
She is a credit to the coding profession.*

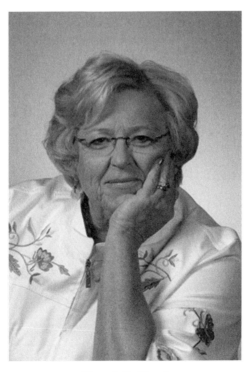

Carol J. Buck

Acknowledgments

There are so many, many people who participated in the development of this text, and only through the effort of all of the team members has it been possible to publish this text. **Karla R. Lovaasen** and **Debbie Kroll,** who have been a steady guiding presence through the development of the text and who never failed to keep the faith during the journey. **Judith Neppel,** whose exceptional knowledge of medical terminology, anatomy, and pathophysiology improved the material greatly.

    Sally Schrefer, Executive Vice President, Nursing and Health Professions, who possesses great listening skills and the ability to ensure the publication of high-quality educational materials. **Andrew Allen,** Vice President and Publisher, Health Professions, who sees the bigger picture and shares the vision. **Michael Ledbetter,** Publisher, who maintains an excellent sense of humor and is a valued member of the team who can always be depended upon for reasoned judgment. **Josh Rapplean,** Developmental Editor, who has taken over the developmental duties of this text with calm, confidence, and tremendous efficiency. **Laura Slown Sullivan,** Production Editor, Graphic World, who assumed responsibility for many projects while maintaining a high degree of professionalism. The employees of Elsevier have participated in the publication of this text and demonstrated the highest levels of professionalism and competence.

Preface

Thank you for purchasing *CCS Coding Exam Review 2009: The Certification Step,* the latest guide to the CCS certification examination. This 2009 edition has been carefully reviewed and updated with the latest content, making it the most current guide for your review. The author and publishers have made every effort to equip you with skills and tools you will need to succeed on the examination. To this end, this review guide endeavors to present essential information about all health care coding systems, anatomy, terminology, and pathophysiology, as well as sample examinations for practice. No other review guide on the market brings together such thorough coverage of all necessary examination material in one source.

ORGANIZATION OF THIS TEXTBOOK

Following a basic outline approach, *CCS Coding Exam Review 2009* takes a practical approach to assisting you with your examination preparations. The text is divided into four units—Anatomy, Terminology, and Pathophysiology; Reimbursement Issues and Data Quality; Overview of CPT, ICD-9-CM, and HCPCS Coding; and Coding Challenge—and there are several appendices for your reference. Additionally, there is a bound-in CD-ROM that is used in conjunction with the text to provide you with examinations to help your progress.

Unit I, Anatomy, Terminology, and Pathophysiology Covers all the essential body systems and terms you'll need to get certified. Organized by body systems, the sections also include illustrations to review each major anatomical area and quizzes to check your understanding and recall.

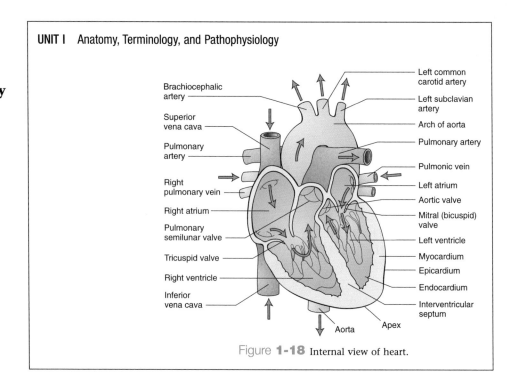

UNIT I   Anatomy, Terminology, and Pathophysiology

Figure **1-18** Internal view of heart.

Unit II, Reimbursement Issues and Data Quality Provides a review of important insurance and billing information to help you review the connections between medical coding, insurance, billing, and reimbursement.

UNIT II   Reimbursement Issues and Data Quality

CPT/ HCPCS	Description	Status Indicator	APC	Relative Weight	Payment Rate	Minimum Unadjusted Copayment
10060	Drainage of skin abscess	T	0006	1.4066	$89.59	$17.92
10061	Drainage of skin abscess	T	0006	1.4066	$89.59	$17.92
1006F	Osteoarthritis assess	M				
1007F	Anti-inflm/anlgsc otc assess	M				
10080	Drainage of pilonidal cyst	T	0006	1.4066	$89.59	$17.92
10081	Drainage of pilonidal cyst	T	0007	11.5594	$736.26	$147.25
1008F	Gi/renal risk assess	M				
P9038	RBC irradiated	K	9505	3.0643	$195.18	$39.04
P9039	RBC deglycerolized	K	9504	5.4516	$347.23	$69.45
P9040	RBC leukoreduced irradiated	K	0969	3.7722	$240.27	$48.05

Figure **2-5** APC payment rate and co-insurance amount.

Unit III, Overview of CPT, ICD-9-CM, and HCPCS Coding
Contains comprehensive coverage of the different coding systems and their applications, making other references unnecessary! Simplified text and clear examples are the highlights of this unit, while illustrations are included to clarify difficult concepts.

Embolectomy and Thrombectomy (34001-34490)

Embolus: Dislodged thrombus

Thrombus: Mass of material in vessel located in place of formation

• May be removed by dissection or balloon

Balloon: Threaded into vessel, inflated under mass, pulled out with mass

• Codes are divided by site of incision and artery/vein

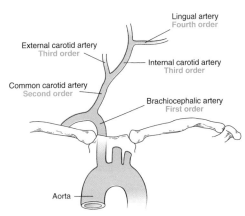

Figure 3-7 Brachiocephalic vascular family with first-, second-, third-, and fourth-order vessels.

Unit IV, Coding Challenge
Contains the types of cases found on the CCS examination. These cases will be used in conjunction with electronic answer sheets, just like the actual examination.

■ PRE-/POST-EXAMINATION

PART II

With the use of a medical dictionary, CPT, and HCPCS and ICD-9-CM coding manuals, assign codes to the following:

1. **CASE 1**

   LOCATION: Inpatient hospital

   PREOPERATIVE DIAGNOSIS: Normal pressure hydrocephalus, obstructed ventriculoperitoneal shunt

   PROCEDURE PERFORMED: Revision of shunt. Replacement of ventricular valve and peritoneal end. Entire shunt replacement.

   PROCEDURE: Under general anesthesia, the patient's head, neck, and abdomen were prepped and draped in the usual manner. An incision was made over the previous site where the shunt had been inserted in the posterior right occipital area. This shunt was found to be nonfunctioning and was removed. The problem was that we could not get the ventricular catheter out without probably producing bleeding, so it was left inside. The peritoneal end of the shunt was then pulled out through the same incision. Having done this, I placed a new ventricular catheter into the ventricle. I then attached this to a medium-pressure bulb valve and secured this with 3-0 silk to the subcutaneous tissue. We then went to the abdomen and made an incision below the previous site, and we were able to trocar the peritoneal end of the shunt by making a stab wound in the neck, then connecting it up to the shunt. This was then connected to the shunt. By pumping on the shunt, we got fluid coming out the other end. I then inserted this end of the shunt into the abdomen by dividing the rectus fascia, splitting the muscle, and dividing the peritoneum and placing the shunt into the abdomen. One 2-0 chromic suture was used around the peritoneum. The wound was then closed with 2-0 Vicryl, 2-0 plain in the subcutaneous tissue, and surgical staples on the skin. The stab wound on the neck was closed with surgical staples. The head wound was closed with 2-0 Vicryl on the galea and surgical staples on the skin. A dressing was applied. The patient was discharged to the recovery room.

ABOUT THE CD-ROM

The companion CD-ROM included in the back of this review guide contains valuable software to assist you with your preparation for the CCS coding certification examination. It includes two timed and scored 73-question examinations, modeled after the actual certification examination that contains two major sections. The Pre-Examination must be completed at the start of your study. After your study is complete, the same examination is to be taken again as the Post-Examination. By comparing the results of both examinations, you can see your improvement after using the review guide. Once you check your scores, you are ready to take the Final Examination.

Summary Screen

When using the program, the Summary screen serves as home base. Here you can find information relating to your progress and performance in different examination sections and subject areas. From this screen, you can choose an examination mode, submit an examination section, check your progress, or review your results.

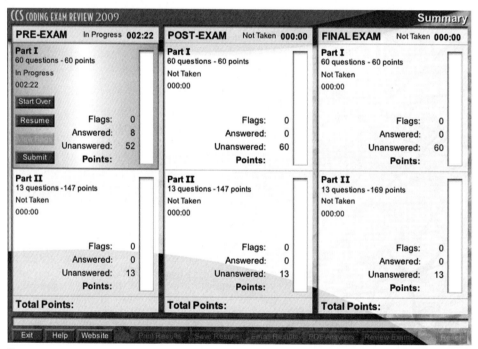

Summary screen.

In addition to displaying your scores for completed sections and tracking the total elapsed time, this screen also shows the answered, unanswered, and flagged questions in each subsection. You can return to the Summary screen at any point while taking or reviewing an examination, and all information related to your answers and position is saved.

Taking the Examination

Part I can be taken using the mouse by clicking the letter buttons to select answers and navigation buttons to move from question to question. You may also use the keyboard to type the letter that corresponds to the answer (A, B, C, D) and the left and right arrow keys to navigate. For Part II, codes can be typed into the electronic answer sheet as you read through the case in the textbook. Your answers will be saved when you close the answer sheet.

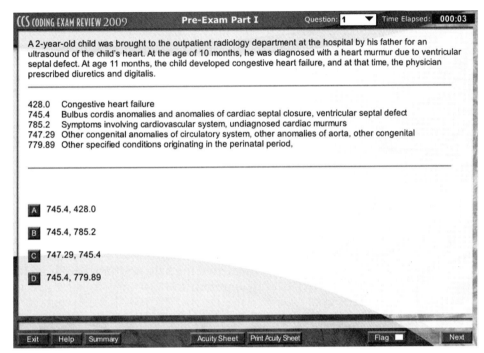

Question screen.

The screen also displays the current question number, which doubles as a pull-down menu that allows you to jump to any question in the current section. An X mark next to a question number in that menu indicates unanswered and flagged questions. The Flag button at the bottom of the screen allows you to mark questions for later reference.

Reviewing Your Results

Once you have taken the Post-Examination on the CD-ROM, you have the option to review all the examination questions with rationales, even the ones you answered correctly. The correct answer is shown for each question, and a rationale is given for each answer option. You can also compare your results on the Pre- and Post-Examinations by viewing the bar graph on the Summary screen or printing out a score sheet.

Additional instructions and help files are included on the CD-ROM to assist you in using the software.

SUPPLEMENTAL RESOURCES

However you decide to prepare for the certification examination, we have developed supplements designed to complement the *CCS Coding Exam Review 2009*. Each of these supplements has been developed with the needs of both students and instructors in mind.

Instructor's Electronic Resource

No matter what your level of teaching experience, this total-teaching solution will help you plan your lessons with ease, and the author has developed all the curriculum materials necessary to use the textbook in the classroom. This CD-ROM includes additional unit quizzes, a course calendar and syllabus, lesson plans, ready-made tests for easy assessment, and PDF files with the questions and answers for the Pre-/Post- and Final Examinations. Also included is a comprehensive PowerPoint collection of the entire text and ExamView test banks. The PowerPoint slides can be easily customized to support your lectures or formatted as overhead transparencies or handouts for student note-taking. The ExamView test generator will help you quickly and easily prepare quizzes and exams from the ready-made test questions, and the test banks can be customized to your specific teaching methods.

Evolve Resources

The Evolve companion website offers many resources that will extend your studies beyond the classroom. Related WebLinks offer you the opportunity to expand your knowledge base and stay current with this ever-changing field, and additional material is available for help and practice. Instructors can also download all materials available from the Instructor's Electronic Resource, as well as content updates.

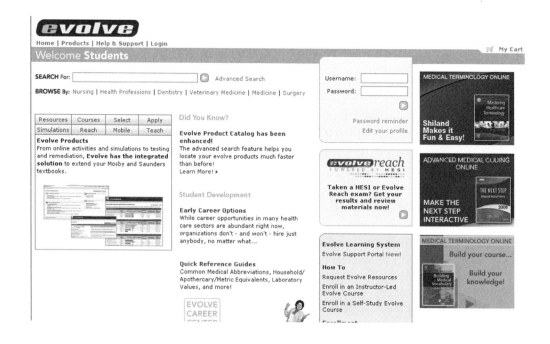

A Course Management System (CMS) is also available free to instructors who adopt this textbook. This web-based platform gives instructors yet another resource to facilitate learning and to make medical coding content accessible to students. In addition to the Evolve Resources available to both faculty and students, there is an entire suite of tools available that allows for communication between instructors and students. Students can log on through the Evolve portal to take online quizzes, participate in threaded discussions, post assignments to instructors, or chat with other classmates, while instructors can use the online grade book to follow class progress.

To access this comprehensive online resource, simply go to the Evolve home page at http://evolve.elsevier.com and enter the user name and password provided by your instructor. If your instructor has not set up a Course Management System, you can still access the free Evolve resources at http://evolve.elsevier.com/Buck/ccs/.

Development of This Edition

This book would not have been possible without a team of educators and professionals, including practicing coders and technical consultants. The combined efforts of the team members have made this text an incredible learning tool.

SENIOR ICD-9-CM CODING REVIEWER

Karla R. Lovaasen, RHIA, CCS, CCS-P*
Coding and Consulting Services
Abingdon, Maryland

*Co-author of: *ICD-9-CM Coding: Theory and Practice, 2009 Edition*, St. Louis, 2009, Saunders.

CODING SPECIALISTS

Patricia Cordy Henricksen, CPC, CCP
Approved PMCC Instructor
President, Lexington Local Chapter of AAPC
Bluegrass Medical Managers Association
Lexington, Kentucky

Jody Klitz, CPC
Coding Reimbursement Specialist
Cancer Center of North Dakota
Grand Forks, North Dakota

Debra Kroll, RHIT
Altru Health System
Grand Forks, North Dakota

Marilyn Rasmussen, RHIA, CPC
Coding, Reimbursement, Compliance Specialist
Albert Lea, Minnesota

Mary Silver-Smith, CCS, CCS-P, CPC, CPC-H, CCP-P
Senior Consultant
KForce
Hampstead, North Carolina

Patricia Harrison Skibbe
Welcoming Officer
AAPC Richardson, Texas, Chapter
Richardson, Texas

Cynthia Stahl, CPC, CCS-P, CPC-H
Reimbursement and Coding Specialist
Lebanon, Indiana

Jane Tuttle, CPC-I, CCS-P
Coding Education Endeavors
Westford, Massachusetts

TERMINOLOGY SPECIALIST

Judith Neppel, RN, MS
Executive Director
Minnesota Rural Health Association
University of Minnesota, Crookston
Crookston, Minnesota

Contents

Success Strategies, S-1

Course Syllabus and Student Calendar, C-1

Unit I   Anatomy, Terminology, and Pathophysiology, 1

1   **Integumentary System**
Integumentary System—Anatomy and Terminology, 2
Integumentary System Anatomy and Terminology Quiz, 7
Integumentary System—Pathophysiology, 9
Integumentary System Pathophysiology Quiz, 27

2   **Musculoskeletal System**
Musculoskeletal System—Anatomy and Terminology, 29
Musculoskeletal System Anatomy and Terminology Quiz, 45
Musculoskeletal System—Pathophysiology, 47
Musculoskeletal System Pathophysiology Quiz, 53

3   **Respiratory System**
Respiratory System—Anatomy and Terminology, 55
Respiratory System Anatomy and Terminology Quiz, 63
Respiratory System—Pathophysiology, 65
Respiratory System Pathophysiology Quiz, 71

4   **Cardiovascular System**
Cardiovascular System—Anatomy and Terminology, 73
Cardiovascular System Anatomy and Terminology Quiz, 83
Cardiovascular System—Pathophysiology, 85
Cardiovascular System Pathophysiology Quiz, 95

5   **Female Genital System and Pregnancy**
Female Genital System and Pregnancy—Anatomy
   and Terminology, 97
Female Genital System and Pregnancy Anatomy and Terminology
   Quiz, 105
Female Genital System and Pregnancy—Pathophysiology, 107
Female Genital System and Pregnancy Pathophysiology Quiz, 121

6   **Male Genital System**
Male Genital System—Anatomy and Terminology, 123
Male Genital System Anatomy and Terminology Quiz, 127

Contents

Male Genital System—Pathophysiology, 129
Male Genital System Pathophysiology Quiz, 139

7   Urinary System
Urinary System—Anatomy and Terminology, 141
Urinary System Anatomy and Terminology Quiz, 147
Urinary System—Pathophysiology, 149
Urinary System Pathophysiology Quiz, 159

8   Digestive System
Digestive System—Anatomy and Terminology, 161
Digestive System Anatomy and Terminology Quiz, 169
Digestive System—Pathophysiology, 171
Digestive System Pathophysiology Quiz, 189

9   Mediastinum and Diaphragm
Mediastinum and Diaphragm—Anatomy and Terminology, 191
Mediastinum and Diaphragm Anatomy and Terminology Quiz, 193

10   Hemic and Lymphatic System
Hemic and Lymphatic System—Anatomy and Terminology, 195
Hemic and Lymphatic System Anatomy and Terminology Quiz, 199
Hemic and Lymphatic System—Pathophysiology, 201
Hemic and Lymphatic System Pathophysiology Quiz, 209

11   Endocrine System
Endocrine System—Anatomy and Terminology, 211
Endocrine System Anatomy and Terminology Quiz, 217
Endocrine System—Pathophysiology, 219
Endocrine System Pathophysiology Quiz, 227

12   Nervous System
Nervous System—Anatomy and Terminology, 229
Nervous System Anatomy and Terminology Quiz, 235
Nervous System—Pathophysiology, 237
Nervous System Pathophysiology Quiz, 251

13   Senses
Senses—Anatomy and Terminology, 253
Senses Anatomy and Terminology Quiz, 261
Senses—Pathophysiology, 263
Senses Pathophysiology Quiz, 269

14   Unit I Quiz Answers, 271

UNIT II   Reimbursement Issues and Data Quality, 277

1   Reimbursement Issues, 278

2   National Correct Coding Initiative (NCCI), 285

3   Ambulatory Payment Classifications (APCs), 285

4   Prospective Payment Systems (PPS), 292

5   Medicare Severity Diagnosis Related Groups (MS-DRG), 293

6   Post Acute Transfer, 305

7   **Present on Admission Indicator (POA), 305**

8   **Revenue Codes, 308**

9   **Data Quality, 309**

10   **Medicare Fraud and Abuse, 310**

11   **Office of the Inspector General (OIG), 312**

12   **Managed Health Care, 312**

13   **Abbreviations, 315**

14   **Reimbursement Terminology, 316**

15   **Reimbursement Quiz, 319**

16   **Reimbursement Quiz Answers, 321**

UNIT III   Overview of CPT, ICD-9-CM, and HCPCS Coding, 323

1   **Introduction to Medical Coding, 324**

2   **CPT, 324**
     A.   Evaluation and Management (E/M) Section, 329
     B.   Surgery Section, 333
          1.   General Subsection, 334
          2.   Integumentary System Subsection, 335
          3.   Musculoskeletal System Subsection, 343
          4.   Respiratory System Subsection, 348
          5.   Cardiovascular (CV) System Subsection, 353
          6.   Hemic and Lymphatic System Subsection, 361
          7.   Mediastinum Subsection, 362
          8.   Diaphragm Subsection, 362
          9.   Digestive System Subsection, 362
          10. Urinary System Subsection, 363
          11. Male Genital System Subsection, 365
          12. Female Genital System Subsection, 366
          13. Maternity Care & Delivery Subsection, 369
          14. Endocrine System Subsection, 370
          15. Nervous System Subsection, 371
          16. Eye and Ocular Adnexa Subsection, 373
          17. Auditory System Subsection, 374

3   **HCPCS Coding, 375**

4   **An Overview of the ICD-9-CM, 376**
     A.   Introduction, 376
     B.   Format of ICD-9-CM, 378
     C.   ICD-9-CM Conventions, 378
     D.   Volume 2, Alphabetic Index, 379
     E.   Sections, 380
     F.   Volume 1, Tabular List, 382

5   **Using the ICD-9-CM, 383**
     A.   General Guidelines, 383
     B.   Steps to Diagnosis Coding (I/O), 383

Contents

C. Selection of Principal Diagnosis (I), 385
D. Selection of Primary Diagnosis (O), 385
E. Diagnosis and Services (I/O), 386
F. V Codes, 387
G. Section I.B.12. Late Effects (I/O), 388
H. ICD-9-CM, Chapter 1, Infectious and Parasitic Diseases (I/O), 388
I. ICD-9-CM, Chapter 2, Neoplasms (I/O), 390
J. ICD-9-CM, Chapter 3, Endocrine, Nutritional, and Metabolic Diseases and Immunity Disorders (I/O), 392
K. ICD-9-CM, Chapter 4, Diseases of Blood and Blood-Forming Organs (I/O), 393
L. ICD-9-CM, Chapter 5, Mental Disorders (I/O), 393
M. ICD-9-CM, Chapter 6, Diseases of Nervous System and Sense Organs (I/O), 394
N. ICD-9-CM, Chapter 7, Diseases of Circulatory System (I/O), 394
O. ICD-9-CM, Chapter 8, Diseases of Respiratory System (I/O), 396
P. ICD-9-CM, Chapter 9, Diseases of Digestive System (I/O), 397
Q. ICD-9-CM, Chapter 10, Diseases of Genitourinary System (I/O), 397
R. ICD-9-CM, Chapter 11, Complications of Pregnancy, Childbirth, and Puerperium (I/O), 398
S. ICD-9-CM, Chapter 12, Diseases of Skin and Subcutaneous Tissue (I/O), 400
T. ICD-9-CM, Chapter 13, Diseases of Musculoskeletal System and Connective Tissue (I/O), 400
U. ICD-9-CM, Chapters 14 and 15, Congenital Anomalies and Conditions Originating in Perinatal Period (I/O), 401
V. ICD-9-CM, Chapter 16, Symptoms, Signs, and Ill-Defined Conditions, 402
W. ICD-9-CM, Chapter 17, Injury and Poisoning, 402
X. Volume 3, Procedures, 407
Y. Volume 3, Table of Contents, 407
Z. Volume 3, Tabular List, 407
AA. Volume 3, Alphabetic Index, 407
BB. Volume 3, Tabular List, 408
CC. Bundling, 408

UNIT IV Coding Challenge, 409

1 Examinations, 410

2 Guidelines, 410

3 Pre-/Post-Examination Cases, Part II, 417

4 Final Examination Cases, Part II, 437

APPENDIX A ICD-9-CM Official Guidelines for Coding and Reporting, A-1

APPENDIX B Medical Terminology, A-94

APPENDIX C Combining Forms, A-114

APPENDIX D Prefixes, A-123

APPENDIX E   **Suffixes, A-125**

APPENDIX F   **Abbreviations, A-128**

APPENDIX G   **Further Text Resources, A-134**

APPENDIX H   **Pharmacology Review, A-137**

Index, I-1

Success Strategies

This review was developed to help you as you prepare for your certification examination. First, congratulations on your initiative. Preparing for a certification examination can seem like a daunting and formidable task. You have already taken the first and hardest step: you have made a commitment. Your steely determination and organizational skills are your best tools as you organize to complete this exciting journey successfully.

How do you prepare for a certification examination? The answers to that question are as varied as the persons preparing for a certification examination. Each person comes to the preparation with different educational, coding, and personal experiences. Therefore, each must develop a plan that meets his or her individual needs and preferences. Success Strategies will help you to develop your individual plan.

THE CERTIFICATION EXAMINATION

This text has been developed to serve as tool in your preparation for the facility-based **CCS** (Certified Coding Specialist) certification examination, offered by the American Health Information Management Association (AHIMA). The certification examination consists of two parts, covering medical terminology, anatomy, pathophysiology, CPT, ICD-9-CM Volumes 1, 2, and 3, and HCPCS. You have 4 hours to complete the computer-based examination. Visit the AHIMA website (www.ahima.org/certification) for the latest information on and content of the examination.

To be successful on the CCS certification examination, you will have to know how to assign medical codes to services and diagnoses. This textbook focuses on providing you with that coding practice as well as anatomy, terminology, pathophysiology, reimbursement, and coding concepts in preparation for the CCS examination.

Date and Location

Although every journey begins with the first step, you have to know where you are going to make a plan to get there. Historically, the CCS examination was administered only twice a year, but with the new computer-based approach, there will be more opportunities throughout the year to the take the test.

- Choose the **date and location** for taking the certification examination. The AHIMA website (www.ahima.org) provides detailed information about the examination sites and dates or contact:

  American Health Information Management Association
  Attn: CCS Examination
  233 North Michigan Avenue, Suite 2150
  Chicago, IL 60601-5800
  Telephone: 312-233-1100

- After you have downloaded the Candidate Handbook, read all the information carefully. Review all competencies outlined in the material to ensure that your study plan contains strategies to address each of these competencies.

- Check the AHIMA website to make certain you have the correct year's coding manuals.

- The questions within this textbook are not the same questions that are in the certification examinations, but the skill and knowledge that you gain through analysis, coding, and recall will increase your ability to be successful on examination day.

- The Candidate Handbook will indicate the coding specifics. For example, the levels of the evaluation and management key components (history, examination, and medical decision-making complexity) are stated in the certification questions so you will not be required to assign the levels.

MANAGING YOUR TIME

Role strain! That is what you get when you have so many different roles in your life and you cannot find time for all of them. Know that feeling? Are you a daughter/son, mother/father, wife/husband, student, friend, worker, volunteer, hobbyist? The list is endless. Each takes time from your schedule, and somehow you now need to fit into the role of successful learner. Because you have only 24 hours in your day, being a successful learner requires a time-balancing act. Maybe you will have to be satisfied with dust bunnies under your bed, dishes in your kitchen sink, or fewer visits with your friends. Whatever you have to do to juggle the time around to give yourself ample time to devote to this important task of examination preparation, you must do and make a plan for in advance; otherwise, life just takes over and you find you do not have adequate study time.

If you are planning a big event in your life—moving, a trip, and so on—think about postponing it until after the examination. Your focus right now has to be on yourself. Make your motto **"It's All About Me!"** Sounds self-centered, I know, and most likely very different from who you are, but just this once, you need to carve out the time you need to accomplish this important goal. This time is for yourself. Make it happen for yourself. Move everything you can out of the way, focus on this preparation, and give this preparation your best effort.

SCHEDULE

Each person has an individual learning style. The coding profession seems to attract those most influenced by logic and facts. The best way for a logical and factual person to learn is to problem-solve and apply the information. Hands-on practice is how you will build your skill and confidence for the examination.

- Choose a location to be your Study Central.
- Gather into Study Central the following study resources:
  - Certification information from www.ahima.org/certification
  - CPT, current edition

- ICD-9-CM Volumes 1, 2, and 3, current edition

- HCPCS, current edition

- ICD-9-CM Official Guidelines for Coding and Reporting (Appendix A of this text)

- Medical dictionary

- Coding textbooks, professional journals, and magazines

- Terminology, anatomy, or pathology text, as needed

- See Appendix G for Further Text Resources

Make Study Central your special place where you can get away from all other responsibilities. Make it a quiet, calm getaway, even if it is a corner of your bedroom. In this quiet place have a comfortable chair, adequate lighting, supplies, and sufficient desktop surface to use all your coding books. This is your place to focus all your attention on preparation for the examination, without distractions.

- Plan your **schedule** from now until the certification examination using a calendar. Make weekly goals so that you have definite tasks to accomplish each week and you can check the tasks off—a great feeling of accomplishment comes from being able to check off a task. In this way, you can see your progress on your countdown to success.

- Choose a specific **time** each day or several times a week when you are going to study, and mark them on your calendar. Make this commitment in writing. After each study session, you should check off that date on the calendar as a visual reminder that you are sticking to your plan and are one step closer to your goal.

- You should plan your study time in advance, know what you are going to be studying the next session, and **be prepared** for that upcoming study session. This will greatly increase the amount of material you are able to cover during the session. At the end of each session, decide what you are going to study next session and ensure that you have all the material and references you will need readily available. At the end of each session, you should be ready for the next study session.

- Your plan should **focus** on those areas where you know you will need improvement. For example, when is the last time you read, not referenced or reviewed, but really read, the CPT Surgery Guidelines? You may not code surgery services often, and as such are not familiar with the information in these guidelines. That is an area for improvement, and your plan should include a thorough reading of all the CPT section guidelines.

- DO THIS BEFORE YOU BEGIN YOUR STUDY: **Assess** your strengths and weaknesses. By making this assessment, you will know where to concentrate your efforts and where to focus your study schedule. You know those areas where you already have strong skills and knowledge and will not need to spend as much time preparing in these areas. The **Pre-Examination** is a 73-question examination that you can use as a tool to assess your current skill level. This examination should be taken before you begin your study and then again immediately after you have completed your entire study schedule. Do not analyze the questions by reviewing the rationales provided; rather, wait until after you have completed your studies and have taken this same examination a second time. If you review the rationales after the first time you take the examination, you will know the answers too well to provide a valid comparison between examinations. See Unit IV of this textbook for the Pre-Examination, Part II cases.

- After you have completed your course of study, take the **Post-Examination**. You should plan to cover the examination in the same amount of time as will be given for the certification examination. Compare your scores with those from the first time you took this examination. Note the areas where you did not demonstrate sufficient skills and knowledge.

- Develop a **second plan** to improve the specific areas where you believe you need further study.

- You are now ready to take the **Final Examination.** Take the examination in the same amount of time that will be allocated for the certification examination. It is best if you complete this final in one sitting, thereby mimicking the actual examination. If your schedule does not allow for taking the examination in one sitting, plan to take it in several sessions, but always keep track of the time used to ensure that you take the examination in the same amount of time allowed for the official examination. Learning to work within the time allocated is part of the skill you are developing. Remember, the certification examinations assess not only your coding knowledge but also your efficiency in completing the test within the allocated time.

USING THIS TEXT

The text is divided into:

- Success Strategies

- Unit I, Anatomy, Terminology, and Pathophysiology

- Unit II, Reimbursement Issues

- Unit III, Overview of CPT, ICD-9-CM, and HCPCS Coding

- Unit IV, Coding Challenge

- Appendix A, ICD-9-CM Official Guidelines for Coding and Reporting

- Appendix B, Medical Terminology

- Appendix C, Combining Forms

- Appendix D, Prefixes

- Appendix E, Suffixes

- Appendix F, Abbreviations

- Appendix G, Further Text Resources

- Appendix H, Pharmacology Review

Appendices B-F are combined lists of Medical Terminology, Combining Forms, Prefixes, Suffixes, and Abbreviations used within Unit I, Anatomy, Terminology, and Pathophysiology.

The material in this review features the following:

- Comprehensive guide in outline format

- Photos and drawings to illustrate key points

- Pre-/Post-Examination—73 questions (60 multiple-choice on CD, 13 cases in text)

- Final Examination—73 questions (60 multiple-choice on CD, 13 cases in text)

- **Unit I** is a review of the anatomy, terminology, and pathophysiology by organ systems designed to provide you with a quick review of that organ system. In addition, there is a list of combining forms, prefixes, suffixes, and abbreviations that are often used in that organ system. At the end of each organ system, there is a quiz that will give you an opportunity to assess your knowledge of anatomy/terminology and pathophysiology.

- **Unit II** is a review of reimbursement and data quality issues and terminology. A quiz is located at the end of the unit to assess your knowledge.

- **Unit III** is a review of CPT, HCPCS, and ICD-9-CM. The CPT and ICD-9-CM material follows the order of the manuals. There is no quiz at the end of this unit because you will be applying this material in the practice examinations and in the Final Examination.

- **Unit IV** contains directions for the examinations. The Pre-/Post-Examination is a 73-question examination located on the CD-ROM (with cases for Part II located in the textbook). The same examination should be taken twice—once before you begin your study and the second time after you have completed your study. You should allow 4 hours (240 minutes) to complete each examination because this is the amount of time you will have for the CCS examination. The computer software stores your scores and compares the results from the first and second time you took the examination; in this way, you can see not only your score on each section but also the improvement from the first to the second examination. The Final Examination is also a 73-question examination on CD-ROM (with cases for Part II located in the textbook), and you should allow 4 hours (240 minutes) to complete the examination. Both examinations are divided into the following sections:

  - **Part 1—60 Questions**

    - Medical Terminology

    - Anatomy

    - ICD-9-CM

    - HCPCS

    - Concepts of Coding and Reimbursement

    - Pathophysiology

  - **Part 2—13 Case Studies**

    - 4 ambulatory surgery cases

    - 1 emergency department case

    - 2 cardiac catheterization/interventional radiology/pain management cases

    - 6 inpatient cases

NOTE: To enable the learner to calculate an examination score, minimums have been identified as "passing" within this text; however, this may or may not be the percentage identified by AHIMA as a "passing" grade. It is your responsibility to review all certification information published by AHIMA as they are the definitive source for information regarding the CCS certification examination.

A passing score for this test is a 74% on each part. There are many ways you could use this text. Whichever way you decide to prepare, you should take the

Pre-Examination before you begin your study to ensure that you develop a study plan that includes time and activities that will increase your knowledge in those areas where your test scores indicate areas of weakness. You could then take the units in the order in which they are presented, or you may want to review the anatomy, terminology, and pathophysiology for a body system and then review the CPT material for that body system. There is no one best way for approaching the use of this text because each individual will have a personal learning style and preferences that will direct how the material is used. Your skills may be very strong in one or more coding or knowledge areas, and you will want to delete those areas from your individual study plan.

This text is not meant to be the only study source; rather, it is just one tool among many that you will use. For example, if your terminology skills need a complete overhaul, the brief overview in this text may not meet your needs. You may want to supplement this text with a terminology text and an in-depth study of terminology.

- **Appendices** are a resource for you as you prepare your study plan.

  - **Appendix A,** Official Guidelines for Coding and Reporting, is the rules for use of ICD-9-CM codes and will be referenced in Unit III during review of the use of ICD-9-CM codes.

  - **Appendix B,** Medical Terminology, is a complete alphabetic list of all the medical terms listed in the Medical Terminology portion of the organ system reviews used in Unit I.

  - **Appendix C,** Combining Forms, is a complete alphabetic list of the combining forms used in Unit I.

  - **Appendix D,** Prefixes, is a complete alphabetic list of the prefixes used in Unit I.

  - **Appendix E,** Suffixes, is a complete alphabetic list of the suffixes used in Unit I.

  - **Appendix F,** Abbreviations, is a complete list of the abbreviations referenced in Unit I.

  - **Appendix G,** Further Text References, is a list of texts that you may want to obtain to supplement your study plan.

  - **Appendix H,** Pharmacology Review, is a list of commonly prescribed pharmaceuticals

DAY BEFORE THE EXAMINATION

- No cramming! Your study time is now over, and cramming the day before the test is not a good idea because it just increases your anxiety level. This day is your day to prepare yourself. Do some things that you enjoy. Take your mind off the examination. Pamper yourself: you deserve it.

- Two forms of picture identification, CPT, ICD-9-CM (Volumes 1, 2, and 3), HCPCS code books, and optionally a medical dictionary, along with your examination admission ticket. It is your responsibility to refer to the AHIMA website to be certain you have the correct identification and books necessary to take the CCS examination. AHIMA is the final source for the examination criteria.

- You cannot have excessive writing, sticky notes, labels, and so forth in your code books. Check the examination details to ensure that your books meet the specifications identified by the testing organization.

- Review the Candidate Handbook one last time to ensure that you have all the required material.

- Listen to the weather and traffic reports. Plan your route to the examination site. If it is in a new location, drive to the location before the big day.

- Eat a light supper and get to bed early. Set the alarm in plenty of time to arrive at the site early. It is a good idea to have a friend or family member give you an early wake-up call to ensure that you do not oversleep.

DAY OF THE EXAMINATION

- Wear comfortable clothes, and be prepared for any room temperature. A short-sleeved shirt with a sweater is a good plan. Dress in layers so you can ensure that you will be comfortable in any environment.

- Take a watch with you.

- Eat a good breakfast. Avoid caffeine because it initially stimulates you but will decrease your concentration in the long run.

- Arrive early. This is a day to be early.

- Ensure that you have the correct room for your examination. Often there are several examinations being administered at one time, so be certain you are in the correct room for your examination.

THE CERTIFICATION EXAMINATION

You are ready for this! You have planned your work and have worked your plan. Now it is time to reap the rewards for all that hard work.

- Choose a good location in which to sit. Choose a location that will not get a lot of traffic from those leaving the room.

- Place approved supplies on the table.

- Have faith in yourself, and visualize yourself being successful. Say to yourself, "I can do this" and then take several deep breaths before you begin to help relax you.

- Some prefer to take the parts of the examination out of order, beginning with those questions about which they are most confident. Others prefer to start at the beginning and work through all questions in order. The approach that you use will depend on your individual test-taking style.

- When you come to a question for which you are unsure of the answer, you may wish to skip over it and come back to all those ones you were unsure of at the end of the examination, depending on the time available. Or you may want to attempt each question and mark those you are unsure of so that you can return to them when you have finished the entire examination. Again, the approach you will use depends on your individual style.

- Read the directions. This may sound too simple, but many persons do not completely read the directions, only to find that the directions gave specific directions about what or what not to code on a certain case (for example, "code only this certain portion of the procedure"). Yet the choices for answers included the full coding of the case as a selection; if you did not read all the directions, you would choose the response with codes for all the items listed in the report. For example, the question may have directed you to code the service only, not the diagnosis, and yet one of the choices would be the correct service and diagnosis codes, which of course would be an incorrect answer based on the directions. So read all of the directions.

- Your speed and accuracy are being tested. You do not have time to labor over each question for a long time if you intend to complete all the questions. Read the directions, read the question, put down your best assessment of the answer, and then move on to the next question.

- Words such as *always, every, never,* and *all* generally indicate broad terms that, with true/false questions, usually indicate a false question.

- If you do not know the answer to the question, first try eliminating those that you know are incorrect and then select the answer that seems most likely to be correct.

- Judge the time as you are moving through the examination. Keep assessing whether you are making sufficient progress or whether you can slow down or need to speed up.

- Answer all questions. Even if you have to guess, at least fill in an answer. The best situation is that you answer all questions and have time left over to go back over the questions about which you are in doubt. For the multiple-choice section of the CCS examination, the computer program has a feature that allows you to mark questions to be returned to later. When you have finished answering all the questions, the computer program gives you the option to return to just the marked questions or to all of the questions. So, fill in the answer with your best hunch and then mark the question to return to later.

- Use every minute of the test time, but it is not a good idea to begin second-guessing yourself. Do not return to those questions for which you did not have serious doubts about the correct answer. Usually, your first answer is the best.

- When the time is finished, pat yourself on the back. You have done an excellent job! Now it is time to go get a good supper and a good night's sleep.

DAYS AFTER THE EXAMINATION

- You will miss the preparation! Okay, maybe not miss it exactly, but your life will be different now without that constant preparation.

- Relax and await the results in confidence. You have done your best. That is always good enough!

- Be proud of yourself; this was no small undertaking, and you did it.

My personal best wishes to you as you prepare for your certification. You can do this!

Best regards,
Carol J. Buck, MS, CPC-I, CPC, CPC-H, CCS-P

Our goals can only be reached through a vehicle of a plan, in which we must fervently believe, and upon which we must vigorously act. There is no other route to success.

Stephen A. Brennen

Course Syllabus and Student Calendar

The following documents are the syllabus and the course calendar that would be used in a classroom setting. It is suggested that these documents be used in development of your personal educational plan.

COURSE SYLLABUS

Course Description

The focus of this class is a review of terminology, anatomy, pathophysiology, reimbursement, and data quality as a preparation to take the **CCS** coding certification examination. A review of CPT, ICD-9-CM, and HCPCS coding will be an integral part of this review course. Two practice certification review examinations will be taken under timed conditions. The course assists the learner in establishing a personal plan for continued development in preparation for a certification examination.

Texts

CCS Coding Exam Review 2009: The Certification Step, by Carol J. Buck, Elsevier

The Extra Step: Facility-Based Coding Practice, by Carol J. Buck, Elsevier

2009 ICD-9-CM, Volumes 1, 2, & 3, by Carol J. Buck, Elsevier

2009 HCPCS Level II, by Carol J. Buck, Elsevier

2009 CPT, American Medical Association

Medical dictionary

Performance Objectives

1. Write a personal plan for preparation for a certification examination.
2. Review the structure, function, terminology, pathophysiology, and abbreviations of the integumentary system.
3. Review the structure, function, terminology, pathophysiology, and abbreviations of the musculoskeletal system.

4. Review the structure, function, terminology, pathophysiology, and abbreviations of the respiratory system.

5. Review the structure, function, terminology, pathophysiology, and abbreviations of the cardiovascular system.

6. Review the structure, function, terminology, pathophysiology, and abbreviations of the female genital system and pregnancy.

7. Review the structure, function, terminology, pathophysiology, and abbreviations of the male genital system.

8. Review the structure, function, terminology, pathophysiology, and abbreviations of the urinary system.

9. Review the structure, function, terminology, pathophysiology, and abbreviations of the digestive system.

10. Review the structure, function, terminology, and abbreviations of the mediastinum and diaphragm.

11. Review the structure, function, terminology, pathophysiology, and abbreviations of the hemic and lymphatic systems.

12. Review the structure, function, terminology, pathophysiology, and abbreviations of the endocrine system.

13. Review the structure, function, terminology, pathophysiology, and abbreviations of the nervous system.

14. Review the structure, function, terminology, and abbreviations of the senses of the body.

15. Demonstrate knowledge of structure, function, terminology, pathophysiology, and abbreviations of organ systems.

16. Review medical reimbursement and data quality issues.

17. Demonstrate knowledge of medical reimbursement issues.

18. Review CPT E/M section.

19. Review CPT Surgery section.

20. Review HCPCS.

21. Review format and conventions of ICD-9-CM.

22. Review assignment of ICD-9-CM codes.

23. Review Official Guidelines for Coding and Reporting.

24. Demonstrate coding ability by assigning CPT codes.

25. Demonstrate ability to assign E/M levels to facility outpatient services.

26. Demonstrate coding ability by assigning HCPCS codes.

27. Demonstrate coding ability by assigning ICD-9-CM codes.

28. Demonstrate ability to apply reimbursement guidelines.

Personal Objectives

The student will:

- Attend class sessions.
- Prepare for class sessions.
- Complete assignments in a timely manner.
- Demonstrate a high level of responsibility.
- Display respect for other members of the class.
- Participate in class discussions.

Evaluation and Grading

- Evaluation is directly related to the performance objectives.
- Performance is measured by examination, assignments, and/or quizzes.
- The letter grade is based on the percentage of the total points earned throughout the semester based on the following scale:
  - A = 93% to 100%
  - B = 85% to 92%
  - C = 79% to 84%
  - D = 70% to 78%
  - F = 69% and below
- Examinations are scheduled in advance. To qualify for the total points on the examinations, the student must take the examination at the scheduled time. Five points will be deducted from each examination if the examination is not taken at the scheduled time. This rule reinforces the need for on-time performance. Any make-up examination must be completed within 3 days of the scheduled examination or no points will be awarded for the examination.
- Assignments are scheduled in advance. To qualify for the total points on the assignment, the student must submit the completed assignment at the scheduled time. Five points are deducted from each assignment if the assignment is not submitted at the scheduled time. This rule reinforces the need for on-time performance. Any late assignment must be completed within 3 days from the date the assignment was due or no points will be awarded for the assignment.
- Cases are due as indicated on the calendar to qualify for the total points for the case. No points will be awarded for late submission of cases.
- Quizzes are scheduled in advance. Quizzes cannot be made up, and no points are awarded for missed quizzes.

Methods of Instruction

The instructional methods used include lecture, class discussion, and assignments.

COURSE CALENDAR

Lesson 1

Reading assignment(s):	Success Strategies, pages S1-S8
Assignment(s):	Complete the Pre-Examination on the CD, and at **Lesson 3** class period, hand in your scores on the two sections for 96 points. The Pre-Examination is NOT graded if each question has been attempted. 2 points will be deducted for each question not attempted.
	Download CCS certification examination information at http://www.ahima.org/certification/
	Print one page to hand in at **Lesson 2** to demonstrate successful access to CCS information from website (10 points—nongraded)

Lesson 2

Student hand in:	One printed page to demonstrate successful access to CCS information from website (10 points—non-graded)
Reading assignment(s):	Unit 1, pages 1-54 (through Musculoskeletal System)
Assignment(s):	Develop a Personal Plan for preparation for Certification Review (20 points—graded) to be submitted at **Lesson 6** class period
	Integumentary Quizzes (24 points)
	Musculoskeletal Quizzes (24 points)
	Prepare results of Pre-Examination for **Lesson 3**
	The Extra Step: Facility-Based Coding Practice, Integumentary, Cases 1-2 (4 points)
	Orthopedic, Case 35 (2 points)

Lesson 3

Student hand in:	Integumentary Quizzes (24 points)
	Musculoskeletal Quizzes (24 points)
	Results of Pre-Examination (96 points—nongraded if each question attempted)
	The Extra Step: Facility-Based Coding Practice, Integumentary, Cases 1-2 (4 points)
	Orthopedic, Case 35 (2 points)
Reading assignment(s):	Unit 1, pages 55-121 (through Female Genital System and Pregnancy)
Assignment(s):	Respiratory Quizzes (24 points)
	Cardiovascular Quizzes (24 points)
	Female Genital System and Pregnancy Quizzes (24 points)
	The Extra Step: Facility-Based Coding Practice, Obstetric and Gynecologic Surgery and Ophthalmology, Case 30 (2 points)
	Otorhinolaryngology, Cases 42-43 (4 points)
	Cardiology, Case 106 (2 points)

Lesson 4

Student hand in:
Respiratory Quizzes (24 points)
Cardiovascular Quizzes (24 points)
Female Genital System and Pregnancy Quizzes
   (24 points)
The Extra Step: Facility-Based Coding Practice,
   Obstetric and Gynecologic Surgery and
   Ophthalmology, Case 30 (2 points)
   Otorhinolaryngology, Cases 42-43 (4 points)
   Cardiology, Case 106 (2 points)

Reading assignment(s):
Unit 1, pages 123-194 (through Mediastinum and
   Diaphragm)

Assignment(s):
Male Genital System Quizzes (24 points)
Urinary System Quizzes (24 points)
Digestive System Quiz (24 points)
Mediastinum and Diaphragm Quiz (12 points)
   (There is NO pathophysiology quiz for Mediastinum
   and Diaphragm.)
The Extra Step: Facility-Based Coding Practice,
   Gastrointestinal, Case 9 (2 points)
   Nephrology, Case 18 (2 points)

Lesson 5

Student hand in:
Male Genital System Quizzes (24 points)
Urinary System Quizzes (24 points)
Digestive System Quizzes (24 points)
Mediastinum and Diaphragm Quiz (12 points)
(There is no pathophysiology quiz for Mediastinum
   and Diaphragm.)
The Extra Step: Facility-Based Coding Practice,
   Gastrointestinal, Case 9 (2 points)
   Nephrology, Case 18 (2 points)

Reading assignment(s):
Unit 1, pages 195-228 (through Endocrine System)

Assignment(s):
Hemic and Lymphatic Quizzes (24 points)
Endocrine Quizzes (24 points)
Prepare to submit Personal Plan for Preparation
   for Certification Examination
The Extra Step: Facility-Based Coding Practice,
   Emergency Department, Cases 67-71 (10 points)

Lesson 6

Student hand in:
Hemic and Lymphatic Quizzes (24 points)
Endocrine Quizzes (24 points)
Submit Personal Plan for Preparation for Certification
   Examination (20 points—graded)
The Extra Step: Facility-Based Coding Practice,
   Emergency Department, Cases 67-71 (10 points)

Reading assignment(s):
Unit 1, pages 229-276 (to end of Unit 1)

Assignment(s):
Nervous System Quizzes (24 points)
Senses Quizzes (24 points)

Prepare for Unit 1, Anatomy, Terminology, and Pathophysiology, Test 1 (50 points, 25 questions, 15 minutes)

The Extra Step: Facility-Based Coding Practice, Neurology/Neurosurgery, Cases 23-25 (6 points)

Lesson 7

UNIT 1: ANATOMY, TERMINOLOGY, AND PATHOPHYSIOLOGY, TEST 1

Student hand in:
Nervous System Quizzes (24 points)
Senses Quizzes (24 points)
The Extra Step: Facility-Based Coding Practice, Neurology/Neurosurgery, Cases 23-25 (6 points)

Reading assignment(s):
Unit 2, pages 279-287 (to Ambulatory Payment Classifications)

Assignment(s):
The Extra Step: Facility-Based Coding Practice, General Surgery, Cases 58-60 (6 points)

Lesson 8

Student hand in:
The Extra Step: Facility-Based Coding Practice, General Surgery, Cases 58-60 (6 points)

Reading assignment(s):
Unit 2, pages 287-291 (to -CA modifier)

Assignment(s):
The Extra Step: Facility-Based Coding Practice, General Surgery, Case 61-64 (8 points)

Lesson 9

Student hand in:
The Extra Step: Facility-Based Coding Practice, General Surgery, Case 61-64 (8 points)

Reading assignment(s):
Unit 2, pages 291-303 (to CMS-1450 Claim Form)

Assignment(s):
The Extra Step: Facility-Based Coding Practice, General Surgery, Cases 65-66 (4 points)

Lesson 10

Student hand in:
The Extra Step: Facility-Based Coding Practice, General Surgery, Cases 65-66 (4 points)

Reading assignment(s):
Unit 2, pages 303-324 (to end of Unit 2)

Assignment(s):
Reimbursement Quiz (10 points)

Lesson 11

Student hand in:
None

Reading assignment(s):
Unit 3, pages 325-327 (to ASC Modifiers)
E/M Guidelines

Assignment(s):
Prepare for Unit 2, Reimbursement, Test 2 (26 points, 20 minutes)
The Extra Step: Facility-Based Coding Practice, Emergency Department, Cases 72-76 (10 points)

Lesson 12

UNIT 2: REIMBURSEMENT, TEST 2

Student hand in: *The Extra Step: Facility-Based Coding Practice,*
                              Emergency Department, Cases 72-76 (10 points)

Reading assignment(s): Unit 3, pages 327-335 (to Surgery Section)

Assignment(s):   None

Lesson 13

Student hand in: None

Reading assignment(s): Unit 3, pages 335-336 (to General Subsection)

                        Read Surgery Guidelines

Assignment(s):   *The Extra Step: Facility-Based Coding Practice,*
                              Integumentary, Cases 3-5 (6 points)

Lesson 14

Student hand in: *The Extra Step: Facility-Based Coding Practice,*
                              Integumentary, Cases 3-5 (6 points)

Reading assignment(s): Unit 3, pages 336-345 (to Musculoskeletal System
                              Subsection)

Assignment(s):   *The Extra Step: Facility-Based Coding Practice,*
                              Integumentary, Cases 6-8 (6 points)

Lesson 15

Student hand in: *The Extra Step: Facility-Based Coding Practice,*
                              Integumentary, Cases 6-8 (6 points)

Reading assignment(s): Unit 3, pages 345-350 (to Respiratory System
                              Subsection)

Assignment(s):   *The Extra Step: Facility-Based Coding Practice,*
                              Orthopedic, Cases 38-39 (4 points)
                              Otorhinolaryngology, Cases 47-48 (4 points)

Lesson 16

Student hand in: *The Extra Step: Facility-Based Coding Practice,*
                              Orthopedic, Cases 38-39 (4 points)
                              Otorhinolaryngology, Cases 47-48 (4 points)

Reading assignment(s): Unit 3, pages 350-355 (to Cardiovascular [CV] System
                              Subsection)

Assignment(s):   *The Extra Step: Facility-Based Coding Practice,*
                              Otorhinolaryngology, Cases 52-57 (12 points)

Lesson 17

Student hand in:	*The Extra Step: Facility-Based Coding Practice,* Otorhinolaryngology, Cases 52-57 (12 points)
Reading assignment(s):	Unit 3, pages 355-362 (to Hemic and Lymphatic System Subsection)
Assignment(s):	*The Extra Step: Facility-Based Coding Practice,* Cardiology, Cases 108-112 (10 points)

Lesson 18

Student hand in:	*The Extra Step: Facility-Based Coding Practice,* Cardiology, Cases 108-112 (10 points)
Reading assignment(s):	Unit 3, pages 363-368 (to Female Genital System Subsection)
Assignment(s):	*The Extra Step: Facility-Based Coding Practice,* Gastrointestinal, Cases 11-14 (8 points)

Lesson 19

Student hand in:	*The Extra Step: Facility-Based Coding Practice,* Gastrointestinal, Cases 11-14 (8 points)
Reading assignment(s):	Unit 3, pages 368-372 (to Endocrine System Subsection)
Assignment(s):	Post-Examination (97 points—nongraded if each question attempted, deduct 2 points for each unattempted question). Due at **Lesson 24** class period. *The Extra Step: Facility-Based Coding Practice,* Gastrointestinal, Cases 15-17 (6 points) Nephrology, Cases 20-22 (6 points)

Lesson 20

Student hand in:	*The Extra Step: Facility-Based Coding Practice,* Gastrointestinal, Cases 15-17 (6 points) Nephrology, Cases 20-22 (6 points)
Reading assignment(s):	Unit 3, pages 372-378 (to An Overview of the ICD-9-CM)
Assignment(s):	Prepare for Unit 3, Test 3, Surgery (26 points, 20 minutes) *The Extra Step: Facility-Based Coding Practice,* Neurology/Neurosurgery, Cases 26-27 (4 points)

Lesson 21

UNIT 3: SURGERY, Test 3

Student hand in: *The Extra Step: Facility-Based Coding Practice*,
Neurology/Neurosurgery, Cases 26-27 (4 points)

Reading assignment(s): Unit 3, pages 378-384 (to Volume 1, Tabular List)

Assignment(s): *The Extra Step: Facility-Based Coding Practice*,
Neurology/Neurosurgery, Cases 28-29 (4 points)

Lesson 22

Student hand in: *The Extra Step: Facility-Based Coding Practice*,
Neurology/Neurosurgery, Cases 28-29 (4 points)

Reading assignment(s): Unit 3, pages 384-392 (to ICD-9-CM, Chapter 2,
Neoplasms [I/O])

Assignment(s): Prepare for Unit 3, Test 4 (16 points, 15 minutes)
(requires ICD-9-CM and CPT manuals)
The Extra Step: Facility-Based Coding Practice,
Diagnostic Radiology, Cases 77-86 (20 points)
Interventional Radiology, Radiation Oncology, and
Nuclear Medicine, Cases 99-101 (6 points)

Lesson 23

UNIT 3, TEST 4

Student hand in: *The Extra Step: Facility-Based Coding Practice*,
Diagnostic Radiology, Cases 77-86 (20 points)
Interventional Radiology, Radiation Oncology, and
Nuclear Medicine, Cases 99-101 (6 points)

Reading assignment(s): Unit 3, pages 392-410 (to end of Unit 3)

Assignment(s): Prepare for Unit 3, Test 5 (15 points, 25 minutes)
(requires ICD-9-CM and CPT manuals)
Prepare Post-Examination for submission
The Extra Step: Facility-Based Coding Practice,
Diagnostic Radiology, Cases 87-88 (4 points)
Interventional Radiology, Radiation Oncology,
and Nuclear Medicine, Cases 102-105 (8 points)

Lesson 24

UNIT 3, TEST 5

Student hand in: Results of Post-Examination (as assigned in
Lesson 1) (97 points—nongraded if each
question attempted)
The Extra Step: Facility-Based Coding Practice,
Diagnostic Radiology, Cases 87-88 (4 points)
Interventional Radiology, Radiation Oncology,
and Nuclear Medicine, Cases 102-105 (8 points)

Reading assignment(s):   None

Assignment(s):   Prepare for Unit 3, Test 6 (15 points, 25 minutes) (requires ICD-9-CM and CPT manuals)
Prepare to begin Final Examination
The Extra Step: Facility-Based Coding Practice, Orthopedic, Cases 36-37 (4 points)
Inpatient, Cases 113-116 (8 points)

Lesson 25

UNIT 3, TEST 6

Begin Final Examination

Student hand in: *The Extra Step: Facility-Based Coding Practice*, Orthopedic, Cases 36-37 (4 points)
Inpatient, Cases 113-116 (8 points)

Reading assignment(s):   None

Assignment(s):   Prepare for Unit 3, Test 7 (20 points, 15 minutes) (requires ICD-9-CM and CPT manuals)
The Extra Step: Facility-Based Coding Practice, Otorhinolaryngology, Cases 44-46 (6 points)

Lesson 26

UNIT 3, TEST 7

Final Examination continues

Student hand in: *The Extra Step: Facility-Based Coding Practice*, Otorhinolaryngology, Cases 44-46 (6 points)

Reading assignment(s):   None

Assignment(s):   *The Extra Step: Facility-Based Coding Practice*, Gastrointestinal, Case 10 (2 points)
Nephrology, Case 19 (2 points)
Obstetric and Gynecologic Surgery and Ophthalmology, Case 31 (2 points)
Cardiology, Case 107 (2 points)

Lesson 27

Final Examination continues

Student hand in: *The Extra Step: Facility-Based Coding Practice*, Gastrointestinal, Case 10 (2 points)
Nephrology, Case 19 (2 points)
Obstetric and Gynecologic Surgery and Ophthalmology, Case 31 (2 points)
Cardiology, Case 107 (2 points)

Reading assignment(s):   None

Assignment(s):   *The Extra Step: Facility-Based Coding Practice*, Diagnostic Radiology, Cases 89-97 (18 points)

Lesson 28

Final Examination continues

Student hand in: *The Extra Step: Facility-Based Coding Practice,* Diagnostic Radiology, Cases 89-97 (18 points)

Reading assignment(s): None

Assignment(s): None

Lesson 29

Final Examination continues

Student hand in: None

Reading assignment(s): None

Assignment(s): *The Extra Step: Facility-Based Coding Practice,* Obstetric and Gynecologic Surgery and Ophthalmology, Cases 32-34 (6 points)

Lesson 30

Final Examination continues

Student hand in: *The Extra Step: Facility-Based Coding Practice,* Obstetric and Gynecologic Surgery and Ophthalmology, Cases 32-34 (6 points)

Reading assignment(s): None

Assignment(s): *The Extra Step: Facility-Based Coding Practice,* Orthopedic, Cases 40-41 (4 points) Otorhinolaryngology, Cases 49-51 (6 points)

Lesson 31

Complete Final Examination

Student hand in: Final Examination results
The Extra Step: Facility-Based Coding Practice, Orthopedic, Cases 40-41 (4 points) Otorhinolaryngology, Cases 49-51 (6 points)

Reading assignment(s): None

Assignment(s): None

Lesson 32

Final grade calculation

Final course evaluation

Anatomy, Terminology, and Pathophysiology

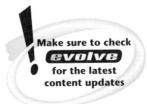

Make sure to check **evolve** for the latest content updates

■ INTEGUMENTARY SYSTEM

INTEGUMENTARY SYSTEM—ANATOMY AND TERMINOLOGY

The skin and accessory organs (nails, hair, and glands)

Layers (Fig. 1–1)

Two layers make up skin: epidermis and dermis

Epidermis. Outermost layer; containing keratin

Stratum corneum, most superficial layer of four layers called stratum

Basal layer, deepest region of epidermis (stratum germinativum or stratum basale), is growth layer

Dermis. The second layer of skin

Two layers are papillare and reticulare and contain:

> Fibrous connective tissue or skin appendages
>
> Blood vessels
>
> Nerves
>
> Hair
>
> Nails
>
> Glands

Subcutaneous Tissue or Hypodermis. Not considered a layer of skin

Contains fat tissue and fibrous connective tissue

AKA: superficial fascia

Connects skin to underlying muscle

Nails

Keratin plates covering dorsal surface of each finger and toe

Lunula—semilunar or half-moon

> White area at base of nail plate is growth area
>
> Thickens and lengthens nail
>
> Eponychium or Cuticle: narrow band of epidermis at base and sides of nail

Paronychium: soft tissue around nail border

Glands

Sebaceous glands located in dermal layer

Secrete sebum that lubricates skin/hair

Influenced by sex hormones so they hypertrophy in adolescence and atrophy in old age

Sudoriferous glands originate in dermis. See Fig. 1–1.

AKA: sweat glands

Extend up through epidermis opening as pores

Secrete mostly water and salts to cool body

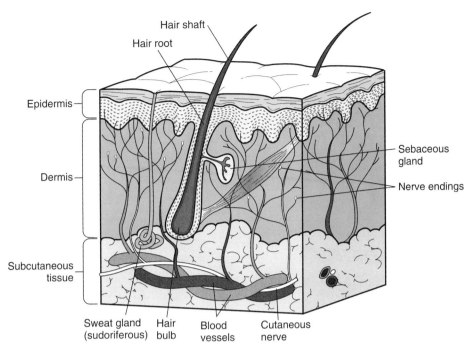

Figure **1-1** Integumentary system.

COMBINING FORMS

1.	aden/o	in relationship to a gland
2.	adip/o	fat
3.	albin/o	white
4.	aut/o	self
5.	bi/o	life
6.	caus/o	burning sensation
7.	cauter/o	burn
8.	crypt/o	hidden
9.	cutane/o	skin
10.	cyan/o	blue
11.	derm/o, dermat/o	skin
12.	diaphor/o	profuse sweating
13.	eosin/o	rosy
14.	erythem/o	red
15.	erythr/o	red
16.	heter/o	different
17.	hidr/o	sweat
18.	ichthy/o	dry/scaly
19.	jaund/o	yellow
20.	kerat/o	hard

21.	leuk/o	white
22.	lip/o	fat
23.	lute/o	yellow
24.	melan/o	black
25.	myc/o	fungus
26.	necr/o	death
27.	onych/o	nail
28.	pachy/o	thick
29.	pht/o	plant
30.	pil/o	hair
31.	poli/o	gray matter
32.	py/o	pus
33.	rhytid/o	wrinkle
34.	rube/o	red
35.	seb/o	sebum/oil
36.	staphyl/o	clusters
37.	steat/o	fat
38.	strept/o	twisted chain
39.	steat/o	fat
40.	squam/o	flat/scalelike
41.	trich/o	hair
42.	ungu/o	nail
43.	xanth/o	yellow
44.	xer/o	dry

PREFIXES

1.	epi-	on/upon
2.	hyper-	over
3.	hypo-	under
4.	intra-	within
5.	para-	beside
6.	per-	through
7.	peri-	surrounding
8.	sub-	under

SUFFIXES

1.	-coccus	spherical bacterium
2.	-ectomy	removal
3.	-ia	condition
4.	-malacia	softening
5.	-opsy	view of
6.	-plasty	surgical repair
7.	-rrhea	discharge
8.	-tome	an instrument to cut
9.	-tomy	to cut

MEDICAL ABBREVIATIONS

1.	bx	biopsy
2.	ca	cancer
3.	derm	dermatology
4.	I&D	incision and drainage
5.	subcu, subq, SC, SQ	subcutaneous
6.	PPD	tuberculin skin test

MEDICAL TERMS

Absence	Without
Adipose	Fatty
Albinism	Lack of color pigment
Allograft	Homograft, same species graft
Alopecia	Condition in which hair falls out
Anhidrosis	Deficiency of sweat
Autograft	From patient's own body
Avulsion	Ripping or tearing away of part either surgically or accidentally
Biopsy	Removal of a small piece of living tissue for diagnostic purposes
Causalgia	Burning pain
Collagen	Protein substance of skin
Debridement	Cleansing of or removal of dead tissue from a wound
Delayed flap	Pedicle of skin with blood supply that is separated from origin over time
Dermabrasion	Planing of skin by means of sander, brush, or sandpaper
Dermatologist	Physician who treats conditions of skin
Dermatoplasty	Surgical repair of skin
Electrocautery	Cauterization by means of heated instrument
Epidermolysis	Loosening of epidermis

Epidermomycosis	Superficial fungal infection
Epithelium	Surface covering of internal and external organs of body
Erythema	Redness of skin
Escharotomy	Surgical incision into necrotic (dead) tissue
Fissure	Cleft or groove
Free full-thickness graft	Graft of epidermis and dermis that is completely removed from donor area
Furuncle	Nodule in skin caused by *Staphylococci* entering through hair follicle
Hematoma	A localized collection of blood, usually result of a break in a blood vessel
Hemograft	Allograft, same species graft
Ichthyosis	Skin disorder characterized by scaling
Incise	To cut into
Island pedicle flap	Contains a single artery and vein that remains attached to origin temporarily or permanently
Leukoderma	Depigmentation of skin
Leukoplakia	White patch on mucous membrane
Lipocyte	Fat cell
Lipoma	Fatty tumor
Melanin	Dark pigment of skin
Melanoma	Tumor of epidermis, malignant and black in color
Mohs' surgery or Mohs' micrographic surgery	Removal of skin cancer in layers by a surgeon who also acts as a pathologist during surgery
Muscle flap	Transfer of muscle from origin to recipient site
Neurovascular flap	Contains artery, vein, and nerve
Pedicle	Growth attached with a stem
Pilosebaceous	Pertains to hair follicles and sebaceous glands
Sebaceous gland	Secretes sebum
Seborrhea	Excess sebum secretion
Sebum	Oily substance
Split-thickness graft	All epidermis and some of dermis
Steatoma	Fat mass in sebaceous gland
Stratified	Layered
Stratum (strata)	Layer
Subungual	Beneath nail
Xanthoma	Tumor composed of cells containing lipid material, yellow in color
Xenograft	Different species graft
Xeroderma	Dry, discolored, scaly skin

INTEGUMENTARY SYSTEM ANATOMY AND TERMINOLOGY QUIZ

1. This is the outermost layer of skin:
   a. basal
   b. dermis
   c. epidermis
   d. subcutaneous

2. Which of the following is NOT a part of skin or accessory organs:
   a. sudoriferous glands
   b. sebaceous gland
   c. nail
   d. arterioles

3. This prefix means beside:
   a. para-
   b. intra-
   c. per-
   d. epi-

4. This combining form means hair:
   a. xanth/o
   b. trich/o
   c. ichthy/o
   d. kerat/o

5. Lunula is the:
   a. narrow band of epidermis at base of nail
   b. opening of pores
   c. outermost layer of epidermis
   d. white area at base of nail plate

6. Subcutaneous tissue is also known as:
   a. dermal
   b. adipose
   c. hypodermis
   d. stratum corneum

7. Which of the following combining forms does not refer to a color?
   a. cyan/o
   b. jaund/o
   c. eosin/o
   d. pachy/o

8. This medical term means surgical incision into dead tissue:
   a. onychomycosis
   b. escharotomy
   c. keratotomy
   d. curettage

9. This suffix means surgical repair:
   a. -opsy
   b. -rrhea
   c. -plasty
   d. -tome

10. Soft tissue around nail border is the:
   a. cuticle
   b. lunula
   c. paronychium
   d. corium

INTEGUMENTARY SYSTEM—PATHOPHYSIOLOGY

Lesions and Other Abnormalities (Fig. 1–2)

Macule
Flat area of color change (mostly reddened)

No elevation or depression

> *Example:* flat moles, freckles

Papule
Solid elevation

Less than 1.0 cm in diameter

May run together and form plaques

> *Example:* warts, lichen planus, elevated mole

Nodule
Solid elevation 1-2 cm in diameter

Extends deeper into dermis than papule

> *Example:* lipoma, erythema nodosum, enlarged lymph nodes

Pustule
Elevated area

Filled with purulent fluid

> *Example:* pimple, impetigo, abscess

Tumor
Solid mass

Uncontrolled, progressive growth of cells

> *Example:* hemangioma, neoplasm, lipoma

Plaque
Flat, elevated surface

Equal or greater than 1.0 cm

> *Example:* psoriasis, seborrheic keratosis

Wheal
Temporary localized elevation of skin

Results in transient edema in dermis

> *Example:* insect bite, allergic reaction

Vesicle
Small blister

Less than 1 cm in diameter

Filled with serous fluid in epidermis

> *Example:* herpes zoster (shingles), varicella (chickenpox)

Bulla
Large blister

Greater than 1.0 cm in diameter

> *Example:* blister

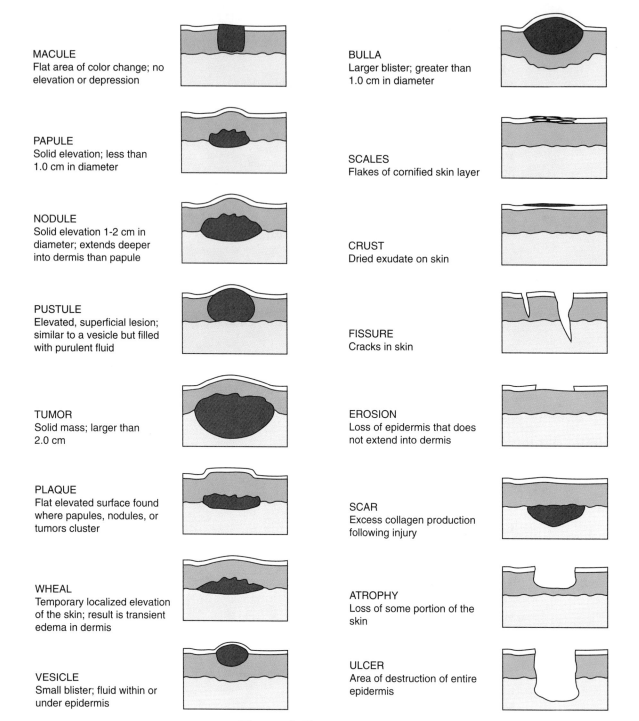

MACULE
Flat area of color change; no elevation or depression

PAPULE
Solid elevation; less than 1.0 cm in diameter

NODULE
Solid elevation 1-2 cm in diameter; extends deeper into dermis than papule

PUSTULE
Elevated, superficial lesion; similar to a vesicle but filled with purulent fluid

TUMOR
Solid mass; larger than 2.0 cm

PLAQUE
Flat elevated surface found where papules, nodules, or tumors cluster

WHEAL
Temporary localized elevation of the skin; result is transient edema in dermis

VESICLE
Small blister; fluid within or under epidermis

BULLA
Larger blister; greater than 1.0 cm in diameter

SCALES
Flakes of cornified skin layer

CRUST
Dried exudate on skin

FISSURE
Cracks in skin

EROSION
Loss of epidermis that does not extend into dermis

SCAR
Excess collagen production following injury

ATROPHY
Loss of some portion of the skin

ULCER
Area of destruction of entire epidermis

Figure **1-2** Lesions of skin.

Scales
Flakes of cornified skin layer

Example: dry skin

Crust
Dried exudate on skin

Example: scab

Fissure
Cracks in skin

Example: athlete's foot, openings in corners of mouth

Erosion
Loss of epidermis

Does not extend into dermis

Example: blisters

Scar
Excess collagen production following surgery or trauma

Example: healed surgical wound

Atrophy
Loss of some portion of skin and appears translucent

Example: aged skin

- Not a lesion, but a physiologic response in aging process

Ulcer
Area of destruction of entire epidermis

Example: missing tissue on heel, decubitus bedsore (pressure sore)

Pressure Ulcer (Decubitis Ulcer) (Fig. 1-3)
Result of pressure or force
Occludes blood flow, causing ischemia and tissue death

Develops over bony prominence

Locations
- Coccygeal (end of spine)

- Sacral (between hips)

- Heel

- Elbow

- Ischial (lower hip)

- Trochanteric (outer hip)

Staging or classification system
- Stage I: erythema (redness) of skin

- Stage II: partial loss of skin (epidermis or dermis)

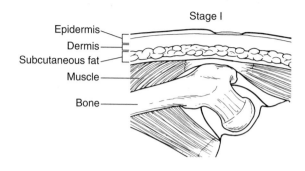

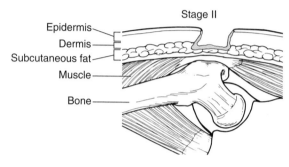

Figure **1-3** Stage I, II, III, and IV of pressure ulcers.

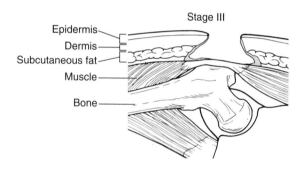

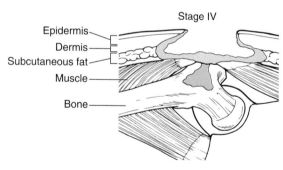

- Stage III: full thickness loss of skin (up to but not through fascia)
- Stage IV: full thickness loss (extensive destruction and necrosis)
  Deep ulcers may require surgical debridement

Keloids

Sharply elevated, irregularly shaped scars that progressively enlarge

Due to excessive collagen in corneum during connective tissue repair

Result of tissue repair or trauma

Familial tendency for formation

Cicatrix
Normal scar left after wound healing

Inflammatory Disorders

Atopic Dermatitis
Unknown etiology

Exogenous (external causes) include
Irritant dermatitis

Allergic contact dermatitis

Endogenous (internal cause) includes
Seborrheic dermatitis

Results in activation of
- Mast cells

- Eosinophils

- T lymphocytes

- Monocytes

Greater in those with family history of
- Asthma

- Dry skin

- Eczema

- Allergic rhinitis

Common in
- Children

- Infants

Results in
- Chronic inflammation

- Scratching

- Erythema

- Thickened, leathery skin (lichenification)

- Secondary *Staphylococcus aureus* infection

Treatment
- Topical steroid

- Antibiotic for secondary infection

- Antihistamines

Allergic Contact Dermatitis
Most common in infants and children

Potential causes
- Hypersensitivity to allergens

  - Microorganisms

  - Drugs

- Foreign proteins

- Chemicals

- Latex

- Metals

- Plants

Manifestations
- Scaling

- Lichenification (leathery, thickened skin)

- Erythema

- Itching (pruritus)

- Vesicular lesions

- Edema

Diagnosis and treatment
- Check medical history

- Patch test

- Avoidance of irritant

- Skin lubrication and hydration

- Steroids

  - Topical

  - Systemic

- Topical tacrolimus (immunosuppressive agent)

Irritant Contact Dermatitis
Response to
- Chemical

- Exposure to irritant

Treatment
- Removal of irritant

- Topical agents

Stasis Dermatitis
Usually on the legs from venous stasis

Associated with
- Phlebitis

- Vascular trauma

- Varicosities

Progress
- Begins with erythema and pruritus

- Progresses to scaling, hyperpigmentation, petechia (small hemorrhagic areas)

- Lesion becomes ulcerated

Treatment

- Elevate legs

- Reduce standing

- No constricting clothes

- Eliminate external compression

- Antibiotics for acute lesions

- Silver nitrate or Burow's solution dressings for chronic lesions

Seborrheic Dermatitis

Common chronic inflammation of sebaceous glands—cause unknown

Periods of remission and exacerbation

Commonly occurs on

- Scalp (cradle cap in infants)

- Ear canals

- Eyelids

- Eyebrow

- Nose

- Axillae

- Chest

- Groin

Lesions are

- Scaly (dry or greasy)

- White or yellowish

- Mildly pruritic

Treatment of mild cases

- Soap/shampoo of

  - Coal tar

  - Sulfur

  - Salicylic acid

Treatment of more severe cases

- Corticosteroid

Papulosquamous Disorders

Conditions associated with

- Scales

- Papules

- Plaque

- Erythema

Three types
- Psoriasis

- Pityriasis

- Lichen planus

Psoriasis
Chronic, relapsing, proliferating skin disorder

Usually begins by age 20

Cause unknown, suggested to be
- Exacerbated by anxiety, appears to run in families

- Immunologic

- Biochemical alterations

- Triggering agent

Commonly occurs on
- Face

- Scalp

- Forearms and elbows

- Knees and legs

Results in
- Thickened dermis and epidermis

- Well-demarcated plaque

- Cell hyperproliferation/scaly

- Inflammation (pruritus)

- Lesions are deep red color

Treatment
- Only palliative (treatment of symptoms)

Mild cases

- Keratolytic agents

- Corticosteroids

- Emollients

Moderate cases

- Interleukin-2 inhibitors

- Psoralens and ultraviolet A (PUVA) light therapy

- Coal tar

- Cyclosporin

- Vitamin D analogs

Severe cases

- Topical agents

- Systemic corticosteroids

- Antimetabolic
- Hospitalization

Pityriasis Rosea
Unknown cause

Self-limiting inflammatory disorder

Occurs most often in young adults

Primary lesion
- Begins with herald patch 3 to 4 cm
- Salmon-pink colored
- Circular and well-defined lesions

Secondary lesions
- 14 to 21 days

Trunk and upper extremities

- Oval lesions
- Severe pruritus

Diagnosis
May be confused with

- Secondary syphilis
- Seborrheic dermatitis
- Psoriasis

Treatment
- Antipruritics
- Antihistamines
- Corticosteroids
- Ultraviolet light
- Sunlight

Lichen Planus
Occurs on skin and mucous membranes

Unknown cause (idiopathic)

Autoimmune inflammatory disorder

Onset ages 30 to 70

Lesions
- Begin as pink lesions that turn into violet-colored pruritic papules
- Results in hyperpigmentation
- 2- to 10-mm flat lesions with central depression
- Last 12 to 18 months
- Tend to reoccur

Treatment
- Antihistamines
- Corticosteroids

  Topical

  Systemic

Acne Vulgaris

Site of lesion is sebaceous (pilosebaceous) follicles

Primarily on face and upper trunk

Occurs in 85% of the population between the ages of 12 and 25

Exact cause: unknown

Causative factor: sebum accumulation/inflammation in pores of skin

Types
Noninflammatory acne

- Whiteheads
- Blackheads

Inflammatory acne

- Follicle walls rupture
- Sebum expels into dermis
- Inflammation begins
  - Pustules, cysts, and papules result

Cause
  Unknown

Treatment
  Topical

- Antibiotics
- Salicylic acid
- Benzoyl peroxide
- Tretinoin

  Systemic

- Antibiotic
- Hormones
- Corticosteroids
- Isotretinoin

Diaper Dermatitis

Variety of disorders

Causes
  Urine

  Feces

  Plastic diaper cover

Allergic reaction

Secondary *Candida albicans* infection

Treatment
Clean, dry area

Expose to air

Topical antifungal medications

Topical steroids

Pruritus (Itching)
Symptom of skin disorder/dermatitis

Can be localized or generalized and is a condition not an inflammation

Results from stimulation of nerves of skin reacting to an allergen or irritation from substances in blood or foreign bodies

Causes
Primary skin disorder

 Example: eczema or lice

Systemic disease

 Example: chronic renal failure

Opiates

Allergic reaction

Treatment is for underlying condition
Antihistamines

Minor tranquilizers

Application of emollients (lotions)

Topical steroids

Skin Infections

■ Bacterial
Impetigo
Most common in infants and children

 Usually on face and begins as small vesicles

 Caused primarily by *Staphylococcus*

• Sometimes by group A beta-hemolytic *Streptococcus*

It is a highly contagious pyoderma

Treatment in mild cases
Topical antibiotics

Topical antiseptics

Treatment in moderate cases
Systemic antibiotics

Local compresses

Analgesics

Cellulitis

Caused primarily by *Staphylococcus*

Often secondary to an injury

Results in
  Erythema, usually of lower trunk and legs

  Fever

  Localized pain

  Lymphangitis

Treatment
  Systemic antibiotics

  Burow's soaks for pain relief

Furuncles (Boils)

Infected hair follicle

Usually caused by *Staphylococcus*

Developed boil drains pus and necrotic tissue

Squeezing spreads infection

Collection of furuncles that have merged is a carbuncle

Folliculitis

Infection of hair follicles

Results in
  Erythema

  Pustules

Causes
  Skin trauma, such as irritation or friction

  Poor hygiene

  Excessive skin moisture

Treatment
  Cleansing of area

  Topical antibiotics

Erysipelas

Infection of skin

Cause
  Group A beta-hemolytic *Streptococci*

  Common occurrence: face, ears, lower legs

Prior to outbreak, presents with

- Fever

- Malaise

- Chills

Lesions appear as
Bright red and hot

- Develops raised borders

- Itching

- Burning

- Tenderness

Acute Necrotizing Fasciitis
Flesh-eating disease
Virulent strain of gram-positive, group A beta-hemolytic *Streptococcus*

Mortality rate of over 40%

Causes
  Skin trauma

  Skin infection

Areas secrete tissue-destroying enzyme, proteases
Extreme inflammation and pain

Rapidly increasing

Dermal gangrene develops

Systemic toxicity may develop with
  Fever

  Disorientation

  Hypotension

  Tachycardia (fast heart rate)

May lead to organ failure

Treatment
  Antimicrobial therapy

  Fluid replacement

  Removal of areas of infection

■ Viral
Herpes Simplex (Cold Sores)
Causes
Herpes simplex virus type 1 (HSV-1)

- Most common type

- Results in fever blisters or cold sores on or near lips or canker sores of the mouth

Herpes simplex virus type 2 (HSV-2)

- Genital and oral type

- Prominent sexually transmitted disease

Primary infections may show no symptoms (asymptomatic)

Virus remains in nerve tissue to later reactivate

Reactivation may be triggered by
Stress

Common cold

Exposure to sun

Presents with
Burning or tingling

Develops painful vesicles that rupture
Causes spreading

May cause secondary infection of eye

- Episode lasts several weeks

- Treatment may include antiviral medication

  · No permanent cure exists

Herpes Zoster (Shingles)
Usually older adult

Caused by varicella-zoster virus (VZV)
Virus was dormant and then reactivates

Result of varicella or chickenpox, usually in childhood

Affects
One cranial nerve or one dermatome (an area of skin supplied with afferent nerve fibers by a posterior spinal root)

Results in
Pain

Rash (unilateral)

Paresthesia (abnormal touch sensation, such as burning)

Course
Several weeks

Pain may continue even after lesion disappears

Treatment
Clears spontaneously

Antiviral medications provide symptomatic relief

Sedatives

Analgesic

Antipruritics

Warts (Verrucae)
Verruca vulgaris (common wart)

Caused by human papillomavirus (HPV)

- Numerous types of HPV

Spread by contact

Appear anywhere on body

Present with a grayish appearance

Variety of shapes and sizes

Transmitted by touch

Plantar warts (verrucae) are located on pressure points of body (such as feet; *plantar* means the bottom surface of foot)

Painful when pressure is applied

Juvenile warts occur on feet and hands of children

Venereal warts occur on genitals/anus

Treatment

Liquid nitrogen

Topical keratolytics

Laser

Electrocautery

Often persist even with treatment

Fungal (Mycoses)

Usually superficial dermatophytes (fungus)

Fungus lives off dead cells

Tinea

Superficial skin infections

Tinea capitis

- Infection of scalp

- Common in children

- Treatment with oral antifungal medication

Tinea corporis (ringworm)

- Infection of body

- Presents as a red ring

- Produces burning sensation and pruritus

- Treatment with topical antifungal medication

Tinea pedis (athlete's foot)

- Involves feet and toes

- Produces pain, inflammation, fissures, and foul odor

- Treatment with topical antifungal medication

Tinea unguium (onychomycosis)

- Nail infection

  - Usually toenails

- Nail turns white then brown, thickens and cracks

- Spreads to other nails

Candidiasis

Caused by *Candida albicans*

Normally on mucous membranes of gastrointestinal tract and vagina

Poor health and certain conditions predispose individuals to overarching infection by candidiasis

- Antibiotic therapy, which changes the balance of the normal flora in the body

Treatment is topical or oral antifungal medications

Tumors of Skin

■ Benign Tumors
Keratosis(es)
Seborrheic keratosis
  Proliferation of basal cells

  Dark colored lesion

  Found on trunk and face

Actinic keratosis
  Pigmented, scaly patch

  Often caused by exposure to sun

  Often in fair-skinned individuals

  Premalignant lesion

  May develop into squamous cell carcinoma

Treatment with cryosurgery (freezing area) or excision

Keratoacanthoma
  Occurs in hair follicles

  Usually in those over 60

  Often of face, neck, back of hands, and other locations exposed to the sun

  Resolve spontaneously or are excised

Moles (Nevi)
  Located on any body part

  Various shapes and sizes

  May become malignant

- Especially if located in area of continual irritation

■ Malignant Tumors
Squamous Cell Carcinoma
Similar to basal cell carcinoma

Grows wherever squamous epithelium is located (mouth, pharynx, esophagus, lungs, bladder)

Most often appears in areas exposed to sun (actinic keratosis—precancerous)

Scaly appearance

Rarely metastatic (spreading)

Easily treated with good prognosis

  Surgical excision

Cryotherapy

Curettage

Electrodesiccation

Radiotherapy

Basal Cell Carcinoma
Common type of skin cancer

Developed in deeper skin layers (basal cells) than squamous cell carcinoma

Often occurs with sun exposure in fair-skinned individuals

Shiny appearance and slow growing

Easily treated with good prognosis

Malignant Melanoma
Originates in cells that produce pigment (melanocytes) or nevi

Increased incidence with
Sun exposure

Fair hair and skin/freckles

Genetic predisposition

Skin nevus (mole) often brown and evenly colored with irregular borders

Grow downward into tissues

- Metastasize quickly

Treatment is removal with extensive border excision

- Depending on extent, chemotherapy or radiation therapy may be used

Kaposi's Sarcoma
Rare form of vascular skin cancer

Associated with
Human immunodeficiency virus (HIV)

Acquired immunodeficiency syndrome (AIDS)

Herpes virus may be found in lesions

Cells originate from endothelium in small blood vessels

Painful lesions develop rapidly, appearing as purple papules; spreads quickly to lymph nodes and internal organs

Treatment

Radiation

Chemotherapy

INTEGUMENTARY SYSTEM PATHOPHYSIOLOGY QUIZ

1. A pimple is an example of a:
   a. papule
   b. vesicle
   c. pustule
   d. nodule

2. A Stage III pressure ulcer involves:
   a. erythema of skin
   b. partial loss of epidermis and dermis
   c. full thickness loss of skin up to but not through fascia
   d. full thickness loss of skin with extensive destruction and necrosis

3. This type of dermatitis may be exogenous or endogenous and is common in children and infants:
   a. atopic
   b. irritant contact
   c. stasis
   d. seborrheic

4. Psoriasis, pityriasis, and lichen planus are three types of this disorder:
   a. dermatitis
   b. inflammatory
   c. acne
   d. papulosquamous

5. This condition begins with a herald spot:
   a. psoriasis
   b. pityriasis
   c. lichen planus
   d. dermatitis

6. This skin infection is caused by group A beta-hemolytic *Streptococci*, and the lesions appear as firm red spots with itching, burning, and tenderness:
   a. furuncles
   b. folliculitis
   c. erysipelas
   d. fasciitis

7. This type of herpes produces cold sores:
   a. herpes zoster
   b. shingles
   c. VZV
   d. herpes simplex

8. This condition is caused by human papillomavirus:
   a. mycoses
   b. verrucae
   c. shingles
   d. folliculitis

9. This type of tumor occurs in hair follicles:
   a. keratoses
   b. nevi
   c. Kaposi's sarcoma
   d. keratoacanthoma

10. This type of superficial carcinoma is rarely metastatic:
   a. squamous cell
   b. basal cell
   c. melanoma
   d. Kaposi's sarcoma

■ MUSCULOSKELETAL SYSTEM
MUSCULOSKELETAL SYSTEM—ANATOMY AND TERMINOLOGY

Skeletal System

Comprises 206 bones, cartilage, and ligaments

Provides organ protection, movement, framework, stores calcium, hematopoiesis (formation of blood cells)

Classification of Bones
Long bones (tubular)
Length exceeds width of bone

Broad at ends, such as thigh, lower leg, upper arm, and lower arm

Short bones (cuboidal)
Cubelike bones, such as carpals (wrist) and tarsals (ankle)

Flat
Thin—flattened with curved surfaces

Cover body parts, such as skull, scapula, sternum, ribs

Irregular
Varied shapes, such as zygoma of face or vertebrae

Sesamoid
Rounded

Found near joint, such as patella (kneecap)

Patella is largest sesamoid bone in body.

Structure

Long Bones (Fig. 1–4)
Diaphysis: shaft

Epiphysis: both ends of long bones—bulbular shape with muscle attachments

• Articular cartilage covers epiphyses and serves as a cushion

Epiphyseal line or plate: growth plate that disappears when fully grown

Metaphysis: flared portion of bone near epiphyseal plate

Periosteum: dense, white outer covering (fibrous)

Cortical or compact bone: hard bone beneath periosteum mainly found in shaft

• Medullary cavity contains yellow marrow (fatty bone marrow)

Cancellous bones: spongy or trabecular

• Contains red bone marrow (blood cell development)

Endosteum is thin epithelial membrane lining medullary cavity of long bone

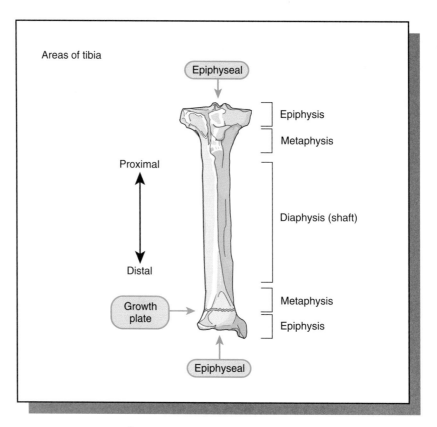

Figure **1-4** Structure of bones.

Two Skeletal Divisions
Axial (trunk)

Appendicular (appendages)

Axial Skeleton, comprised of 80 bones
Skull, hyoid bone, vertebral column, sacrum, ribs, and sternum

Skull (Fig. 1–5)
Cranial
Frontal (forehead)

Parietal (sides and top)

Temporal (lower sides)

Occipital (posterior of cranium)

Sphenoid (floor of cranium)

Ethmoid (area between orbits and nasal cavity)

Styloid process (below ear)

Zygomatic process (cheek)

Middle ear bones (Fig. 1–6)
Malleus (hammer)

Incus (anvil)

Stapes (stirrup)

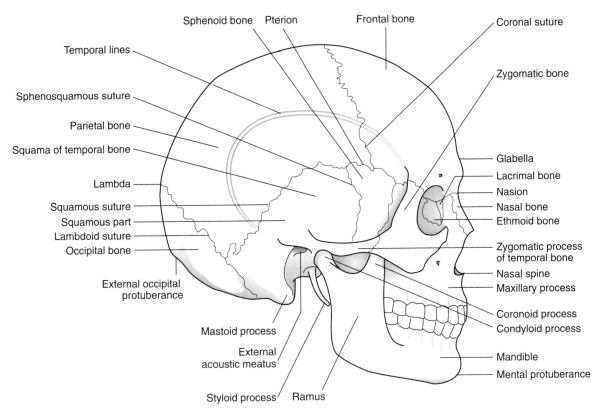

Figure **1-5** Lateral view of skull.

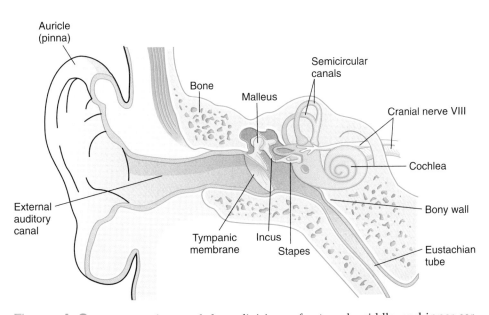

Figure **1-6** Structure of ear and three divisions of external, middle, and inner ear.

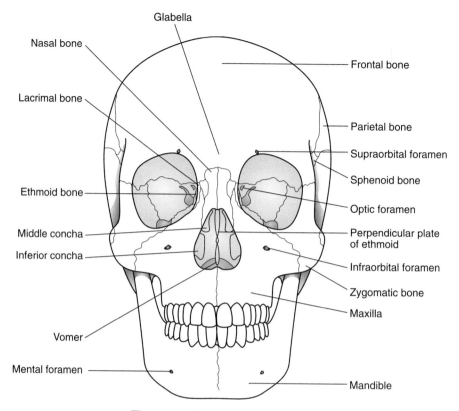

Figure **1-7** Frontal view of skull.

Face (Fig. 1–7)

Nasal (bridge of nose)

Maxilla (upper jaw)

Zygomatic (arch of cheekbone)

Mandible (lower jawbone)

Lacrimal (near orbits)

Palate (separates oral and nasal cavities)

Vomer (base, nasal septum)

Nasal conchae (turbinates)

   Interior

   Middle

   Superior

Hyoid

Supports tongue

U shaped

Attached by ligaments and muscles to larynx and skull

Spine (33 vertebrae) (Fig. 1–8)

Cervical vertebrae (7)

- C1-7
- (C1)-atlas
- (C2)-axis

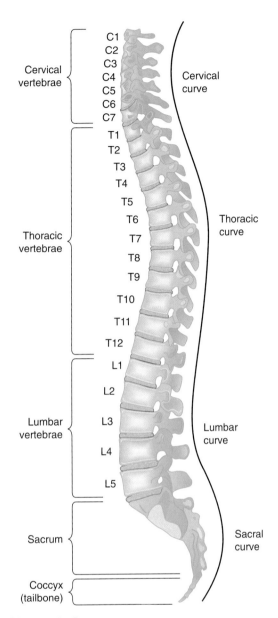

Figure **1-8** Anterior view of vertebral column.

Thoracic vertebrae (12) (T1-12)

Lumbar vertebrae (5) (L1-5)

Sacrum (5)—fused in adults

Coccyx (4)—fused in adults

Thorax (Fig. 1–9)
Ribs, 12 pairs

- True ribs, 1-7

- False ribs, 8-10

- Floating ribs, 11 and 12

Sternum

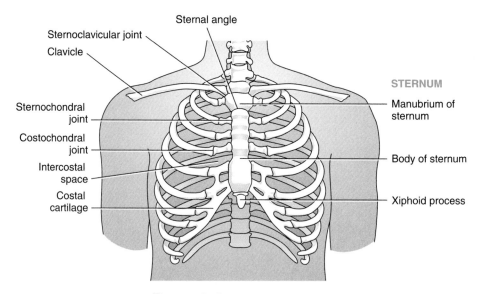

Figure **1-9** The thoracic cage.

Appendicular Skeleton, comprised of 126 bones (Fig. 1–10)
Shoulder, girdle, pelvic girdle, and extremities
Pelvis
Ilium (uppermost part) wing shaped

• Acetabulum, depression on lateral hip surface into which head of femur fits

Ischium (posterior part)

Pubis (anterior part)

Pubis symphysis (cartilage between pubic bones)

Lower extremities
Femur (thighbone)
Trochanter (processes at neck of femur)

Head fits into acetabulum

Patella (kneecap)

Tibia (shinbone)

Fibula (smaller lateral bone in lower leg)

Talus (ankle bone)

Calcaneus (heel bone)

Metatarsals (foot instep)

Phalanges (toes)

Lateral malleolus (lower part of fibula)

Medial malleolus (lower part of tibia)

Upper extremities
Clavicle (collarbone)

Scapula (shoulder blade)

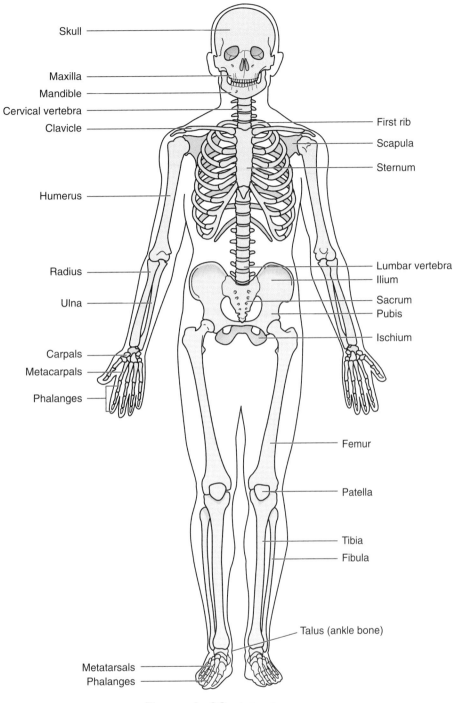

Figure **1-10** Skeletal system.

Humerus (upper arm)

Radius (forearm, thumb side)

Ulna (forearm, little finger side)

Olecranon (projection of ulna at elbow)

Carpals (wrist)—eight bones bound by ligaments in two rows with 4 bones in each

Metacarpals (hand)—framework or palm of hand (5 bones)

Phalanges (finger)

Olecranon (tip of elbow)

Joints (Articulations)
Condyle, rounded end of bone

Classified by degree of movement

- Synarthrosis (immovable and fibrous)

  Example: joint between cranial bones

- Amphiarthrosis (slightly movable and cartilaginous)

  Example: intervertebral (joint between bodies of vertebra)

- Diarthrosis (considerably movable and synovial)

Types

  - Uniaxial—hinge and pivot joints

      Example—elbow (hinge and pivot) and cervical 2 (axis) (pivot)

  - Biaxial—saddle and condyloid joints

      Example—thumb and joints between radius and carpal bones

  - Multiaxial—ball and socket and gliding

      Example—shoulder and hip/joints between articular surfaces of vertebrae

  Example: elbow, hip

  - Bursa, sac of synovial fluid located in the tissues to prevent friction

Muscular System

Functions
Heat production

Movement

Posture

Protection

Shape

Muscle Tissue Types

Skeletal—600 muscles constituting 40% to 50% of body weight
Striated (cross stripes) (Figs. 1–11 and 1–12)

Move body

Voluntary

Attaches to bones

- Most attach to two bones with a joint in between

- Origin, point where muscle attaches to stationary bone

- Insertion, where muscle attaches to movable bone

- Body of muscle, main part of muscle

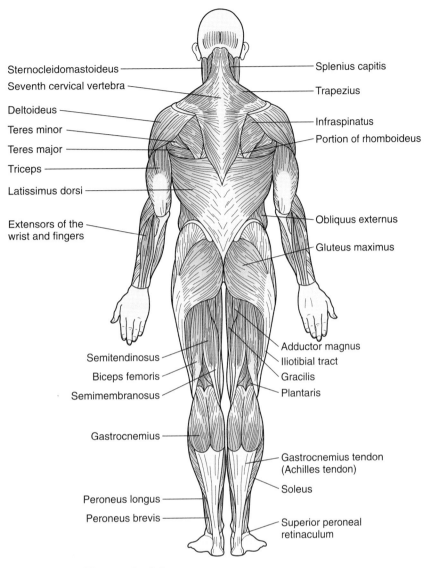

Figure **1-11** Muscular system, posterior view.

Cardiac/Heart Muscle
Striated and smooth muscle

Specialized cells which interlock so that muscle cells contract together

Involuntary

Moves blood by means of contractions

Smooth/Visceral
Linings such as bowel, urethra, blood vessels

Nonstriated

Involuntary

Tendons Anchor Muscle to Bone

Ligaments Anchor Bones to Bones

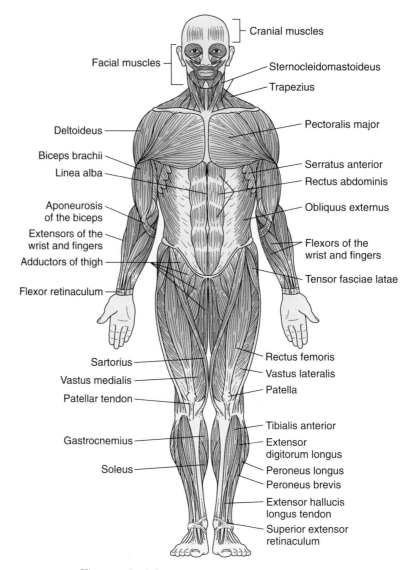

Figure **1-12** Muscular system, anterior view.

Muscle Action

Muscle Capabilities

Stretches

Contracts

Receives and responds to stimulus

Returns to original shape and length

Muscle Movement

Prime mover, responsible for movement (agonist)

Synergist, assists prime mover

Antagonist, relaxes as prime mover and synergists contract, resulting in movement

Fixator, acts as joint stabilizer

Terms of Movement—from midline of body

Flexion (bend)

Extension (straighten)

Abduction (away)

Adduction (toward)

Rotation (turn on axis)

Circumduction (circular)

Supination (turning palm upward or forward [anteriorly] or lying down with face upward)

Pronation (turning palm downward or backward or act of lying face down)

Hyperextension (overextension)

Inversion (inward)

Eversion (outward)

Names of Muscles

Head and neck
Facial expression

- Occipitofrontalis (raises eyebrows and wrinkles forehead horizontally)

- Corrugator supercilii (wrinkles forehead vertically)

- Orbicularis oris (opens mouth)

- Zygomaticus (elevates corners of mouth)

- Orbicularis oculi (opens and closes eyelid)

- Buccinator (smiling and blowing)

Mastication (chewing)

- Masseter (used to chew closing jaw)

- Temporalis (closes jaw)

- Pterygoids (grates teeth)

Muscles moving head

- Sternocleidomastoid (flexes head)

- Semispinalis capitis (complexus) (extends head)

- Splenius capitis (extends head, bends and rotates head to side where muscle is contracting)

- Longissimus capitis (trachelomastoid muscle) (extends head, bends and rotates to contracting side)

Trapezius (extends head)

Upper extremities
Biceps brachii (flexes elbow)

Triceps brachii and anconeus (extends elbow)

Brachialis (flexes prone forearm)

Brachioradialis (flexes semi-prone/supinated forearm)

Deltoid (abducts upper arm)

Latissimus dorsi (extends upper arm)

Pectoralis major (flexes upper arm)

Trapezius (raises/lowers shoulder)

Trunk
External oblique (compresses abdomen)

Internal oblique (compresses abdomen)

Transversus abdominis (compresses abdomen)

Rectus abdominis (flexes trunk)

Quadratus lumborum (flexes vertebral column laterally)

Respiratory
Diaphragm (enlarges thorax/inspiration)

External intercostals (raise ribs)

Internal intercostal (depress ribs)

Lower extremities
Thigh

- Gluteus group, maximus, medius, minimus (abducts thigh)

- Tensor fasciae latae (abducts thigh)

- Abductor group, brevis, longus, magnus (adducts thigh)

- Gracilis (adducts thigh)

- Iliopsoas (flexes thigh)

- Rectus femoris (flexes thigh)

Hamstring group, biceps femoris, semitendinosus, semimembranosus (extends thigh)

Quadriceps group, rectus femoris, vastus lateralis, vastus medialis, vastus intermedius (extends lower leg)

Sartorius (flexes, abducts, and rotates leg)

Lower leg

Tibialis anterior (dorsiflexes foot)

Peroneus group, longus, brevis, tertius (everts foot)

Gastrocnemius (calf, with soleus extends foot, also flexes knee)

Soleus (calf, extends foot)

Extensor digitorum longus (extends toes, flexes foot)

Achilles tendon (largest tendon, extending from gastrocnemius to calcaneus)

COMBINING FORMS

1.	acetabul/o	hip socket
2.	ankyl/o	bent, fused

3.	aponeur/o	tendon type
4.	arthr/o	joint
5.	articul/o	joint
6.	burs/o	fluid-filled sac in a joint
7.	calc/o, calci/o	calcium
8.	calcane/o	calcaneus (heel)
9.	carp/o	carpals (wrist bones)
10.	chondr/o	cartilage
11.	clavic/o, clavicul/o	clavicle (collar bone)
12.	cost/o	rib
13.	crani/o	cranium (skull)
14.	disk/o	intervertebral disk
15.	femor/o	thighbone
16.	fibul/o	fibula
17.	humer/o	humerus (upper arm bone)
18.	ili/o	ilium (upper pelvic bone)
19.	ischi/o	ischium (posterior pelvic bone)
20.	kinesi/o	movement
21.	kyph/o	hump
22.	lamin/o	lamina
23.	lord/o	curve
24.	lumb/o	lower back
25.	malleol/o	malleolus (process on lateral ankle)
26.	mandibul/o	mandible (lower jawbone)
27.	maxill/o	maxilla (upper jawbone)
28.	menisc/o	meniscus
29.	menisci/o	meniscus
30.	metacarp/o	metacarpals (hand)
31.	metatars/o	metatarsals (foot)
32.	myel/o	bone marrow
33.	my/o, muscul/o	muscle
34.	olecran/o	olecranon (elbow)
35.	orth/o	straight
36.	oste/o	bone
37.	patell/o	patella (kneecap)
38.	pelv/i	pelvis (hip)
39.	perone/o	fibula

40.	petr/o	stone
41.	phalang/o	phalanges (finger or toe)
42.	plant/o	sole of foot
43.	pub/o	pubis
44.	rachi/o	spine
45.	radi/o	radius (lower arm)
46.	rhabdomy/o	skeletal (striated muscle)
47.	rheumat/o	watery flow (collection of fluids in joints)
48.	sacr/o	sacrum
49.	scapul/o	scapula (shoulder)
50.	scoli/o	bent
51.	spondyl/o	vertebra
52.	stern/o	sternum (breast bone)
53.	synovi/o	synovial joint membrane
54.	tars/o	tarsal (ankle/foot)
55.	ten/o	tendon
56.	tend/o	tendon (connective tissue)
57.	tendin/o	tendon (connective tissue)
58.	tibi/o	shin bone
59.	uln/o	ulna (lower arm bone)
60.	vertebr/o	vertebra

PREFIXES

1.	inter-	between
2.	supra-	above
3.	sym-	together
4.	syn-	together

SUFFIXES

1.	-asthenia	weakness
2.	-blast	embryonic
3.	-clast, -clasia, -clasis	break
4.	-desis	bind together
5.	-listhesia	slipping
6.	-malacia	softening
7.	-physis	to grow
8.	-porosis	passage, cavity formation
9.	-schisis	split
10.	-stenosis	narrowing

| 11. -tome | instrument that cuts |
| 12. -tomy | incision |

MEDICAL ABBREVIATIONS

1. ACL	anterior cruciate ligament
2. AKA	above-knee amputation
3. BKA	below-knee amputation
4. C1-C7	cervical vertebrae
5. CTS	carpal tunnel syndrome
6. fx	fracture
7. L1-L5	lumbar vertebrae
8. OA	osteoarthritis
9. RA	rheumatoid arthritis
10. T1-T12	thoracic vertebrae
11. TMJ	temporomandibular joint

MEDICAL TERMS

Arthrocentesis	Injection and/or aspiration of joint
Arthrodesis	Surgical immobilization of a joint
Arthrography	Radiography of joint
Arthroplasty	Reshaping or reconstruction of a joint
Arthroscopy	Use of scope to view inside joint
Arthrotomy	Incision into a joint
Articular	Pertains to a joint
Aspiration	Use of a needle and a syringe to withdraw fluid
Atrophy	Wasting away
Bunion	Hallux valgus, abnormal increase in size of metatarsal head that results in displacement of great toe
Bursitis	Inflammation of bursa (joint sac)
Chondral	Referring to the cartilage
Carpal tunnel syndrome	Compression of medial nerve
Closed fracture repair	Not surgically opened with/without manipulation and with/without traction
Closed treatment	Fracture site that is not surgically opened and visualized
Colles' fracture	Fracture at lower end of radius that displaces bone posteriorly
Dislocation	Placement in a location other than original location
Endoscopy	Inspection of body organs or cavities using a lighted scope that may be inserted through an existing opening or through a small incision

Fasciectomy	Removal of band of fibrous tissue
Fissure	Groove
Fracture	Break in a bone
Ganglion	Knot or knotlike mass
Internal/External fixation	Application of pins, wires, screws, placed externally or internally to immobilize a body part
Kyphosis	Humpback
Lamina	Flat plate
Ligament	Fibrous band of tissue that connects cartilage or bone
Lordosis	Anterior curve of spine
Lumbodynia	Pain in lumbar area
Lysis	Releasing
Manipulation or reduction	Alignment of a fracture or joint dislocation to normal position
Open fracture repair	Surgical opening (incision) over or remote opening as access to a fracture site
Osteoarthritis	Degenerative condition of articular cartilage
Osteoclast	Absorbs or removes bone
Osteotomy	Cutting into bone
Percutaneous	Through skin
Percutaneous fracture repair	Repair of a fracture by means of pins and wires inserted through the fracture site
Percutaneous skeletal fixation	Considered neither open nor closed; fracture is not visualized, but fixation is placed across fracture site under x-ray imaging
Reduction	Replacement to normal position
Scoliosis	Lateral curve of spine
Skeletal traction	Application of pressure to bone by means of pins and/or wires inserted into bone
Skin traction	Application of pressure to bone by means of tape applied to the skin
Spondylitis	Inflammation of vertebrae
Subluxation	Partial dislocation
Supination	Supine position—lying on back, face upward
Synchondrosis	Union between two bones (connected by cartilage)
Tendon	Attaches a muscle to a bone
Tenodesis	Suturing of a tendon to a bone
Tenorrhaphy	Suture repair of tendon
Traction	Application of pressure to maintain normal alignment
Trocar needle	Needle with a cannula that can be removed; used to puncture and withdraw fluid from a cavity

MUSCULOSKELETAL SYSTEM ANATOMY AND TERMINOLOGY QUIZ

1. Tubular is another name for these bones:
   a. short
   b. long
   c. flat
   d. irregular

2. These bones are found near joints:
   a. irregular
   b. flat
   c. sesamoid
   d. broad

3. Zygoma is an example of this type of bone:
   a. irregular
   b. flat
   c. sesamoid
   d. broad

4. Diaphysis is this part of bone:
   a. end
   b. surface
   c. shaft
   d. marrow

5. Which is NOT a part of cranium?
   a. condyle
   b. sphenoid
   c. ethmoid
   d. parietal

6. This is NOT an ear bone:
   a. malleus
   b. stapes
   c. incus
   d. styloid

7. This term describes growth plate:
   a. endosteum
   b. epiphyseal
   c. metaphysis
   d. periosteum

8. This is a depression on lateral hip surface into which head of femur fits:
   a. ilium
   b. ischium
   c. patella
   d. acetabulum

9. Tip of elbow is the:
   a. olecranon
   b. trapezium
   c. humerus
   d. tarsal

10. This term describes an immovable joint:
    a. amphiarthrosis
    b. diarthrosis
    c. synarthrosis
    d. ischium

MUSCULOSKELETAL SYSTEM—PATHOPHYSIOLOGY

Injuries

■ Fractures

Classification of fractures

Open/closed

Open (compound): broken bone penetrates skin

Closed (simple): broken bone does not penetrate skin

Complete/incomplete

Complete: bone is broken all way through

> *Example:* oblique, linear, spiral, and transverse

Incomplete: bone is not broken all way through

> *Example:* greenstick, bowing, torus, stress, and transchondral

Treatment

Closed reduction (realignment of bone fragments by manipulation)

Reduction (the returning of the bone to normal alignment)

Immobilization (returns to normal alignment and holds in place)

Traction (application of pulling force to hold bone in alignment)

- Skeletal traction uses internal devices (pins, screws, wires, etc.) inserted into bone with ends sticking out through skin for attachment of traction device (Fig. 1–13)

- Skin traction is use of strapping, elastic wrap, or tape attached to skin to which weights are attached (Fig. 1–14)

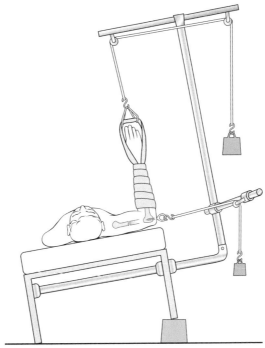

Figure **1-13** Skeletal traction uses patient's bones to secure internal devices to which traction is attached.

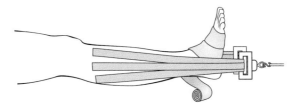

Figure **1-14** Skin traction utilizes strapping, wraps, or tape to which traction is attached.

Improper union

Nonunion: failure of bone ends to grow together

Malunion: incorrect alignment of bone ends

Delayed union: delay of bone union 8 or 9 months

Dislocations

Bone and soft tissue damage usually caused by trauma

Any part of bone is displaced

Can result in nerve and tissue damage

Treatment

Reduction

Immobilization

Sprains and strains

Soft tissue damage usually caused by trauma to tendons and ligaments

Strain: partial tear of a tendon

Sprain results from overuse or overextension/tearing or rupture of some part of musculature

Bone Disorders

Osteomyelitis

Bone infection

Usually caused by bacteria

- Exogenous osteomyelitis is caused by bacteria that enter from outside body

- Hematogenous osteomyelitis (endogenous) is caused from a bacterial infection within body

Osteoporosis

Common disorder in postmenopausal women and elderly and most common metabolic disease

- Malabsorption of calcium and magnesium; certain trace elements and vitamins C and D contribute to bone loss

Decreased bone mass and density

- Fractures more common due to decrease in strength of bone

Treatment

Increased intake of calcium, magnesium, and vitamin D

Increased weight-bearing activity

Osteomalacia and Rickets

Osteomalacia is softened adult bones, while rickets is softened growing bones in children

Caused by vitamin D and phosphate deficiency

Osteitis Deformans (Paget's Disease)

Abnormal bone remodeling and resorption resulting in enlarged, soft bones

Unknown cause but strong genetic considerations

Treatment

Calcitonin and biophosphates

Spinal Curvatures

Lordosis: swayback

- Inward curvature of spine

Kyphosis: humpback

- Outward curvature of spine

Scoliosis

- Lateral curvature of spine

Spina Bifida

Congenital abnormality in which vertebrae do not close correctly around the spinal cord

Joint Disorders

Bursitis: inflammation of bursa (joint sac)

Arthritis: inflammation of joints

Osteoarthritis (OA)

This is degenerative or wear/tear arthritis

- DJD, degenerative joint disease

Chronic inflammation of joint

Increased pain on weightbearing or movement

Affects weight-bearing joints

- Loss of articular cartilage
- Sclerosis of bone—eburnation

    Turning bone into ivorylike mass—polished

- Osteophytes (bone spurs)

Symptoms

Pain and stiffness

Crepitation (bone on bone creates characteristic grinding sound)

Classifications
Primary (idiopathic)

- No known cause

Secondary

- Associated with joint instability, joint stress, or congenital abnormalities

Treatment
Symptomatic

Arthroplasty

Rheumatoid Arthritis (RA)
Inflammatory connective tissue in joints disease that is progressive

Systemic autoimmune disease

- Can invade arteries, lung, skin, and other organs with nodules

Affects small joints

- Destroys synovial membrane, articular cartilage, and surrounding tissues

Leads to loss of function due to fixation and deformity

Treatment
Pharmaceuticals to modify autoimmune and inflammatory processes

Gene therapy and stem cell transplantation are being researched

Symptomatic

Arthroplasty

Infectious and Septic Arthritis
Infectious process

Usually affects single joint

Without antimicrobial intervention, permanent joint damage results

Example: Lyme disease

Treatment
Antibiotics—early intervention

Gout (Gouty Arthritis)
Inflammatory arthritis

Often affects the joint of the great toe

Caused by excessive amounts of uric acid that crystallizes in connective tissue of joints

Leads to inflammation and destruction of joint

Treatment
Pharmaceuticals—nonsteroidal antiinflammatory drugs

Ankylosing Spondylitis (AS)
Inflammatory disease that is progressive

Affects vertebral joints and insertion points of ligaments, tendons, and joint capsules

Leads to rigid spinal column and sacroiliac joints

Treatment
    Nonsteroidal anti-inflammatory drugs relieve symptoms

    Analgesics for pain

Tendon, Muscle, and Ligament Disorders

Muscular Dystrophy—Familial Disorder
Progressive degenerative muscle disorder

Multiple types of muscular dystrophy

Most often affects boys

- Genetic predisposition—Duchenne MD

Primary Fibromyalgia Syndrome
Symptoms
    Generalized aching and pain

    Tender points

    Fatigue

    Depression

Usually appears in
    Middle-aged women

Polymyositis
General muscle inflammation causing weakness

- With skin rash = dermatomyositis

Tumors

Bone Tumors
Origin of bone tumors
    Osteogenic (bone cells)

    Chondrogenic (cartilage cell)

    Collagenic (fibrous tissue cell)

    Myelogenic (marrow cell)

Osteoma
    Benign

    Abnormal outgrowth of bone

Chondroblastoma
    Rare

    Usually benign

Osteosarcoma
    Malignant tumor of long bones

    Usually in young adults

    Typically causes bone pain

Multiple myeloma

Malignant plasma cells in skeletal system and soft tissue

Progressive and generally fatal

Usually in those over 40

Chondrosarcoma

Malignant cartilage tumor

Usually in middle-aged and older individuals

In late stages, symptoms include local swelling and pain

• Worsens with time

Surgical excision is usually treatment of choice

If diagnosed in early stages, it is treatable with long-term survival possible

Muscle Tumors

Rare

Rhabdomyosarcoma

Aggressive, invasive carcinoma with widespread metastasis

MUSCULOSKELETAL SYSTEM PATHOPHYSIOLOGY QUIZ

1. A compound fracture is also known as:
   a. complete
   b. incomplete
   c. closed
   d. open

2. This is a common bone disorder in postmenopausal women resulting from lower levels of calcium and potassium:
   a. Paget's disease
   b. lordosis
   c. osteoporosis
   d. rheumatoid arthritis

3. This inflammatory disease is progressive and leads to a rigid spinal column:
   a. polymyositis
   b. ankylosing spondylitis
   c. primary fibromyalgia syndrome
   d. septic arthritis of spine

4. This type of tumor arises from bone cells:
   a. osteogenic
   b. chondrogenic
   c. collagenic
   d. myelogenic

5. This type of tumor is the most common type of malignant bone tumor that occurs in those over 40 and is progressive and generally fatal:
   a. rhabdomyosarcoma
   b. chondrosarcoma
   c. osteosarcoma
   d. multiple myeloma

6. A general muscle inflammation with an accompanying skin rash is:
   a. muscular dystrophy
   b. dermatologic arthritis
   c. ankylosing spondylitis
   d. dermatomyositis

7. A cartilage tumor that usually occurs in middle-aged and older individuals:
   a. chondrosarcoma
   b. osteosarcoma
   c. chondroblastoma
   d. rhabdomyosarcoma

8. Returning of bone to normal alignment is:
   a. immobilization
   b. traction
   c. reduction
   d. manipulation

9. Result of overuse or overextension of a ligament is:
   a. strain
   b. sprain
   c. fracture
   d. displacement

10. Primary osteoarthritis is also known as:
    a. secondary
    b. functional
    c. congenital
    d. idiopathic

■ RESPIRATORY SYSTEM
RESPIRATORY SYSTEM—ANATOMY AND TERMINOLOGY

Supplies oxygen to body and helps clean body of waste (carbon dioxide)

Two tracts (Fig. 1–15A)

- Upper respiratory tract (nose, naso/oro/larngo, pharynx, and larynx)

- Lower respiratory tract (trachea, bronchial tree, and lungs)

Lined with ciliated mucosa

- Purifies air by trapping irritants

Warms and humidifies air

Upper Respiratory Tract (URT)

Nose
Sense of smell (olfactory)

Moistens and warms air

Nasal septum divides interior

Sinuses (Paranasal or Accessory Sinuses) (4 pair)
Frontal

Ethmoid

Maxillary

Sphenoid

Turbinates (Conchae)
Bones on inside of nose

Divided into inferior, middle, and superior (Fig. 1–15B)

Warms and humidifies air

Pharynx (Throat)
Passageway for both food and air

Nasopharynx contains adenoids

Oropharynx contains tonsils

Laryngopharynx leads to larynx

Larynx (Voice Box) (opening to trachea)
Contains vocal cords

- Cartilages of larynx, thyroid, epiglottis, and arytenoid

Lower Respiratory Tract (LRT)

Trachea (Windpipe)—Air-Conducting Structure
Mucus-lined tube with C-shaped cartilage rings to hold windpipe open

Segmental Bronchi
Trachea divides into right and left main bronchus which further divide into lobar bronchii—3 on right, 2 on left

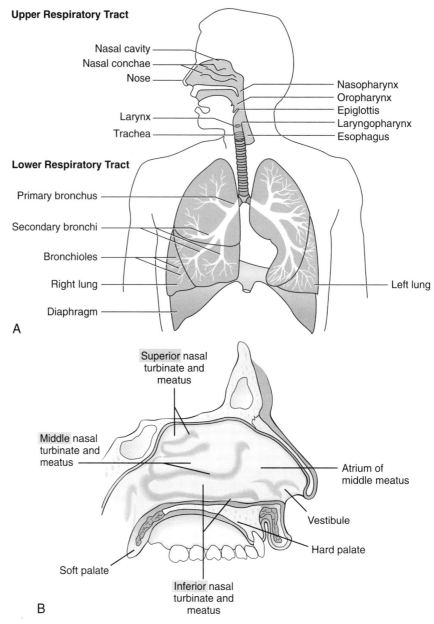

Figure **1-15 A,** Upper and lower respiratory system. **B,** Superior, inferior, and middle nasal turbinates.

Bronchioles
Branches divide into secondary bronchi, then smaller bronchioles

Alveolar Ducts (minute branches of bronchial tree)
End in alveoli (sacs) of simple squamous cells

• Primary gas-exchange units

Surrounded by capillaries and where exchange of oxygen and carbon dioxide takes place

Lungs

Covered by pleura

Cone-shaped organs filling thoracic cavity

Base rests on diaphragm and apex (top of lungs) extends to above clavicles

Hilum is medial surface of lung where pulmonary artery, pulmonary veins, nerves, lymphatics, and bronchial tubes enter and exit

Left lung contains two lobes divided by fissures

Right lung contains three lobes

Respiration

Inspiration—oxygen moves in, downward movement of lungs enlarging thoracic cavity

Expiration—carbon dioxide moves out, upward movement of diaphragm decreasing lung space

COMBINING FORMS

1.	adenoid/o	adenoid
2.	alveol/o	alveolus
3.	atel/o	incomplete
4.	bronch/o	bronchus
5.	bronchi/o	bronchus
6.	bronchiol/o	bronchiole
7.	capn/o	carbon dioxide
8.	coni/o	dust
9.	cyan/o	blue
10.	diaphragmat/o	diaphragm
11.	epiglott/o	epiglottis
12.	laryng/o	larynx
13.	lob/o	lobe
14.	mediastin/o	mediastinum
15.	muc/o	mucus
16.	nas/o	nose
17.	orth/o	straight
18.	ox/o	oxygen
19.	oxy/o	oxygen
20.	pector/o	chest
21.	pharyng/o	pharynx
22.	phon/o	voice

23.	phren/o	diaphragm
24.	pleur/o	pleura
25.	pneum/o	lung/air
26.	pneumat/o	air
27.	pneumon/o	lung/air
28.	pulmon/o	lung
29.	py/o	pus
30.	rhin/o	nose
31.	sept/o	septum
32.	sinus/o	sinus
33.	spir/o	breath
34.	tel/o	complete
35.	thorac/o	thorax
36.	tonsill/o	tonsil
37.	trache/o	trachea

PREFIXES

1.	a-	not
2.	an-	not
3.	endo-	within
4.	eu-	good
5.	dys-	difficult
6.	pan-	all
7.	poly-	many

SUFFIXES

1.	-algia	pain
2.	-ar	pertaining to
3.	-ary	pertaining to
4.	-capnia	carbon dioxide
5.	-centesis	puncture to remove (drain)
6.	-dynia	pain
7.	-eal	pertaining to
8.	-ectasis	stretching
9.	-emia	blood
10.	-gram	record

11.	-graph	recording instrument
12.	-graphy	recording process
13.	-itis	inflammation
14.	-meter	measurement or instrument that measures
15.	-metry	measurement of
16.	-osmia	smell
17.	-oxia	oxygen
18.	-pexy	fixation
19.	-phonia	sound
20.	-pnea	breathing
21.	-ptysis	spitting
22.	-rrhage, -rrhagia	abnormal, excessive flow
23.	-scopy	to examine
24.	-spasm	contraction of muscle
25.	-sphyxia	pulse
26.	-stenosis	blockage, narrowing
27.	-stomy	opening
28.	-thorax	chest
29.	-tomy	cutting, incision

MEDICAL ABBREVIATIONS

1.	ABG	arterial blood gas
2.	AFB	acid-fast bacillus
3.	ARDS	adult respiratory distress syndrome
4.	BiPAP	bi-level positive airway pressure
5.	COPD	chronic obstructive pulmonary disease
6.	CPAP	continuous positive airway pressure
7.	DLCO	diffuse capacity of lungs for carbon monoxide
8.	FEF	forced expiratory flow
9.	FEV_1	forced expiratory volume in 1 second
10.	FEV_1:FVC	maximum amount of forced expiratory volume in 1 second
11.	FRC	functional residual capacity
12.	FVC	forced vital capacity
13.	HHN	hand-held nebulizer
14.	IPAP	inspiratory positive airway pressure
15.	IRDS	infant respiratory distress syndrome

16. MDI	metered-dose inhaler
17. MVV	maximum voluntary ventilation
18. PAWP	pulmonary artery wedge pressure
19. PCWP	pulmonary capillary wedge pressure
20. PEAP	positive end-airway pressure
21. PEEP	positive end-expiratory pressure
22. PFT	pulmonary function test
23. PND	paroxysmal nocturnal dyspnea
24. RDS	respiratory distress syndrome
25. RSV	respiratory syncytial virus
26. RV	respiratory volume
27. RV:TLC	ratio of respiratory volume to total lung capacity
28. TLC	total lung capacity
29. TLV	total lung volume
30. URI	upper respiratory infection
31. V/Q	ventilation/perfusion scan

MEDICAL TERMS

Ablation	Removal or destruction by cutting, chemicals, or electrocautery
Adenoidectomy	Removal of adenoids
Apnea	Cessation of breathing
Asphyxia	Lack of oxygen
Asthma	Shortage of breath caused by contraction of bronchi
Atelectasis	Incomplete expansion of lung, collapse
Auscultation	Listening to sounds, such as to lung sounds
Bacilli	Plural of bacillus, a rod-shaped bacteria
Bilobectomy	Surgical removal of two lobes of a lung
Bronchiole	Smaller division of bronchial tree
Bronchoplasty	Surgical repair of bronchi
Bronchoscopy	Inspection of bronchial tree using a bronchoscope
Catheter	Tube placed into body to put fluid in or take fluid out
Cauterization	Destruction of tissue by use of cautery
Cordectomy	Surgical removal of vocal cord(s)
Crackle	Abnormal sound when breathing (heard on auscultation)
Croup	Acute viral infection (obstruction of larynx), stridor
Cyanosis	Bluish discoloration

Drainage	Free flow or withdrawal of fluids from a wound or cavity
Dysphonia	Speech impairment
Dyspnea	Shortage of breath, difficult breathing
Emphysema	Air accumulated in organ or tissue
Epiglottidectomy	Excision of covering of larynx
Epistaxis	Nose bleed
Glottis	True vocal cords
Hemoptysis	Bloody sputum
Intramural	Within organ wall
Intubation	Insertion of a tube
Laryngeal web	Congenital abnormality of connective tissue between vocal cords
Laryngectomy	Surgical removal of larynx
Laryngoplasty	Surgical repair of larynx
Laryngoscope	Fiberoptic scope used to view inside of larynx
Laryngoscopy	Direct visualization and examination of interior of larynx with a laryngoscope
Laryngotomy	Incision into larynx
Lavage	Washing out
Lobectomy	Surgical excision of a lobe of lung
Nasal button	Synthetic circular disk used to cover a hole in the nasal septum
Orthopnea	Difficulty in breathing, relieved by assuming upright position
Percussion	Tapping with sharp blows as a diagnostic technique
Pertussis	Whooping cough—highly contagious bacterial infection of pharynx, larynx, and trachea
Pharyngolaryngectomy	Surgical removal of pharynx and larynx
Pleura	Covers lungs and lines thoracic cavity
Pleurectomy	Surgical excision of pleura
Pleuritis	Inflammation of pleura
Pneumocentesis/ pneumonocentesis	Surgical puncturing of a lung to withdraw fluid
Pneumonia	Inflammation of lungs with consolidation
Pneumonolysis/ pneumolysis	Surgical separation of lung from chest wall to allow lung to collapse
Pneumonotomy/ pneumotomy	Incision of lung
Pulmonary edema	Accumulation of fluid in pulmonary tissues and air spaces
Pulmonary embolism	Thrombus or other foreign material lodged in pulmonary artery or one of its branches
Rales	An abnormal respiratory sound heard in auscultation, indicating some pathologic condition

Rhinoplasty	Surgical repair of nose
Rhinorrhea	Free discharge of a thin nasal mucous
Sarcoidosis	Chronic inflammatory disease with nodules developing in lungs, lymph nodes, other organs
Segmentectomy	Surgical removal of the smaller subdivisions (segment) of lobes of a lung
Septoplasty	Surgical repair of nasal septum
Sinusotomy	Surgical incision into a sinus
Spirometry	Measuring breathing capacity
Tachypnea	Quick, shallow breathing
Thoracentesis/ thoracocentesis (pleuracentesis/ pleurocentesis)	Surgical puncture of thoracic cavity, usually using a needle, to remove fluids
Thoracoplasty	Surgical procedure that removes rib(s) and thereby allows collapse of a lung
Thoracoscopy	Use of a lighted endoscope to view pleural spaces and thoracic cavity or to perform surgical procedures
Thoracostomy	Surgical incision into chest wall and insertion of a chest tube
Thoracotomy	Surgical incision into chest wall
Total pneumonectomy	Surgical removal of an entire lung
Tracheostomy	Creation of an opening into trachea
Tracheotomy	Incision into trachea
Transtracheal	Across trachea
Tuberculosis	Infection of the lungs caused by bacteria (tubercle bacillus)

RESPIRATORY SYSTEM ANATOMY AND TERMINOLOGY QUIZ

1. This is NOT a part of lower respiratory tract:
   a. trachea
   b. larynx
   c. bronchi
   d. lungs

2. Another name for voice box is:
   a. oropharynx
   b. pharynx
   c. laryngopharynx
   d. larynx

3. This is the windpipe:
   a. pharynx
   b. larynx
   c. trachea
   d. sphenoid

4. Interior of nose is divided by the:
   a. septum
   b. sphenoid
   c. oropharynx
   d. apical

5. This combining form means incomplete:
   a. atel/o
   b. alveol/o
   c. ox/i
   d. pneumat/o

6. This combining form means breath:
   a. py/o
   b. lob/o
   c. spir/o
   d. pleur/o

7. This prefix means all:
   a. a-
   b. an-
   c. pan-
   d. poly-

8. This abbreviation refers to a syndrome that involves difficulty in breathing:
   a. ABG
   b. ARDS
   c. BiPAP
   d. FEF

9. This abbreviation refers to amount of air patient can expel from the lungs in 1 second:
   a. PFT
   b. PND
   c. RDS
   d. FEV_1

10. This suffix means breathing:
    a. -stenosis
    b. -spasm
    c. -pexy
    d. -pnea

RESPIRATORY SYSTEM—PATHOPHYSIOLOGY

Signs and Symptoms of Pulmonary Disorders

Dyspnea
Difficult breathing (sense of air hunger)

Increased respiratory effort

Hypoventilation
Decreased alveolar ventilation

Hyperventilation
Increased alveolar ventilation

Hemoptysis
Bloody sputum

Hypoxia
Reduced oxygenation of tissue cells

Cough
Caused by irritant

Protective reflex

Acute cough is up to 3 weeks

Chronic cough is over 3 weeks

Tachypnea
Rapid breathing

Apnea
Lack of breathing

Orthopnea
Requiring sitting upright to facilitate breathing

Pulmonary Diseases and Disorders

Hypercapnia
Increased carbon dioxide in arterial blood

Caused by inadequate ventilation of alveoli

Can result in respiratory acidosis

Hypoxemia
Reduced oxygenation of arterial blood

Acute Respiratory Failure
Inadequate gas exchange

Hypoxemia

Can result from trauma or disease

Adult Respiratory Distress Syndrome (ARDS)
Acute injury to alveolocapillary membrane

Results in edema and atelectasis

In infants, infant respiratory distress syndrome (IRDS)

Pulmonary Edema
Accumulation of fluid in lung tissue

Most common cause is left ventricular failure

Aspiration
Passage of fluid and solid particles into lung

Can cause severe pneumonitis

- Localized inflammation of lung

Atelectasis
Collapse of lung

Three most common types are:

- Adhesive
- Compression
- Obstruction

May be chronic or acute

- Acute, such as compression as a result of an automobile accident
- Chronic from structural defect

Absorption Atelectasis
Results from absence of air in alveoli

Caused by

   Foreign body

   Tumor

   Abnormal external pressure

Bronchiectasis
Chronic, irreversible dilation of bronchi

Common types that describe severity of condition
- Cylindrical
- Varicose
- Sacular or cystic

Respiratory Acidosis
Decreased level of pH

   Due to excess retention of carbon dioxide

Bronchiolitis
Inflammation and obstruction of bronchioles

Usually in children less than 2—preceded by URI

Viral infection (respiratory syncytial virus, or RSV)

Common types
- Constrictive
- Proliferative
- Obliterative

Pneumothorax

Air collected in pleural cavity

Leads to lung collapse

Communicating pneumothorax is barometric air pressure in pleural space

Spontaneous pneumothorax is spontaneous rupture of visceral pleura

Secondary pneumothorax is a result of trauma to chest

Pneumoconiosis

Dust particles or other particulate matter in lung

Common types
- Coal
- Asbestos
- Fiberglass

Pleural Effusion-Fluid in Pleural Space

Common types
- Hemothorax—hemorrhage into pleural cavity
- Empyema—Infectious materials in pleural space
- Exudate—Fluid remaining after infection, inflammation, malignancy

Empyema

Infectious pleural effusion

Pus in pleural space

Is a complication of respiratory infection

Commonly follows pneumonia and is treated like pneumonia

Pulmonary Embolism

Air, tissue, or clot occlusion

Lodges in pulmonary artery or branch of artery

Risk with congestive heart failure

Most clots originate in leg veins

Cor Pulmonale

Hypertrophy or failure of right ventricle

Result of lung, pulmonary vessels, or chest wall disorders

Acute is secondary to pulmonary embolus

Chronic is secondary to obstructive lung disease

Pleurisy (Pleuritis)

Inflammation of pleura

Often preceded by an upper respiratory infection

Infectious Disease
Upper respiratory infection (URI)

Acute inflammatory process of mucous membranes in trachea and above

Common types
- Common cold

- Croup

- Sinusitis

- Laryngitis

Lower Respiratory Infection (LRI)

Pneumonia

Inflammation of lungs with consolidation

Categorized according to causative organism

Can be caused by

Aspiration

Bacteria

Protozoa

Fungi

Chlamydia

Virus

Common types

Aspiration pneumonia

Bacterial

Chlamydial

Drug resistant

Eosinophil

Fungal

Hospital acquired (nosocomial)

Legionnaire's

Mycoplasma

Pneumococcal

Viral

Tuberculosis

Communicable lung disease—airborne droplet

Caused by *Mycobacterium tuberculosis (bacilli)*

Chronic Obstructive Pulmonary Disease (COPD)

Irreversible airway obstruction that decreases expiration

Includes

Chronic bronchitis

- Bronchial spasms

- Dyspnea

- Wheezing

- Productive cough

- Cyanosis

- Chronic hypoventilation

- Polycythemia

- Cor pulmonale

- Prolonged expiration

Emphysema

- Loss of elasticity and enlargement of alveoli

- Mimics symptoms of chronic bronchitis but more exaggerated

RESPIRATORY SYSTEM PATHOPHYSIOLOGY QUIZ

1. Acute injury to alveolocapillary membrane that results in edema and atelectasis:
   a. hypoxemia
   b. adult respiratory distress syndrome
   c. bronchiolitis
   d. pneumoconiosis

2. Condition in which pus is in pleural space and is often a complication of pneumonia:
   a. empyema
   b. cor pulmonale
   c. pneumothorax
   d. atelectasis

3. Which of the following is NOT one of the most common types of atelectasis?
   a. adhesive
   b. compression
   c. obstruction
   d. expansion

4. This condition is a result of accumulation of dust particles in lung:
   a. pleurisy
   b. tuberculosis
   c. chronic obstructive pulmonary disease
   d. pneumoconiosis

5. An irreversible airway obstructive disease in which symptoms are bronchial spasm, dyspnea, and wheezing:
   a. pleurisy
   b. empyema
   c. bronchiolitis
   d. COPD

6. Cylindrical, varicose, and secular/cystic are examples of:
   a. bronchiectasis
   b. cor pulmonale
   c. pneumothorax
   d. atelectasis

7. Condition in which there is a loss of elasticity and enlargement of alveoli:
   a. chronic bronchitis
   b. asthma
   c. emphysema
   d. empyema

8. Definition of a chronic cough is one that lasts for over this number of weeks:
   a. 2
   b. 3
   c. 4
   d. 5

9. A condition marked by an increase in carbon dioxide in arterial blood and decreased ability to breathe that can result in respiratory acidosis:
   a. hypercapnia
   b. hypoxemia
   c. acute respiratory failure
   d. pulmonary edema

10. This condition often follows a viral infection and occurs in children under 2 years of age. Examples of various types of this condition are constrictive, proliferating, and obliterative.
   a. pneumoconiosis
   b. pulmonary edema
   c. bronchiolitis
   d. bronchiectasis

■ CARDIOVASCULAR SYSTEM
CARDIOVASCULAR SYSTEM—ANATOMY AND TERMINOLOGY

Consists of blood, blood vessels, and heart

Blood (function is to maintain a constant environment)

Composed of cells suspended in plasma (clear, straw-colored liquid)

Carries
Oxygen and nutrients to cells

Waste and carbon dioxide to kidneys, liver, and lungs

Hormones from endocrine system

Regulates
Temperature by circulating blood

Protection
White cells (leukocytes) produce antibodies

Composed of Two Parts
Liquid part (extracellular) is plasma

Water 91%

Protein 1%, albumin, globulins, fibrinogen, ferritin, transferrin

2% ions, nutrients, waste products, gases, regulating substances

Cellular structures

Leukocytes (WBCs) granular and agranular—fight infections

- Neutrophils
- Lymphocytes
- Monocytes
- Eosinophils
- Basophils

Erythrocytes (red blood cells)—hemoglobin carries oxygen

Thrombocytes (platelets)—important for hemostasis

Blood types: A, B, AB, and O are genetically endowed

- Blood type O negative is known as universal donor (no Rh and no red cell antigens present)

Vessels—Circulatory System

Function

To carry blood delivering nutrients and oxygen (arterial system) and carry away cell waste and carbon dioxide (venous system)

Types
Arteries (Fig. 1–16) carrying oxygenated blood

Inner layer, endothelium

Lead away from heart

Branches are arterioles

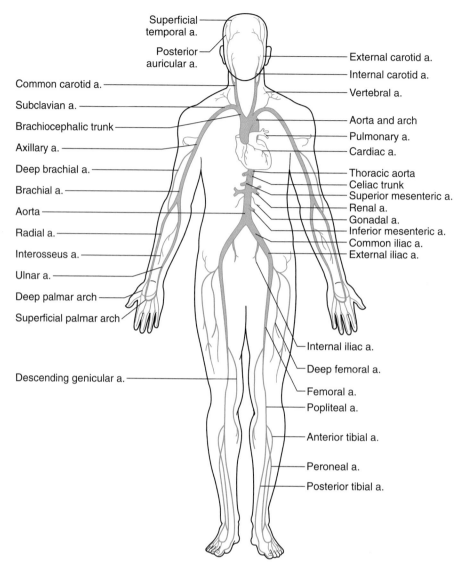

Figure **1-16** Arteries of circulatory system.

Capillaries

Connection between arterioles and venules

Exchange structure (oxygen and carbon dioxide, nutrients, and waste)

Veins (Fig. 1–17) carrying deoxygenated blood
Carry blood to heart

Venules are small branches

Heart

Circulates blood

Four Chambers (Fig. 1–18)
Two upper
Right and left atria (singular: atrium) receive blood

Two lower
Right and left ventricles discharge blood (pump)

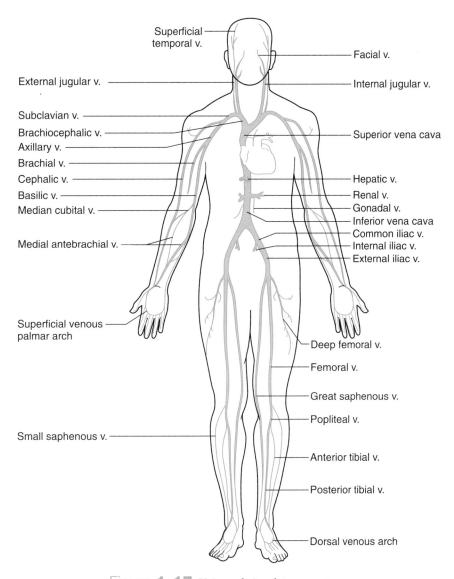

Figure **1-17** Veins of circulatory system.

Chamber Walls
Composed of three layers

- Endocardium: smooth inner layer

- Myocardium: middle muscular layer

- Epicardium: outer layer

Septa (singular: septum)
Divide chambers

- Interatrial septum

    Separates two upper chambers

- Interventricular septum

    Separates two lower chambers

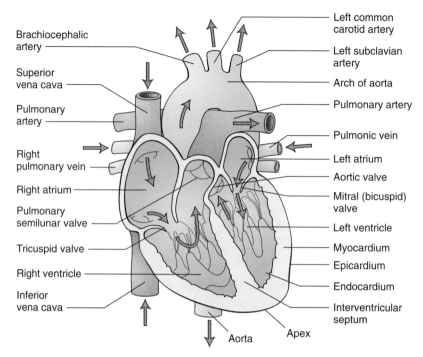

Figure **1-18** Internal view of heart.

Major Blood Vessels

Inferior vena cava—carries deoxygenated blood from lower extremities, pelvic and abdominal viscera to right atrium

Superior vena cava—drains deoxygenated blood from head, neck, upper extremities, and chest to right atrium

Pulmonary artery bifurcates and becomes right and left pulmonary artery—carries deoxygenated blood from right ventricle to lungs

Right and left pulmonary veins (4)—carry oxygenated blood from lungs to left atrium

Aorta—carries oxygenated blood from left side of heart to body

Pericardium

Sac comprised of two layers that covers heart

- Parietal pericardium: outermost covering

- Visceral pericardium: innermost (epicardium)

- Pericardial cavity: contains about 30 cc of fluid

Valves (4 in heart)

Tricuspid: between right atrium and right ventricle

Pulmonary: at entrance of pulmonary artery leading from right ventricle

Aortic: at entrance of aorta leading from left ventricle

Bicuspid (mitral): between left atrium and left ventricle

Conduction System (Fig. 1–19)

Sinoatrial node: SAN, nature's pacemaker, sends impulses to atrioventricular node

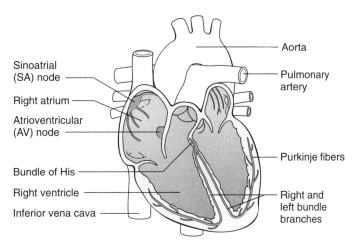

Figure **1-19** Electrical system of heart.

Atrioventricular node (AVN): located on interatrial septum and sends impulses to bundle of His

Bundle of His: divides into right bundle branch (RBB) and left bundle branch (LBB) in septum

Purkinje fibers: merge from bundle branches into specialized cells of myocardium, located at base of heart

Heartbeat

Two Phases—Correspond to Blood Pressure Readouts

Systole: contraction—top number reading

Diastole: relaxation—lower number reading

Trace a drop of blood from trunk of body (deoxygenated) to trunk of body (oxygenated)

Inferior vena cava to right atrium

Through tricuspid valve to right ventricle

From right ventricle to pulmonary artery to lung capillaries

From lung capillaries to pulmonary veins

To left atrium through mitral (bicuspid) valve to left ventricle

Though aortic valve to aorta

COMBINING FORMS

1.	angi/o	vessel
2.	aort/o	aorta
3.	ather/o	yellow plaque (fat)
4.	arter/o	artery
5.	arteri/o	artery
6.	atri/o	atrium
7.	brachi/o	arm

8. cardi/o   heart
9. cholesterol/o   cholesterol
10. coron/o   heart
11. cyan/o   blue
12. my/o, muscul/o muscle
13. myx/o   mucous
14. ox/o   oxygen
15. pericardi/o   pericardium
16. phleb/o   vein
17. sphygm/o   pulse
18. steth/o   chest
19. thromb/o   clot
20. valv/o   valve
21. valvul/o   valve
22. vascul/o   vessel
23. vas/o   vessel
24. ven/o   vein
25. ventricul/o   ventricle

PREFIXES

1. a-   not
2. an-   not
3. bi-   two
4. brady-   slow
5. de-   lack of
6. dys-   bad, difficult, painful
7. endo-   in
8. hyper-   over
9. hypo-   under
10. inter- between
11. intra- within
12. meta-   change, after
13. peri-   surrounding
14. tachy- fast
15. tetra- four
16. tri-   three

SUFFIXES

1.	-dilation	widening, expanding
2.	-emia	blood
3.	-graphy	recording process
4.	-lysis	separation
5.	-megaly	enlargement
6.	-oma	tumor
7.	-osis	condition
8.	-plasty	repair
9.	-sclerosis	hardening
10.	-stenosis	blockage, narrowing
11.	-tomy	cutting, incision

MEDICAL ABBREVIATIONS

1.	ASCVD	arteriosclerotic cardiovascular disease
2.	ASD	atrial septal defect
3.	ASHD	arteriosclerotic heart disease
4.	AV	atrioventricular
5.	CABG	coronary artery bypass graft
6.	CHF	congestive heart failure
7.	CK	creatine kinase
8.	CPK	creatine phosphokinase
9.	CVI	cerebrovascular insufficiency
10.	DSE	dobutamine stress echocardiography
11.	HCVD	hypertensive cardiovascular disease
12.	LBBB	left bundle branch block
13.	LVH	left ventricular hypertrophy
14.	MAT	multifocal atrial tachycardia
15.	MI	myocardial infarction
16.	NSR	normal sinus rhythm
17.	PAC	premature atrial contraction
18.	PAT	paroxysmal atrial tachycardia
19.	PST/PSVT	paroxysmal supraventricular tachycardia
20.	PTCA	percutaneous transluminal coronary angioplasty
21.	PVC	premature ventricular contraction
22.	RBBB	right bundle branch block
23.	RSR	regular sinus rhythm

24. RVH	right ventricular hypertrophy
25. SVT	supraventricular tachycardia
26. TEE	transesophageal echocardiography
27. TST	treadmill stress test

MEDICAL TERMS

Acute Coronary Syndrome (ACS)	An umbrella term used to cover clinical symptoms compatible with acute myocardial ischemia
Anastomosis	Surgical connection of two tubular structures, such as two pieces of the intestine
Aneurysm	Abnormal dilation of vessels, usually an artery
Angina	Spasmotic, choking, or suffocative pain
Angiography	Radiography of blood vessels
Angioplasty	Procedure in a vessel to dilate vessel opening
Atherectomy	Removal of plaque from an artery (can be done by a percutaneous or open procedure)
Auscultation	Listening for sounds within body
Bundle of His	Muscular cardiac fibers that provide heart rhythm to ventricles
Bypass	To go around
Cardiopulmonary	Refers to heart and lungs
Cardiopulmonary bypass	Blood bypasses heart through a heart-lung machine
Cardioverter-defibrillator	Surgically placed or wearable device that directs an electric shock to the heart to restore rhythm
Circumflex	A coronary artery that circles heart
Cutdown	Incision into a vessel for placement of a catheter
Edema	Swelling due to abnormal fluid collection in tissue spaces
Electrode	Lead attached to a generator that carries electric current from the generator to atria or ventricles
Electrophysiology	Study of electrical system of heart, including study of arrhythmias
Embolectomy	Removal of blockage (embolism) from vessel
Endarterectomy	Incision into an artery to remove inner lining
Epicardial	Over heart
False aneurysm	Sac of clotted blood that has completely destroyed vessel and is being contained by tissue that surrounds vessel
Fistula	Abnormal opening from one area to another area or to outside of the body
Hematoma	Mass of blood that forms outside vessel
Hemolysis	Breakdown of red blood cells
Hypoxemia	Low level of oxygen in blood

Hypoxia	Low level of oxygen in tissue
Intracardiac	Inside heart
Invasive	Entering body, breaking skin
Noninvasive	Not entering body, not breaking skin
Nuclear cardiology	Diagnostic specialty that uses radiologic procedures to aid in diagnosis of cardiologic conditions
Order	Shows subordination of one thing to another; family or class
Pericardiocentesis	Procedure in which a surgeon withdraws fluid from pericardial space by means of a needle inserted percutaneously
Pericardium	Membranous sac enclosing heart and ends of great vessels
Swan Ganz catheter	A catheter that measures pressure in right side of heart and in pulmonary artery
Thoracostomy	Incision into chest wall and insertion of a chest tube
Thromboendarterectomy	Removal of thrombus and atherosclerotic lining from an artery (percutaneous or open procedure)
Transvenous	Through a vein

CARDIOVASCULAR SYSTEM ANATOMY AND TERMINOLOGY QUIZ

1. These carry blood to the heart:
   a. capillaries
   b. arteries
   c. arterioles
   d. veins

2. Relaxation phase of heartbeat:
   a. diastole
   b. systole

3. Nature's pacemaker is this node:
   a. atrioventricular
   b. Bundle of His
   c. sinoatrial
   d. mitral

4. Node located on interatrial septum:
   a. atrioventricular
   b. Bundle of His
   c. sinoatrial
   d. Purkinje

5. Which of following is NOT one of the three layers of chamber walls of the heart?
   a. endocardium
   b. myocardium
   c. epicardium
   d. parietal

6. Septum that divides upper two chambers of heart:
   a. intraventricular
   b. interatrial
   c. tricuspid
   d. myocardium

7. Valve between right atrium and right ventricle:
   a. pulmonary
   b. aortic
   c. bicuspid
   d. tricuspid

8. Outer two-layer covering of heart:
   a. pericardium
   b. mitral
   c. myocardium
   d. epicardium

9. These are chambers that receive blood:
   a. right and left ventricle
   b. left ventricle and right atrium
   c. right atrium and right ventricle
   d. right and left atria

10. This combining form means plaque:
    a. atri/o
    b. brachi/o
    c. cyan/o
    d. ather/o

CARDIOVASCULAR SYSTEM—PATHOPHYSIOLOGY
Vascular Disorders

Coronary Artery Disease (CAD)/Ischemic Heart Disease (IHD)
Thickening and hardening of arterial intima (innermost layer) with lipid and fibrous plaque (atherosclerosis)

- Produces narrowing and stiffening of vessel

Location of lesions leads to various vascular diseases

- Femoral and popliteal arteries = peripheral vascular disease
- Carotid arteries = stroke
- Aorta = aneurysms (dilation/weakening of vessel walls)
- Coronary arteries = ischemic heart disease or myocardial infarction

Resulting in decreased oxygen supply

Risk factors increased by:

- Age
- Family history of CAD
- Hyperlipidemia
- Low HDL-C (good cholesterol)
- Hypertension
- Cigarette smoking
- Diabetes mellitus
- Obesity, particularly abdominal

Ischemia
Deficiency of oxygenated blood

- Often due to constriction or obstruction of blood vessel

Localized myocardial ischemia—most common cause: atherosclerosis of vessels
Oxygen demand of tissues greater than supply

Presenting symptoms

- Chest pain (angina pectoris)
- Hypotension
- Changes in ECG

Transient ischemia
Heart muscle begins to perform at a low level due to lack of oxygen (reversible ischemia)

Irreversible ischemia—is cause of an MI (myocardial infarction)
Heart muscle dies—necrosis (myocardial infarction)

- Prolonged ischemia of 30 minutes or more
- Reestablishment of blood flow reduces residual necrosis
  - Thrombolytic agents to dissolve or split up thrombus
  - Primary percutaneous transluminal coronary angioplasty (PTCA)

Cardiac enzymes are released from damaged cells

- Blood test reveals elevation of enzymes, confirming myocardial infarction

Hypertension (HTN)

Normal is less than 120/80 for adults

- Fig. 1–20 illustrates new hypertension classifications

Leading cause of death in United States, due to damage to brain, heart, kidneys, eyes, and arteries of the lower extremities

Cause is unknown in 95% of cases

- Known as
  - Primary hypertension
  - Essential hypertension

5% of cases are secondary to underlying disease

Increased resistance damages heart and blood vessels

- Retinal vascular changes are monitored to assess therapy and disease progression

Chronic hypertension often leads to end-stage renal disease

- Result of progressive sclerosis of renal vessels

Treatment
Medications

- ACE (angiotensin-converting enzyme) inhibitor
- Alpha-adrenergic or beta-adrenergic receptor blocker
- Diuretic
- Calcium channel blocker

Lifestyle changes

Classification of blood pressure for
adults aged 18 years or older[1]

Category	Systolic (mm Hg)	Diastolic (mm Hg)
Normal	<120	<80
Prehypertension (stays between)	120–139	80–89
Hypertension[2]		
Stage 1 (mild)	140–159	90–99
Stage 2 (moderate)	160–179	100–109
Stage 3 (severe)	≥180	≥110

[1] Not taking antihypertensive drugs and not acutely ill. When systolic and diastolic pressures fall into different categories, the higher category should be selected.

[2] Based on the average of two or more readings taken at each of two or more visits after an initial screening.

Figure **1-20** Classification of blood pressure.

Hypotension
Abnormally low blood pressure

Types

Orthostatic (postural) hypotension

- Fall in both systolic and diastolic arterial blood pressure on standing
- Associated with
  - Dizziness
  - Blurred vision
  - Fainting (syncope)
- Caused by insufficient oxygenated blood flow through brain
- Can be acute (temporary) or chronic

Chronic orthostatic hypotension—types

- Primary of unknown cause
- Secondary to certain disease processes
- Such as:
  - Endocrine
  - Metabolic
  - Central nervous system disorders
- Treatment for secondary hypotension is correction of underlying disease

Aneurysm
Dilation of an arterial blood vessel wall or cardiac chamber

- Danger is rupture of aneurysm

Atherosclerosis is common cause

Arteriosclerosis and hypertension also common in persons with aneurysms

True aneurysm

Involves all three layers of arterial wall

Causes weakening and ballooning of arterial wall

False or psuedoaneurysm

Usually result of trauma

Also known as saccular

Separation of arterial wall layers (dissecting) in artery wall (crisis situation—a medical emergency)

Bleeds into dissected space and is contained by arterial connective tissue wall

Thrombus
Blood clot that remains attached to vessel wall and occludes vessel

Dislodged thrombus is a thromboembolus

Causes

Trauma

Interior wall lining irritation/roughening

Infection

Inflammation

Low blood pressure/blood stagnation

Obstruction

Atherosclerosis

Risks related to thrombus
Dislodge/moving to lungs, brain, heart

Grow to occlude blood flow

Treatment
Pharmacologic, anticoagulants

Heparin

Warfarin derivatives

Non-invasive intervention
Balloon-tipped catheter to remove or compress thrombus

Thrombophlebitis Caused by Inflammation (Phlebitis)
Causes
Trauma

Infection

Immobility

Commonly associated with
Endocarditis

Rheumatic heart disease

Embolism
Mass that is present and circulating in blood

Common types
Air bubble

Fat

Bacterial mass

Cancer cells

Foreign substances

Dislodged thrombus

Amniotic fluid

Obstructs vessel
Pulmonary emboli travel through venous side or right side of heart to the pulmonary artery

Systemic or arterial emboli originate in left side of the heart

Associated with

- Myocardial infarction
- Left-side heart failure

- Endocarditis

- Valvular conditions

- Dysrhythmias

Peripheral Arterial Disease
Thromboangiitis obliterans (Buerger's disease)
Occurs most often in young men who are heavy smokers

Inflammatory disease of peripheral arteries creating thombi and vasospasms

Involves small or medium arteries of feet and often hands

- May necessitate amputation

Raynaud's disease
Vasospasms and constriction of small arterioles of fingers and toes

Affects young women as a secodary condition

Triggered by cold temperatures, emotional stress, cigarette smoking

Fingertips thicken and nails become brittle

Raynaud's phenomenon is secondary to primary disease, such as

- Scleroderma

- Pulmonary hypertension

Treatment of underlying condition
No known origin or treatment

Varicose Veins
Blood pools in veins, distending them

Tends to be progressive/vein valve failure

Occurs most commonly in saphenous veins

Hemorroids are varicose veins of anus

Leads to
Swelling and discomfort

Fatigue when in legs

Possible ulcerations

Heart Disorders

Congestive Heart Failure (CHF)—heart cannot pump required amounts of blood
Can be left-sided or right-sided heart failure

Left-sided heart failure (systolic); cannot generate adequate output, causing pulmonary edema

Common causes:

Myocardial infarction

Myocarditis

Cardiomyopathies leading to ischemia

Symptoms of left-sided congestive heart failure include:

Shortness of breath

Fatigue

Exercise intolerance

Right-sided heart failure (diastolic) results in right ventricle stasis, inadequate pulmonary circulation, and peripheral edema/hepatosplenomegaly

Abnormal Heart Rhythms (Conduction Irregularities)

Bradycardia and heart block (atrioventricular block)

Inadequate conduction impulses from SA node though AV node to AV bundle

Treatment

Cardiac pacemaker to maintain proper heart rate

Flutter—rapid regular contractions (most commonly of atria)

Symptoms—palpitations

Treatment

Cardioversion (electronic shock to heart)

Ablation (radiofrequency catheter destroying tissue causing arrhythmia)

Fibrillation—rapid, erratic, inefficient contractions of atria and ventricles

Atrial fibrillation—most common (electrical impulses move randomly in atria)

Symptoms—palpitation, risk of stroke due to clot formations from poor atrial outputs

Treatment

Cardioversion

Ablation

Ventricular fibrillation—life-threatening, random electrical impulses throughout ventricles

Symptoms

Cardiac death or arrest without immediate treatment

Treatment

Cardioversion

Digoxin—drug used to slow heart rate

Implantable cardioverter-defibrillator (ICD)

Emergency treatment—automatic external defibrillators (AEDs)

Radiofrequency catheter ablation (RFA) is a minimally invasive technique used to treat cardiac arrhythmias

Infective Endocarditis

Inflammation of interior most lining of heart

Leads to destruction and permanent damage to heart valves

Caused by

> Bacteria (most common streptococci and staphlococci)
>
> Virus
>
> Fungi
>
> Parasites

Patients with heart defects or damage usually take antibiotics prior to invasive procedures

Pericarditis
Inflammation of pericardium of heart

Common types
- Acute

- Pericardial effusion

- Constrictive

Rheumatic Fever/Rheumatic Heart Disease
Results in formation of scar tissue of the endocardium and heart valves

In 10% of cases leads to rheumatic heart disease

Family tendency to develop

Begins as carditis (inflammation of all layers of heart wall)

Long-term effect:

Mitral and/or aortic valve disease

> Stenosis
>
> Regurgitation
>
> Insuffiency

Tricuspid valve

> Affected in about 10% of cases

Pulmonary valve

> Rarely affected

Valvular Heart Disease

Valves are extensions of endocardial tissue

Endocardial damage can be congenital or acquired

Damage leads to stenosis and/or incompetent valve

Includes

- Valvular stenosis is narrowing, stiffness, thickening, fusion, or blockage of valve, creating resistance, resulting in increased pressure in cardiac chamber behind valve

- Valvular regurgitation is failure of valve leaflet to close tightly, allowing backflow of blood

  - Result of lesions causing valve leaflets to shrink

  - Functional valvular regurgitation results in increased chamber size (cardiomegaly)

Stenosis
Aortic valve stenosis

Caused by

Congenital malformation

Degeneration

Infection

Results in slowing blood circulatory rate

Symptoms

Bradycardia

Faint pulse

May lead to heart murmur and hypertrophy

Mitral valve stenosis

Impaired flow from left atrium to left ventricle

Caused by

Rheumatic fever

Bacterial infections

Symptom

Decreased cardiac output

May lead to

- Pulmonary hypertension
- Right ventricular heart failure
- And/or edema

Valvular Regurgitation
Flow in opposite direction from normal

Mitral regurgitation (MR)

Backflow of blood from left ventricle into left atrium

Aortic regurgitation (AR)

Backflow of blood from aorta into the left ventricle

Pulmonic regurgitation (PR)

Backflow of blood from pulmonary artery into right ventricle

Tricuspid regurgitation (TR)

Backflow of blood from right ventricle into the right atrium

Heart Wall Disorders

Acute Pericarditis
Roughening and inflammation of pericardium (sac around heart)

Treatment

Antiinflammatory drugs and pain medication

Constrictive Pericarditis (Restrictive Pericarditis)

Forms fibrous lesions that encase heart

Compresses heart—thickened pericardial sac prevents heart from expanding when blood enters it

Tamponade occurs when fluid builds up in pericardial space

Pressure stops heart from beating—pericardial effusion or bleeding after heart surgery

Reduces output

Pericardial Effusion

Accumulation of fluid in pericardial cavity

Results in pressure on heart

- Sudden development of pressure on heart is tamponade

Cardiomyopathies

Myocardium: muscular wall (middle layer) of heart musculature

Group of diseases that affect myocardium

Cause

Idiopathic (most common)

Underlying condition

Types of Cardiomyopathy

Dilated cardiomyopathy (congestive cardiomyopathy)

- Ventricular distention and impaired systolic function

Hypertrophic cardiomyopathy

- Cause is often hypertensive or valvular heart disease
- Results in thickened interventricular septum (septum between the ventricle chambers)

Restrictive cardiomyopathy

- Myocardium becomes stiffened
- Heart enlarges (cardiomegaly)
- Dysrhythmias common
- Caused by infiltrative diseases such as amyloidosis

Congenital Heart Defects

Coarctation of aorta (CoA)—narrowing of the aorta

- Treatment

Surgical removal of narrow segment/end to end anastomosis

Patent ductus arteriosus (PDA)—opening between aorta and pulmonary artery

- Treatment

Drugs to close/embolize or plug ductus or tying off surgically

Tetralogy of Fallot—malformation of heart including four defects

- Pulmonary artery stenosis—narrowing/obstruction

Ventricular septal defect

- Hole between two ventricles

Shift of aorta to right—aorta overrides the interventricular septum

- Hypertrophy of right ventricle

- Myocardium enlarges to pump blood through narrowed pulmonary artery

Septal defect—holes in the septa (wall) between the atria (atrial septal defect) or the ventricles (ventricular septal defect)

- Treatment

    Close hole using open heart technique and heart lung machine support or percutaneous transcatheter closure is used to close hole in septum

CARDIOVASCULAR SYSTEM PATHOPHYSIOLOGY QUIZ

1. Lesion of carotid artery may lead to:
   a. heart attack
   b. stroke
   c. peripheral vascular disease
   d. ischemic heart disease

2. This blood pressure is hypertension:
   a. 120/80
   b. 130/70
   c. 140/90
   d. 110/70

3. Tachyarrhythmia or fast heart rate is that in excess of _____bpm.
   a. 60
   b. 80
   c. 90
   d. 100

4. Angina pectoris is:
   a. heart block
   b. heart murmur
   c. chest pain
   d. barrel chest

5. In this type of regurgitation there is a backflow of blood from left ventricle into left atrium:
   a. aortic
   b. pulmonic
   c. tricuspid
   d. mitral

6. In this type of heart wall disorder, fibrous lesions form and encase heart:
   a. constrictive pericarditis
   b. acute pericarditis
   c. pericardial effusion
   d. cardiomyopathy

7. Which of the following terms means "of unknown cause"?
   a. etiology
   b. manifestation
   c. idiopathic
   d. late effect

8. This condition is also known as congestive cardiomyopathy:
   a. hypertrophic
   b. valvular
   c. dilated
   d. restrictive

9. This peripheral arterial disease most often occurs in young men who are heavy smokers:
   a. Buerger's
   b. Pick's
   c. Addison's
   d. Glasser's

10. This cardiomyopathy results in a thickened interventricular septum:
    a. restrictive
    b. congestive
    c. dilated
    d. hypertrophic

■ FEMALE GENITAL SYSTEM AND PREGNANCY

FEMALE GENITAL SYSTEM AND PREGNANCY—ANATOMY AND TERMINOLOGY

Terminology

Ovaries (Pair)
Produce ova (single female gamete) and hormones; ova: plural; ovum: singular (Fig. 1–21). Each ova/gamete contains 23 chromosomes.

Fallopian Tubes (Uterine Tubes or Oviducts)
Ducts from ovary to uterus

Uterus (Womb)
Muscular organ that holds embryo

Three layers
- Endometrium: inner mucosa
- Myometrium: middle layer/muscle
- Perimetrium/Uterine serosa: outer layer
  - Cervix: lower narrow portion of uterus
  - Fundus: the upper rounded part of the uterus

Vagina
Tube from uterus to outside of body

Vulva
External genitalia
- Clitoris: erectile tissue
- Labia majora: outer lips of vagina
- Labia minora: inner lips of vagina
- Urinary meatus: opening to urethra
- Bartholin's gland: glands on either side of vagina
- Hymen: membrane partially or wholly occludes entrance to vagina

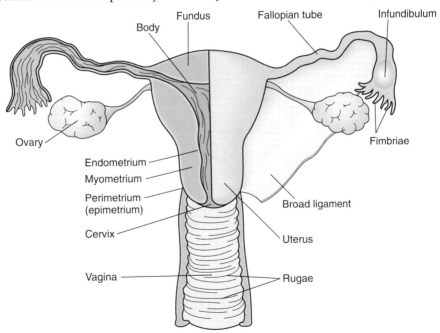

Figure **1-21** Female reproductive system.

Perineum

Area between anus and vaginal orifice

Accessory Organs (Fig. 1–22)

Breasts

Mammary glands

Composed of glandular tissue containing milk glands/lactiferous ducts

In response to hormones from pituitary gland, milk is produced in acini (also known as alveolua) (lactation)

Lactiferous ducts transfer milk to nipple

Nipple, surrounded by areola

Menstruation and Pregnancy

Proliferation Phase

Menstruation (Days 1-5): discharge of blood fluid containing endometrial cells, blood cells, and glandular secretions from endometrium

Endometrium repair (Days 6-12): maturing follicle in ovary produces estrogen (hormone) which causes endometrium to thicken and ovum (egg) to mature in graafian follicle

Secretory Phase

Ovulation (Days 13-14): occurs when graafian follicle ruptures and ovum travels down fallopian tube

Usually only one graffian follicle develops each month

Premenstruation (Days 15-28): a period of time in which graafian follicle converts to corpus luteum secreting progesterone to stimulate build-up of uterine lining. If after 5 days no fertilization occurs, cycle repeats.

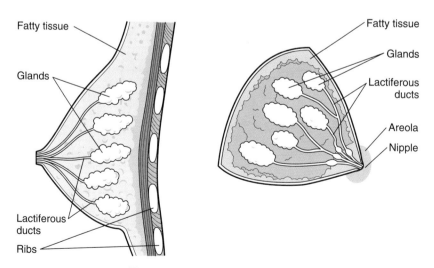

Figure **1-22** Breast structure.

Pregnancy

Prenatal stage of development from fertilization to birth (39 weeks)

Fertilized ovum or zygote develops in a double cavity: yolk sac (produces blood cells) and amniotic cavity (contains amniotic fluid)

Embryo, stage of development from 4th to 8th week

Fetus, unborn offspring, 9 weeks until birth

Placenta Forms Within Uterine Wall and Produces Hormone—Human Chorionic Gonadotropin (HCG)

HCG is horomone tested in urine pregnancy tests

HCG stimulates corpus luteum to produce estrogen and progesterone until the third month of pregnancy

Placenta then produces hormones

Expelled after delivery (afterbirth)

Gestation, Approximately 266 Days

280 days used when calculating Estimated Date of Delivery (EDD) or that time from last menstrual period (LMP)

Three trimesters

- First   LMP-12 weeks
- Second   13-27 weeks
- Third   28 weeks-EDD

COMBINING FORMS

1.	amni/o	amnion
2.	arche/o	first
3.	cephal/o	head
4.	cervic/o	cervix
5.	chori/o	chorion
6.	colp/o	vagina
7.	crypt/o	hidden
8.	culd/o	cul-de-sac
9.	episi/o	vulva
10.	fet/o	fetus
11.	galact/o	milk
12.	gynec/o	female
13.	gyn/o	female
14.	hymen/o	hymen
15.	hyster/o	uterus
16.	lact/o	milk

17. lapar/o   abdominal wall
18. mamm/o   breast
19. mast/o   breast
20. men/o   menstruation, month
21. metr/o   uterus, measure
22. metr/i   uterus
23. my/o, muscul/o muscle
24. nat/a   birth
25. nat/i   birth
26. obstetr/o   pregnancy/childbirth
27. olig/o   few
28. oo/o   egg
29. oophor/o   ovary
30. ov/o   egg
31. ovari/o   ovary
32. ovul/o   ovulation
33. perine/o   perineum
34. peritone/o   peritoneum
35. phor/o   to bear
36. salping/o   uterine tube, fallopian tube
37. top/o   place
38. uter/o   uterus
39. vagin/o   vagina
40. vulv/o   vulva

PREFIXES

1. ante-   before
2. dys-   painful
3. ecto-   outside
4. endo-   in
5. extra-   outside
6. in-   into
7. intra-   within
8. multi-   many
9. neo-   new
10. nulli- none
11. nulti- none

12. post-   after
13. primi-   first
14. pseudo-   false
15. retro-   backwards
16. uni-   one

SUFFIXES

1. -arche   beginning
2. -cyesis   pregnancy
3. -gravida   pregnancy
4. -rrhexis   rupture
5. -para   woman who has given birth
6. -parous   to bear
7. -rrhea   discharge
8. -salpinx   uterine tube
9. -tocia   labor
10. -version   turning

MEDICAL ABBREVIATIONS

1. AFI   amniotic fluid index
2. AGA   appropriate for gestational age
3. ARM   artificial rupture of membrane
4. BPD   biparietal diameter
5. BPP   biophysical profile
6. BV   bacterial vaginosis
7. CHL   crown-to-heel length
8. CNM   certified nurse midwife
9. CPD   cephalopelvic disproportion
10. CPP   chronic pelvic pain
11. D&C   dilation and curettage
12. D&E   dilation and evacuation
13. DUB   dysfunctional uterine bleeding
14. ECC   endocervical curettage
15. EDC   estimated date of confinement
16. EDD   estimated date of delivery
17. EFM   electronic fetal monitoring
18. EFW   estimated fetal weight

19.	EGA	estimated gestational age
20.	EMC	endometrial curettage
21.	ERT	estrogen replacement therapy
22.	FAS	fetal alcohol syndrome
23.	FHR	fetal heart rate
24.	FSH	follicle-stimulating hormone
25.	HPV	human papillomavirus
26.	HSG	hysterosalpingogram
27.	HSV	herpes simplex virus
28.	IVF	in vitro fertilization
29.	LEEP	loop electrosurgical excision procedure
30.	LGA	large for gestational age
31.	PID	pelvic inflammatory disease
32.	PROM	premature rupture of membranes
33.	SHG	sonohysterogram
34.	SROM	spontaneous rupture of membrane
35.	SUI	stress urinary incontinence
36.	TAH	total abdominal hysterectomy
37.	VBAC	vaginal birth after cesarean

MEDICAL TERMS

Abortion	Termination of pregnancy
Amniocentesis	Percutaneous aspiration of amniotic fluid
Amniotic sac	Sac containing fetus and amniotic fluid
Antepartum	Before childbirth
Cesarean	Surgical opening through abdominal wall for delivery
Chorionic villus sampling	CVS, biopsy of outermost part of placenta
Cordocentesis	Procedure to obtain a fetal blood sample; also called a percutaneous umbilical blood sampling
Curettage	Scraping of a cavity using a spoon-shaped instrument
Cystocele	Herniation of bladder into vagina
Delivery	Childbirth
Dilation	Expansion (of cervix)
Ectopic	Pregnancy outside uterus (i.e., in fallopian tube)
Hysterectomy	Surgical removal of uterus
Hysterorrhaphy	Suturing of uterus
Hysteroscopy	Visualization of canal and cavity of uterus using a scope placed through vagina

Introitus	Opening or entrance to vagina
Ligation	Binding or tying off, as in constricting blood flow of a vessel or binding fallopian tubes for sterilization
Multipara	More than one pregnancy
Oophorectomy	Surgical removal of ovary(ies)
Perineum	Area between vulva and anus; also known as pelvic floor
Placenta	A structure that connects fetus and mother during pregnancy
Postpartum	After childbirth
Primigravida	First pregnancy
Primipara	First delivered infant/given birth to only one child
Salpingectomy	Surgical removal of uterine tube
Salpingostomy	Creation of a fistula into uterine tube
Tocolysis	Repression of uterine contractions
Vesicovaginal fistula	Abnormal opening/channel between vagina and bladder

FEMALE GENITAL SYSTEM AND PREGNANCY ANATOMY AND TERMINOLOGY QUIZ

1. This is NOT one of three layers of uterus:
   a. perimetrium
   b. endometrium
   c. myometrium
   d. barametrium

2. Located at the lower end of uterus is the:
   a. cervix
   b. vagina
   c. perineum
   d. labia majora

3. Approximate gestation of a human fetus is:
   a. 266 days
   b. 276 days
   c. 290 days
   d. 292 days

4. LMP is the:
   a. later maternity phase
   b. last menstrual period
   c. low metabolic pregnancy
   d. late menstruation phase

5. Name of stage that describes development of fetus from fertilization to birth is:
   a. postpartum
   b. antepartum
   c. prenatal
   d. natal

6. Which of the following correctly identifies three trimesters of gestation?
   a. LMP-12 weeks, 13-27 weeks, 28-EDD
   b. LMP-14 weeks, 15-27 weeks, 28-EDD
   c. LMP-14 weeks, 15-28 weeks, 29-EDD
   d. LMP-11 weeks, 12-26 weeks, 27-EDD

7. Combining form meaning few:
   a. oopho/o
   b. olig/o
   c. nati/i
   d. top/o

8. Combining form meaning hidden:
   a. amni/o
   b. crypt/o
   c. chori/o
   d. fet/o

9. Suffix meaning beginning:
   a. -cyesis
   b. -rrhea
   c. -arche
   d. -orrhexis

10. Prefix meaning within:
    a. ante-
    b. dys-
    c. ecto-
    d. endo-

Dysmenorrhea
Painful menstruation

Common types
- Primary and secondary

Primary dysmenorrhea
No underlying condition but begins with commencement of ovulation

Cramping is caused by excess of prostaglandin

- Causes contractions and uterine ischemia
- Develops 24 to 48 hours prior to menstruation

Treatment
- Nonsteroidal antiinflammatory agents
- Progesterone

Secondary dysmenorrhea
Caused by an underlying disorder, such as

- Polyps
- Tumors
- Endometriosis
- Pelvic inflammatory disease

Treatment
Directed at underlying disorder

Amenorrhea
Amenorrhea is absence of menstruation

Common types
- Primary and secondary

Primary amenorrhea
Menstruation has never occurred

May be genetic disorder

- Turner's syndrome (ovaries do not function)

Secondary amenorrhea
Cessation of menstruation for 3 cycles or 6 months

- Individual has previously menstruated

Various causes of annovulation/amenorrhea

Examples:
- Tumors
- Stress
- Eating disorders
- Competitive sports participation

Dysfunctional Uterine Bleeding (DUB)

Abnormal bleeding patterns

Occurs when no organic cause can be identified

Abnormal Menstruation Types

Oligomenorrhea: in excess of 6 weeks between periods

Polymenorrhea: less than 3 weeks between periods

Metrorrhagia: bleeding between cycles

Menorrhagia: increase in amount and duration of flow

Hypomenorrhea: light or spotty flow

Menometrorrhagia: irregular cycle with varying amounts and duration

Menorrhea: lengthy menstrual flow

Dysmenorrhea: painful menstruation

Premenstrual Syndrome (PMS)

Also known as premenstrual tension (PMT)

Occurs before onset of menses (luteal phase) and ends at onset of menses

Cluster of common symptoms

Weight gain

Breast tenderness

Sleep disturbances

Headache

Irritability

Cause is unknown

Treatment

- Vary depending on individual symptoms

Endometriosis

Endometrial tissue (uterine lining) develops outside the uterus (on ovaries, fallopian tubes, small intestine, etc.)

Responses to hormone cycle

Ectopic (out of place) endometrial tissue degenerates, sheds, and bleeds

Causes

- Irritation

- Inflammation

- Pain

Continued cycles produce fibrous tissue

- Adhesions and obstructions can then form

- Interferes with normal bodily function

- For example, fallopian tube endometriosis may lead to obstructed tubes

Primary symptom is dysmenorrhea

- May also cause painful intercourse (dyspareunia)

Risks
Increased risk for cancers

- Breast

- Ovaries

- Non-Hodgkin lymphoma

Treatment Includes
Hormonal suppression

Surgical removal of endometrial tissue

- May require hysterectomy and BSO (bilateral salpingo-oophorectomy)

Infection, Inflammation, and Sexually Transmitted Diseases

Pelvic Inflammatory Disease (PID)

Infection and inflammation of reproductive tract

- Primarily ovaries and fallopian tubes

- Usually originates in cervix or vagina

  - Migrates up through reproductive tract

Types
Acute

Chronic

Commonly forms adhesions and strictures

- May lead to infertility

Candidiasis

Yeast infection

- *Candida albicans (Monilia)*

Not sexually transmitted

Opportunistic infection may follow

- Infection treated with antibiotics

- Period of reduced resistance

- Increased glucose or glycogen levels (often associated with diabetes mellitus)

Affects mucous membranes

Produces a white, thick, curd-type discharge

Result may be dyspareunia and dysuria

Treatment
Antifungal substances such as nystatin

Identification and treatment of underlying condition

Chlamydia

Most common sexually transmitted disease (STD)

Cause
Bacteria, *Chlamydia trachomatis*

Symptoms
Asymptomatic or mild discharge and dysuria

Treatment
Antimicrobial

Genital Herpes
Cause
Virus, herpes simplex 2 (HSV-2)

Symptoms
Ulcers and vesicles

Treatment
Antiviral, manage outbreaks

There is no cure for genital herpes

Genital Warts
Cause
Virus, human papillomavirus

Symptoms
Polyps or grey lesions

Treatment
Excision

Prevention
Vaccine

There is no cure for genital warts

Gonorrhea
Cause
Bacteria, *Neisseria gonorrhoeae*

Some strains are drug-resistant

Symptoms
Dysuria

Discharge

Treatment
Antibacterial drugs

Syphilis
Cause
Bacteria, *Treponema pallidum*

Symptoms
Primary syphilis

- Ulcer or chancre at site of entry

Secondary syphilis

- Headache

- Fever

- Rash

- Tertiary

  - Affects cardiovascular and nervous systems

Treatment
Penicillin

Trichomoniasis
Cause
Protozoa, *Trichomonas vaginalis*

Symptoms
Usually asymptomatic

Treatment
Antimicrobial drugs

Benign Lesions

Leiomyomas—Uterine Fibroids
Well-defined, solid uterine tumor

Also known as

- Uterine fibroids

- Fibromyoma

- Fibroma

- Myoma

- Fibroid

Classification is based on location of tumor within uterine wall

Submucous: beneath endometrium

Subserous: beneath serosa

Intramural: in muscle wall

Symptoms
May be asymptomatic

Abnormal uterine bleeding

Pressure on nearby structures, such as bladder and rectum

Constipation

Pain

Sensation of heaviness

Treatment
Surgical excision of lesions

Hysterectomy may be necessary

Adenomyosis
Within uterine myometrium

Symptoms
Usually asymptomatic

Abnormal menstrual bleeding

Enlarged uterus

Commonly develops in late reproductive years

Common in those taking Tamoxifen

Treatment
Symptomatic in mild cases

Surgical in severe cases

- Excision of adenomyosis or hysterectomy

Malignant Lesions

Carcinoma of Breast
Accessory of reproductive system

Most often develops in upper outer quadrant

- Due to location, often spreads to lymph nodes

- May metastasize to lungs, brain, bone, liver, etc.

Majority arise from epithelial cells of ducts and lobules

Second most common cancer of women

Most are adenocarcinoma

- Invasive ductal carcinoma most common type

- Invasive lobular carcinoma second most common type

- Lymph node spread is determined by biopsying sentinel node (SNB)

- Small primary tumors are excised in a lumpectomy (tumor and immediate surrounding tissue only)

- Mastectomy is alternative surgical procedure removing entire breast

- Chemotherapy and radiation may be indicated to prevent reoccurrence

If neoplasm is responsive to hormone, hormone-blocking agents are administered

Increased risks
- Heredity

  - Especially history of mother or sister who developed breast cancer

  - Mutated breast cancer gene (BRCA-1)

  - Familial breast cancer syndrome associated with BRCA-2

- Lower socioeconomic status

- Radiation exposure

Carcinoma of Uterus (Endometrial Cancer)

Most frequent pelvic cancer

Usually postmenopausal

Associated with higher levels of estrogen

Increases risk

Obesity (estrogen produced by fat tissue)

Early menarche

Delayed menopause

Hypertension

Diabetes mellitus

Nulliparity (no viable births)

Some types of colorectal cancer

Oral contraceptives (estrogen)

Estrogen-producing tumors

Symptoms

Abnormal, excessive uterine bleeding

Postmenopausal bleeding

No simple screening test available

- Uterine cells may be aspirated for evaluation

Staging of endometrial, cervical, and ovarian malignancies

I—Confined to corpus

II—Involves corpus and cervix

III—Extends outside uterus but not outside true pelvis

IV—Extends outside true pelvis or involves rectum or bladder

Treatment

Pharmaceutical

Surgical

Irradiation

Chemotherapy

Combination of above

Carcinoma of Cervix

Routinely found on Papanicolaou smear

Dysplasia is an early change in cervical epithelium

Increases risks

Herpes simplex virus type 2 (HSV-2)

Human papillomavirus (HPV)

Young age of sexual activity

Smoking

Lower socioeconomic status

Stages of cervical cancer

Stage 1 Carcinoma of cervix

Stage 2 Carcinoma spread from cervix to upper vagina

Stage 3 Carcinoma spread to lower portion of vagina/pelvic wall

Stage 4 Most invasive stage spreading to other body parts

Symptoms

Early stages asymptomatic

Later stages

- Bleeding

- Discharge

Biopsy is used to confirm

Treatment

Pharmaceutical

Surgical

Irradiation

Chemotherapy

Combination of above

Carcinoma of Ovary

Cause is unknown—considered silent killer

Increased risks

Genetic factors (BRCA-1)

Endocrine

- Nulliparous

- Early menarche

- Late menopause

- Non-breast feeding

- Late first pregnancy

- Postmenopausal estrogen replacement therapy (ERT)

Tumor categories

Germ cell tumors

Arise from primitive germ cells, usually the testis and ovum

Types

- Germinoma

- Yolk sac

- Endodermal sinus tumor
- Teratoma
- Embryonal carcinoma
- Polyembryoma
- Gonadoblastoma
- Some types of choriocarcinoma

Categories

- Dermoid cysts (benign)
- Malignant tumors
- Primitive malignant
  - Embryonic
  - Extraembryonic cells

Epithelial tumors
Most common gynecologic cancer

Gonadal stromal tumors
Symptoms
   Pelvic heaviness

   Dysuria

   Increased urinary frequency

   Sometimes vaginal bleeding

Treatment
   Excision

      Hysterectomy, including bilateral salpingo-oophorectomy with omentectomy (fold of peritoneum)

   Chemotherapy

   Radiation therapy

   Combination of above

Carcinoma of Fallopian Tubes

Primary fallopian tube tumors
Rare

Must be located within tube to be considered primary

- Adenocarcinoma most common primary tumor

Most tumors are secondary

Symptoms
   Often asymptomatic

   Bleeding or discharge

   Irregular menstruation

   Pain

Treatment

Hysterectomy, including bilateral salpingo-oophorectomy with any necessary omentectomy (fold of peritoneum)

Chemotherapy

Radiation therapy

Combination of above

Carcinoma of Vulva

Usually squamous cell carcinoma (90%)

Increased risk with STDs

Symptoms

Can be asymptomatic

Pruritic vulvular lesion

Treatment

Radical vulvectomy with node dissection

Wide local excision

Carcinoma of Vagina

Usually squamous cell carcinoma

Increased risk

Human papillomavirus (HPV)

Postmenopausal hysterectomy

History of abnormal Pap

History of other carcinomas

Symptoms

Often asymptomatic

Vaginal pain, discharge, or bleeding

Treatment

Squamous cell—radiation

Early tumors may be excised

Vaginectomy

Hysterectomy

Lymph node dissection

Pregnancy

Placenta Previa

Opening of cervix is obstructed by displaced placenta

Types (Fig. 1–23)

Marginal

Partial

Total

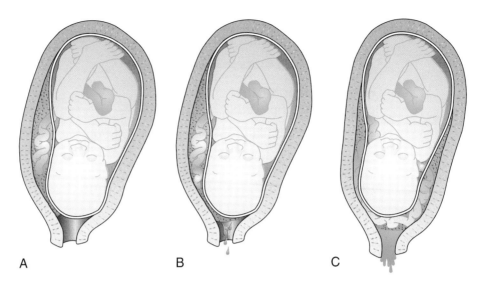

Figure **1-23** **A,** Marginal placenta previa. **B,** Partial placenta previa. **C,** Total placenta previa.

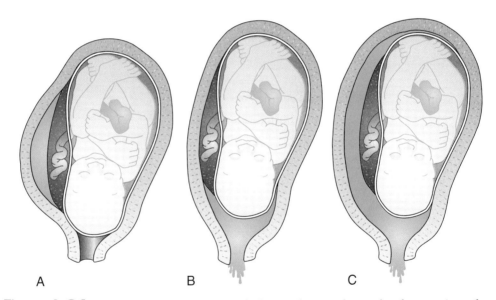

Figure **1-24** Abruptio placentae is classified according to the grade of separation of the placenta from uterine wall. **A,** Mild separation in which hemorrhage is internal. **B,** Moderate separation in which there is external hemorrhage. **C,** Severe separation in which there is external hemorrhage and extreme separation.

Abruptio Placentae (Fig. 1–24)
Premature separation of placenta from uterine wall

Eclampsia
Serious condition of pregnancy characterized by

- Hypertension
- Edema
- Proteinuria

Ectopic Pregnancy (Extrauterine) (Fig. 1–25)
Implantation of fertilized ovum outside uterus

- Often fallopian tubes (tubal pregnancy)

Hydatidiform Mole
Benign tumor of placenta

Secretes hormone (chorionic gonadotropic hormone, CGH)

Indicates positive pregnancy test

Malpositions and Malpresentations (Fig. 1–26)
Vaginal Delivery

Breech

Vertex

Face

Brow

Shoulder

Abortion
Types

Spontaneous

- Miscarriage
- Happens naturally
- Uterus completely empties

Incomplete

- Uterus does not completely empty
- Requires intervention to remove remaining fetal material

Missed

- Fetus dies naturally
- Requires intervention to remove fetal material

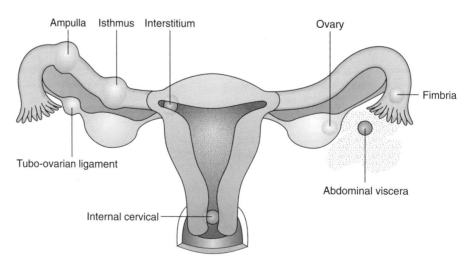

Figure **1-25** Ectopic pregnancy most often occurs in fallopian tube. Pregnancy outside the uterus may end in life-threatening rupture.

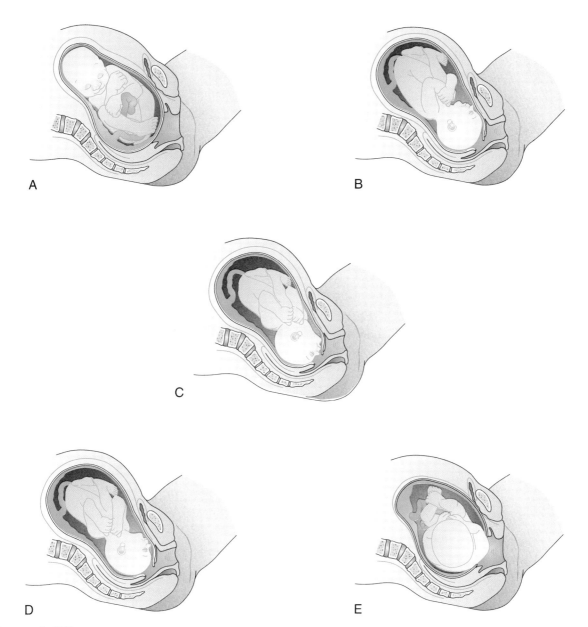

Figure **1-26** Five types of malposition and malpresentation of fetus: **A,** Breech. **B,** Vertex. **C,** Face. **D,** Brow. **E,** Shoulder.

Septic

- Similar to missed

- Has added complication of infection

- Requires intervention to remove fetal material

- Vigorous treatment of infection

Methods
D&C

- Dilation and curettage (scraping)

Evacuation (suction)

Intra-amniotic injections

- Saline (salt) solution

Vaginal suppositories

- Such as prostaglandin

FEMALE GENITAL SYSTEM AND PREGNANCY PATHOPHYSIOLOGY QUIZ

1. Most common solution used for intra-amniotic injections is:
   a. prostaglandin
   b. saline
   c. estrogen
   d. chorionic gonadotropic hormone

2. This type of dysmenorrhea is treated with nonsteroidal antiinflammatory agents and progesterone:
   a. secondary
   b. constrictive
   c. periodic
   d. primary

3. In this type of amenorrhea there is a cessation of menstruation:
   a. secondary
   b. constrictive
   c. periodic
   d. primary

Match the abnormal menstruation type with correct definition.

4. oligomenorrhea _____   a. increased amount and duration of flow

5. metrorrhagia _____   b. bleeding between cycles

6. menorrhagia _____   c. in excess of 6 weeks

7. Increased risks of breast cancer, ovarian cancer, and non-Hodgkin lymphoma exist with this condition:
   a. endometriosis
   b. pelvic inflammatory disease
   c. sexually transmitted disease
   d. dysfunctional uterine bleeding

8. This benign lesion is also known as uterine fibroids:
   a. adenomyosis
   b. squamous cell
   c. leiomyoma
   d. extraembryonic cell primitive

9. Marginal, partial, and total are types of this condition:
   a. abruptio placentae
   b. placenta previa
   c. ectopic pregnancy
   d. hydatidiform mole

10. Which of the following is NOT a malposition of fetus?
    a. breech
    b. shoulder
    c. back
    d. brow

■ MALE GENITAL SYSTEM
MALE GENITAL SYSTEM—ANATOMY AND TERMINOLOGY

Function, reproduction

Structure, essential organs, and accessory organs (Fig. 1–27)

Essential Organs

Testes (Gonads)
Produce sperm (male gamete with 23 chromosomes) in seminiferous tubules

Covered by tunica albuginea, located in scrotum

Produce testosterone in Leydig cells

Vas Deferens
Is a tube

End of epididymis

Accessory Organs

Ducts (carry sperm from testes to exterior), sex glands (produce solutions that mix with sperm), and external genitalia

Seminal vesicles produce most seminal fluid

Prostate gland produces some seminal fluid and activates sperm

Bulbourethral gland (Cowper's glands) secretes a very small amount of seminal fluid

External genitalia: penis and scrotum

• Penis contains three columns of erectile tissue: two corpora cavernosa and one spongiosum

• Urethra passes through corpora spongiosum

• Scrotum encloses testes

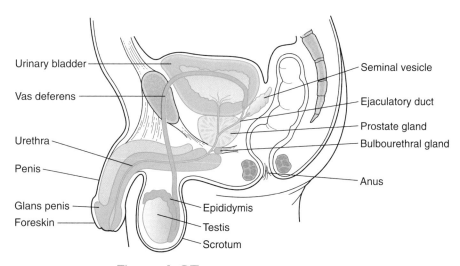

Figure **1-27** Male reproductive system.

Passage of sperm from production to exterior

Sperm are produced in seminiferous tubules (testes) and pass into

Epididymis then to vas deferens (within seminal vesicles) to

Ejaculatory duct then through urethra (prostate gland and Cowper's [bulbourethral] gland)

Passes though penis to outside of body

COMBINING FORMS

1.	andr/o	male
2.	balan/o	glans penis
3.	cry/o	cold
4.	crypt/o	hidden
5.	epididym/o	epididymis
6.	gon/o	seed
7.	hydr/o	water, fluid
8.	orch/i	testicle
9.	orch/o	testicle
10.	orchi/o	testicle
11.	orchid/o	testicle
12.	prostat/o	prostate gland
13.	semin/i	semen
14.	sperm/o	sperm
15.	spermat/o	sperm
16.	test/o	testicle
17.	varic/o	varicose veins
18.	vas/o	vessel, vas deferens
19.	vesicul/o	seminal vesicles

SUFFIXES

1.	-one	hormone
2.	-pexy	fixation
3.	-ectomy	removal
4.	-stomy	new opening

MEDICAL ABBREVIATIONS

1.	BPH	benign prostatic hypertrophy
2.	PSA	prostate-specific antigen
3.	TURBT	transurethral resection of bladder tumor
4.	TURP	transurethral resection of prostate

MEDICAL TERMS

Cavernosa	Connection between cavity of penis and a vein
Cavernosography	Radiographic recording of a cavity, e.g., pulmonary cavity or main part of penis
Cavernosometry	Measurement of pressure in a cavity, e.g., penis
Chordee	Condition resulting in penis being bent downward
Corpora cavernosa	The two cavities of penis
Epididymectomy	Surgical removal of epididymis
Epididymis	Tube located at the top of testes that stores sperm
Epididymovasostomy	Creation of a new connection between vas deferens and epididymis
Meatotomy	Surgical enlargement of opening of urinary meatus
Orchiectomy	Castration, removal of testes
Orchiopexy	Surgical procedure to release undescended testis and fixate within scrotum
Penoscrotal	Referring to penis and scrotum
Plethysmography	Determining changes in volume of an organ part or body
Priapism	Painful condition in which penis is constantly erect
Prostatotomy	Incision into prostate
Transurethral resection, prostate	Procedure performed through urethra by means of a cystoscopy to remove part or all of prostate
Tumescence	State of being swollen
Tunica vaginalis	Covering of testes
Varicocele	Swelling of a scrotal vein
Vas deferens	Tube that carries sperm from epididymis to ejaculatory duct and seminal vesicles
Vasectomy	Removal of segment of vas deferens
Vasogram	Recording of the flow in vas deferens
Vasotomy	Incision in vas deferens
Vasorrhaphy	Suturing of vas deferens
Vasovasostomy	Reversal of a vasectomy
Vesiculectomy	Excision of seminal vesicle
Vesiculotomy	Incision into seminal vesicle

MALE GENITAL SYSTEM ANATOMY AND TERMINOLOGY QUIZ

1. This gland activates sperm and produces some seminal fluid:
   a. seminal vesicle
   b. bulbourethral gland
   c. prostate gland
   d. scrotum

2. Carries sperm from testes to ejaculatory duct:
   a. vans deferens
   b. sex gland
   c. tunica
   d. seminal

3. Penis contains these erectile tissues:
   a. one corpora cavernosa and two spongiosa
   b. two corpora cavernosa and two spongiosa
   c. one corpora cavernosa and one spongiosum
   d. two corpora cavernosa and one spongiosum

4. Also known as Cowper's gland:
   a. seminal vesicles
   b. bulbourethral gland
   c. prostate gland
   d. scrotum

5. Which of the following is NOT an accessory organ?
   a. gonads
   b. seminal vesicles
   c. prostate
   d. penis

6. Combining form meaning male:
   a. andr/o
   b. balan/o
   c. orchi/o
   d. test/o

7. Combining form meaning glans penis:
   a. balan/o
   b. vas/o
   c. vesicul/o
   d. orch/o

8. Testes are covered by the:
   a. seminal vesicles
   b. androgen
   c. chancre
   d. tunica albuginea

9. This abbreviation describes a surgical resection of prostate that is accomplished by means of an endoscope inserted into urethra:
   a. TURBT
   b. BPH
   c. UPJ
   d. TURP

10. This abbreviation describes a condition of prostate in which there is an enlargement that is benign:
    a. TURBT
    b. BPH
    c. UPJ
    d. TURP

MALE GENITAL SYSTEM—PATHOPHYSIOLOGY

Male Genital System Disorders

Disorders of Scrotum, Testes, and Epididymis

Cryptorchidism

Undescended testes—condition at birth

- Unilateral or bilateral
- Primarily result from obstruction
- Risk neoplastic processes

Treatment

- May descend spontaneously
- Administration of hormone to stimulate testosterone production
- Surgical intervention (orchiopexy) near age 1 to avoid risk of infertility

Orchitis

Inflammation of testes

Most common cause is virus

- Such as mumps orchitis
- Atrophy with irreversible loss of sperm production at risk

May be associated with

- Mumps or epidemic parotitis
- Gonorrhea
- Syphilis
- Tuberculosis

Symptoms

- Mild to severe pain in testes
- Mild to severe edema
- Feeling of weight in testicular area

Treatment

- Depends upon presence of underlying condition

Epididymitis

Inflammation of epididymis

Inflammatory response to trauma or infection

Abscess may form

Types

Sexually transmitted epididymitis

- Gonorrhea
- *T. pallidum*
- *T. vaginalis*

Nonspecific bacterial epididymitis

- *E. coli*

- *Streptococci*

- *Staphylococci*

- Associated with underlying urological disorder

Symptoms
Scrotal pain

Swelling

Erythema

Perhaps hydrocele formation

Treatment
Antibiotic

Bed rest

Ice packs

Scrotal support

Analgesics

Hydrocele (Fig. 1–28)
Collection of fluid in membranes of tunica vaginalis

May be congenital or acquired (response to infection or tumors)

Congenital hydrocele may reabsorb due to a communication between the scrotal sac and peritoneal cavity and require no intervention

Symptoms
Scrotal enlargement

Usually painless

- Unless infection is present

Varicocele
Abnormal dilation of plexus of veins

Decreases sperm production and motility

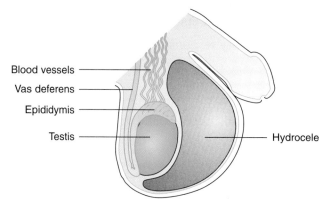

Figure **1-28** Hydrocele.

Symptoms
Usually painless

In elderly, may signal renal tumor

Treatment
Surgical intervention

Torsion of testes (Fig. 1-29)
Twisting of testes

Congenital abnormal development of tunica vaginalis and spermatic cord

Trauma may precipitate

Symptoms
Sudden onset of severe pain

Nausea

Vomiting

Scrotal edema and tenderness

Fever

Treatment
Immediate surgical intervention

Cancer of testes
Rare form of cancer

Cure rate high (95%)

Cause unknown

Usually occurs in younger men

Two main groups

• Germ cell tumors (GCT)—90% testicular tumors

• Sex cord-stromal tumors

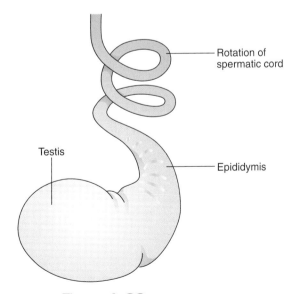

Figure **1-29** Torsion of testis.

Cancer of scrotum
Rare form of cancer

- Squamous cell carcinoma

Symptoms
Asymptomatic in early stages

Ulcerations in later stages

Treatment
Wide local excision

Mohs micrographic surgery

- Precise removal of tumor

- Layers are removed until no further microscopic evidence of abnormal cells is seen

Laser therapy

Lymph nodes are examined for metastasis

Disorders of Urethra
Epispadias
Congenital anomaly

Urethral meatus is located on dorsal side of penis

Usually occurs in conjunction with other abnormalities

Treatment
Surgical reconstruction

Hypospadias
Most common abnormality of penis

Urethral opening on ventral side of penis

Results in curvature of penis

- Due to chordee

Treatment
Surgical reconstruction

Urethritis
Inflammation of urethra

Infectious urethritis can be gonococcal or nongonococcal

Nongonococcal organisms

- *C. trachomatis*

- *U. urealyticum*

Symptoms
Discharge

Inflammation of meatus

Burning

Itching

Urgent and frequent urination

In nongonococcal, symptoms are less

Treatment
Antibiotics based on organism

Disorders of Penis
Balanitis
Inflammation of glans

Causes
Syphilis

Trichomoniasis

Gonorrhea

Candida albicans

Tinea

Underlying disease diabetes mellitus and candidiasis

No circumcision

Symptoms
Irritation

Tenderness

Discharge

Edema

Ulceration

Swelling of lymph nodes

Treatment
Culture of discharge

Saline irrigation

Antibiotics

Phimosis and paraphimosis
Phimosis
Condition in which prepuce (foreskin) is constricted

• Prepuce cannot be retracted over glans penis

Can occur at any age

Associated with poor hygiene and chronic infection in uncircumcised males

Symptoms
Erythema

Edema

Tenderness

Purulent discharge

Treatment
Surgical circumcision

Paraphimosis
Condition in which prepuce (foreskin) is constricted

Prepuce is retracted over glans penis and cannot be moved forward

Symptom
Edema

Treatment
Surgical

Peyronie's disease
Also known as bent nail syndrome

Fibrotic condition

- Results in lateral curvature of penis during erection

Occurs most often in middle-aged men

Cause is unknown but associated with

- Diabetes

- Keloid development

- Dupuytren's contracture (flexion deformity of toes and fingers)

Treatment
Sometimes spontaneous remission

Pharmacologic oxygenation increasing therapies

Surgical resection of fibrous bands

Cancer of penis
Rare form of cancer

Occurs most often in men over 60

Squamous cell carcinoma

Increased risks

- More common in uncircumcised men

- Sexual partner with cervical carcinoma

- Human papillomavirus

Usually begins with small lesion beneath prepuce

Intraepithelial neoplasia is also known as

- Bowen's disease

- Erythroplasia of Queyrat

- Begins as noninvasive

Progresses to invasive if untreated

Metastasis to lymph nodes

Treatment

Excision

Mohs micrographic surgery

Radiation therapy

Laser therapy

Cryosurgery

Advanced tumors are treated with partial or total penectomy and chemotherapy

Disorders of Prostate Gland

Benign prostatic hyperplasia/hypertrophy (BPH)

Multiple fibroadenomatous nodules; usually located on outside of gland so easily palpable on digital exam

- Related to aging; common in men over 60 years of age

- Enlarging prostate obstructs bladder neck and urethra

- Decreases urine flow

It is thought that increased levels of estrogen/androgen cause BPH

Symptoms

Increased frequency and urgency of urination

Nocturia

Incontinence

Hesitancy

Diminished force

Postvoiding dribble

Screening

Prostate-specific antigen (PSA)

Digital rectal examination (DRE)

Treatment

Partial prostatectomy

Transurethral resection of prostate (TURP)

Excision of nodules

Hormone therapy

Placement of urethral stents

Pharmaceuticals—those that inhibit production of testosterone and those that relax smooth muscle of gland and neck of bladder

Prostatitis

Inflammation of prostate

- Acute or chronic bacterial prostatitis

Causes

Escherichia coli

Enterococci

Staphylococci

Streptococci

Chlamydia trachomatis

Ureaplasma urealyticum

Neisseria gonorrhea

Nonbacterial
Spontaneous

Prostatodynia

Symptoms
Acute prostatitis
Fever and chills

Lower back pain

Perineal pain

Dysuria

Tenderness, suprapubic

Urinary tract infection

Chronic prostatitis
Recurring

Same as acute only with no infection in urinary tract

Treatment
Acute
Antibiotic based on culture

Chronic
No treatment available

Cancer of prostate
Most common diagnosed malignancy in men, occuring in men over age 60

Indications are cause is related to androgens

Predominately adenocarcinoma (95%)

No relationship between BPH and cancer of prostate

Symptoms
Asymptomatic in early stages

Later symptoms include

• Dysuria

• Back pain

• Hematuria

• Frequent urination

- Urinary retention

- Increased incidence of uremia

Stages
Two systems used to stage prostate cancer

- Whitmore-Jewett stages as indicated in Fig. 1–30

- Tumor node metastasis (TNM) as indicated in Fig. 1–31

Treatment
Dependent upon stage

WHITMORE-JEWETT STAGES:

Stage A is clinically undetectable tumor confined to the gland and is an incidental finding at prostate surgery.
A1: well-differentiated with focal involvement
A2: moderately or poorly differentiated or involves multiple foci in the gland
Stage B is tumor confined to the prostate gland.
B0: nonpalpable, PSA-detected
B1: single nodule in one lobe of the prostate
B2: more extensive involvement of one lobe or involvement of both lobes
Stage C is a tumor clinically localized to the periprostatic area but extending through the prostatic capsule; seminal vesicles may be involved.
C1: clinical extracapsular extension
C2: extracapsular tumor producing bladder outlet or ureteral obstruction
Stage D is metastatic disease.
D0: clinically localized disease (prostate only)
but persistently elevated enzymatic serum acid phosphatase
D1: regional lymph nodes only
D2: distant lymph nodes, metastases to bone or visceral organs
D3: D2 prostate cancer patients who relapse after adequate endocrine therapy

Figure **1-30** Whitmore-Jewett stages.

TNM STAGES:

Primary Tumor (T)

TX: Primary tumor cannot be assessed

T0: No evidence of primary tumor

T1: Clinically inapparent tumor not palpable or visible by imaging

  T1a: Tumor incidental histologic finding in 5% or less of tissue resected

  T1b: Tumor incidental histologic finding in more than 5% of tissue resected

  T1c: Tumor identified by needle biopsy (e.g., because of elevated PSA)

T2: Tumor confined within the prostate

  T2a: Tumor involves half a lobe or less

  T2b: Tumor involves more than half of a lobe, but not both lobes

  T2c: Tumor involves both lobes; extends through the prostatic capsule

T3a: Unilateral extracapsular extension

T3b: Bilateral extracapsular extension

T3c: Tumor invades the seminal vesicle(s)

T4: Tumor is fixed or invades adjacent structures other than the seminal vesicle(s)

  T4a: Tumor invades any of bladder neck, external sphincter, or rectum

  T4b: Tumor invades levator muscles and/or is fixed to the pelvic wall

Regional lymph nodes (N)

NX: Regional lymph nodes cannot be assessed

N0: No regional lymph node metastasis

N1: Metastasis in a single lymph node, 2 cm or less in greatest dimension

N2: Metastasis in a single lymph node, more than 2 cm but not more than 5 cm in greatest dimension; or multiple lymph node metastases, none more than 5 cm in greatest dimension

N3: Metastasis in a single lymph node more than 5 cm in greatest dimension

Distant metastases (M)

MX: Presence of distant metastasis cannot be assessed

M0: No distant metastasis

M1: Distant metastasis

  M1a: Nonregional lymph node(s)

  M1b: Bone(s)

  M1c: Other site(s)

Figure **1-31** TNM stages.

MALE GENITAL SYSTEM PATHOPHYSIOLOGY QUIZ

1. What is the condition in which testes do not descend?
   a. cryptorchidism
   b. Bowen's disease
   c. torsion
   d. hypospadias

2. Orchitis is most often caused by a:
   a. bacteria
   b. virus
   c. parasite
   d. fungus

3. A condition that can be either congenital or acquired through trauma and that involves twisting of testes is:
   a. hydrocele
   b. hypospadias
   c. cryptorchidism
   d. torsion

4. Cancer of _____ is divided into two main groups of germ cell tumors and sex stromal cord tumors.
   a. testes
   b. penis
   c. scrotum
   d. prostate

5. This type of surgical technique involves excision of a lesion in layers until no further evidence of abnormality is seen:
   a. Bowen's
   b. Addison's
   c. Mohs
   d. laser

6. Epispadias is a disorder of urethra in which urethral meatus is located on _____ side of penis:
   a. ventral
   b. dorsal
   c. lateral
   d. medial

7. Inflammation of glans is:
   a. phimosis
   b. paraphimosis
   c. urethritis
   d. balanitis

8. This disease is also known as bent nail syndrome:
   a. Bowen's
   b. Peyronie's
   c. Addison's
   d. Whitmore-Jewett

9. Condition in which multiple fibroadenomatous nodules form and lead to decreased urine flow. Condition is thought to be related to increased levels of estrogen/androgen.
   a. BPH
   b. DRE
   c. GCT
   d. TNM

10. Cancer of prostate is predominately this type of cancer:
    a. sex cord
    b. adenocarcinoma
    c. squamous cell
    d. seminoma

■ URINARY SYSTEM
URINARY SYSTEM—ANATOMY AND TERMINOLOGY

Removes metabolic waste materials (nitrogenous waste: urea, creatinine, and uric acid)

Conserves nutrients and water

Balances: electrolytes (acids/bases balance)

Electrolytes are electronically charged molecules required for nerve and muscle function

Assists liver in detoxification

Organs (Fig. 1–32)

Kidneys

Ureters

Urinary bladder

Urethra

Kidneys (Fig. 1–33)
Electrolytes and fluid balance

Controls pH balance (acid/base)

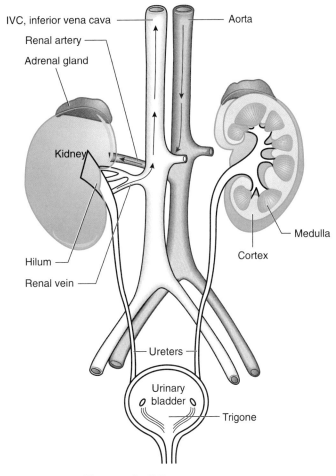

Figure **1-32** Urinary system.

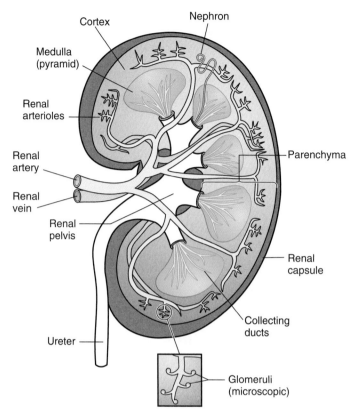

Figure **1-33** Kidney.

Secrete berenin which affects blood pressure and erythropoietin which stimulates red blood cell production in bone marrow

Secrete active vitamin D required for calcium absorption from intestines

Two organs located behind peritoneum (retroperitoneal space)

Kidney Structure
    Cortex (outer layer)

    Medulla (inner portion)

    Hilum (depression on medial border through which blood ressels and nerves pass)

    Pyramids (divisions of medulla)

    Papilla (inner part of pyramids)

    Pelvis (receptacle for urine within kidney)

    Calyces surround top of renal pelvis

    Nephrons (3 types) are operational units of kidney

Ureters
Narrow tubes transporting urine from kidneys to bladder

Urinary Bladder
Reservoir for urine

Shaped like an upside down pear with three surfaces

- Posterior (base)
- Anterior (neck)
- Superior (peritoneum)

Trigone

- Smooth triangular area inside bladder—size never changes
- Formed by openings of ureters and urethra

Urethra
Canal from bladder to exterior of body

Urinary meatus, outside opening of urethra

COMBINING FORMS

1.	albumin/o	albumin
2.	azot/o	urea
3.	bacteri/o	bacteria
4.	cali/o	calyx
5.	cyst/o	urinary
6.	dips/o	thirst
7.	glomerul/o	glomerulus
8.	glyc/o	sugar
9.	glycos/o	sugar
10.	hydr/o	water
11.	ket/o	ketone bodies/ketoacidosis
12.	lith/o	stone
13.	meat/o	meatus
14.	nephr/o	kidney
15.	noct/i	night
16.	olig/o	scant, few
17.	pyel/o	renal pelvis
18.	ren/o	kidney
19.	son/o	sound
20.	tripsy	to crush
21.	tryg/o	trigone region/kidney
22.	ur/o	urine
23.	ureter/o	ureter
24.	urethr/o	urethra
25.	uria	urination/urinary condition
26.	urin/o	urine
27.	vesic/o	bladder

PREFIXES

1.	dys-	painful
2.	peri-	surrounding
3.	poly-	many
4.	retro-	behind

SUFFIXES

1.	-eal	pertaining to
2.	-lithiasis	condition of stones
3.	-lysis	separation
4.	-plasty	repair
5.	-rrhaphy	suture
6.	-tripsy	crush

MEDICAL ABBREVIATIONS

1.	ARF	acute renal failure
2.	BUN	blood urea nitrogen
3.	ESRD	end-stage renal disease
4.	HD	hemodialysis
5.	IVP	intravenous pyelogram
6.	KUB	kidney, ureter, bladder
7.	pH	symbol for acid/base level
8.	PKU	phenylketonuria
9.	sp gr	specific gravity
10.	UA	urinalysis
11.	UPJ	ureteropelvic junction
12.	UTI	urinary tract infection

MEDICAL TERMS

Bulbocavernosus	Muscle that constricts vagina in a female and urethra in a male
Bulbourethral	Gland with duct leading to urethra
Calculus	Concretion of mineral salts, also called a stone
Calycoplasty	Surgical reconstruction of recess of renal pelvis
Calyx	Recess of renal pelvis
Cystolithectomy	Removal of a calculus (stone) from urinary bladder
Cystometrogram	CMG, measurement of pressures and capacity of urinary bladder
Cystoplasty	Surgical reconstruction of bladder
Cystorrhaphy	Suture of bladder

144

Cystoscopy	Use of a scope to view bladder
Cystostomy	Surgical creation of an opening into bladder
Cystotomy	Incision into bladder
Cystourethroplasty	Surgical reconstruction of bladder and urethra
Cystourethroscopy	Use of a scope to view bladder and urethra
Dilation	Stretching or expansion
Dysuria	Painful urination
Endopyelotomy	Procedure involving bladder and ureters, including insertion of a stent into renal pelvis
Extracorporeal	Occurring outside of body
Fundoplasty	Repair of the bottom of bladder
Hydrocele	Sac of fluid
Kock pouch	Surgical creation of a urinary bladder from a segment of the ileum
Nephrocutaneous fistula	An abnormal channel from kidney to skin
Nephrolithotomy	Removal of a kidney stone through an incision made into the kidney
Nephrorrhaphy	Suturing of kidney
Nephrostomy	Creation of a channel into renal pelvis of kidney
Transureteroureterostomy	Surgical connection of one ureter to other ureter
Transvesical ureterolithotomy	Removal of a ureter stone (calculus) through bladder
Ureterectomy	Surgical removal of a ureter, either totally or partially
Ureterocutaneous fistula	Channel from ureter to exterior skin
Ureteroenterostomy	Creation of a connection between intestine and ureter
Ureterolithotomy	Removal of a stone from ureter
Ureterolysis	Freeing of adhesions of ureter
Ureteroneocystostomy	Surgical connection of ureter to a new site on bladder
Ureteropyelography	Ureter and renal pelvis radiography
Ureterotomy	Incision into ureter
Urethrocystography	Radiography of bladder and urethra
Urethromeatoplasty	Surgical repair of urethra and meatus
Urethropexy	Fixation of urethra by means of surgery
Urethroplasty	Surgical repair of urethra
Urethrorrhaphy	Suturing of urethra
Urethroscopy	Use of a scope to view urethra
Vesicostomy	Surgical creation of a connection of viscera of bladder to skin

URINARY SYSTEM ANATOMY AND TERMINOLOGY QUIZ

1. The outer covering of kidney:
   a. medulla
   b. pyramids
   c. cortex
   d. papilla

2. Which is not a division of kidneys?
   a. pelvis
   b. pyramids
   c. cortex
   d. trigone

3. The inner portion of kidneys:
   a. medulla
   b. pyramids
   c. cortex
   d. papilla

4. The smooth area inside bladder:
   a. pyramids
   b. calyces
   c. trigone
   d. cystocele

5. The narrow tube connecting kidney and bladder:
   a. urethra
   b. ureter
   c. meatus
   d. trigone

6. Which of the following is NOT a surface of urinary bladder?
   a. posterior
   b. anterior
   c. superior
   d. inferior

7. Combining form that means stone:
   a. azot/o
   b. cyst/o
   c. lith/o
   d. olig/o

8. Term meaning painful urination:
   a. pyuria
   b. dysuria
   c. diuresis
   d. hyperemia

9. Combining form meaning scant:
   a. glyc/o
   b. hydr/o
   c. meat/o
   d. olig/o

10. Term that describes renal failure that is acute:
    a. ARF
    b. ESRD
    c. HD
    d. BPH

URINARY SYSTEM—PATHOPHYSIOLOGY

Renal Failure

Acute Renal Failure
Sudden onset of renal failure

Cause
Extreme hypotension

Trauma

Infection

Inflammation

Toxicity

Obstructed vascular supply

Symptoms
Uremia

Oliguria (decreased output) or anuria (no output)

Hyperkalemia (high potassium in blood)

Pulmonary edema

Types
Prerenal
- Associated with poor systemic perfusion
- Decreased renal blood flow
  - Such as with congestive heart failure

Intrarenal
- Associated with renal parenchyma disease (functional tissue of kidney)
  - Such as acute interstitial nephritis, glomerulopathies, and malignant hypertension

Postrenal
- Resulting from urine flow obstruction outside kidney (ureters or bladder neck)

Treatment
Underlying condition

Dialysis

Monitoring of fluid and electrolyte balance

Chronic Renal Failure
Gradual loss of function
- Progressively more severe renal insufficiency until end stage of
  - Renal disease
  - Irreversible kidney failure

Stages—based on level of creatinine clearance
Stage I: Blood flow through kidney increases, kidney enlarges

Stage II: (mild) Small amounts of blood protein (albumin) leak into urine (microalbuminuria)

Stage III: (moderate) Albumin and other protein losses increase; patient may develop high blood pressure and kidney loses ability to filter waste

Stage IV: (severe) Large amounts of urine pass through kidney; blood pressure increases

Stage V: End-stage renal failure. Ability to filter waste nearly stops; dialysis or transplant only option

Cause

Long-term exposure to nephrotoxins

Diabetes

Hypertension

Symptoms

No symptoms until well advanced

Polyuria

Nausea or anorexia

Dehydration

Neurologic manifestations

Stages of nephron loss

Decreased reserve

- 60% loss

Renal insufficiency

- 75% loss

End-stage renal failure

- 90% loss

Treatment

No cure

Dialysis

Kidney transplant

Urinary Tract Infections (UTI)

Cystitis—Bacterial

Cause

Bacteria, usually *E. coli*

Symptoms

Lower abdominal pain

Dysuria

Lower back pain

Urinary frequency and urgency

Cloudy, foul-smelling urine

Systemic signs

Fever

Malaise

Nausea

Treatment
Antibiotics

Increased fluid intake

Cystitis—Nonbacterial
Cause
Unknown

May later produce bacterial infection

Symptoms
Urinary frequency and urgency

Dysuria

Negative urine culture

Treatment
No known treatment

Acute Pyelonephritis (Fig. 1–34)
Bacterial infection with multiple abcesses of renal pelvis and medullary tissue

• May involve one or both kidneys

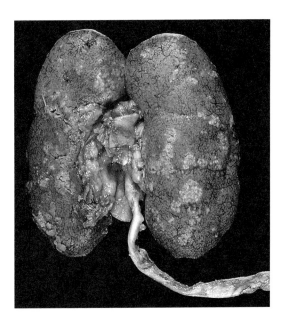

Figure **1-34** Acute pyelonephritis. Cortical surface exhibits grayish white areas of inflammation and abscess formation. (From Kumar V, Abbas AK, Fausto N: *Robbins and Cotran Pathologic Basis of Disease*, ed 7, Philadelphia, 2005, Saunders.)

Cause
E. coli

Proteus

Pseudomonas

Obstruction and reflux of urine from bladder

Symptoms
Fever

Chills

Groin or flank pain

Dysuria

Pyuria

Nocturia

Treatment
Antibiotics

Surgical correction of obstruction

Chronic Pyelonephritis
Recurrent infection that causes scarring of kidney

Cause is difficult to determine

- Repeated infections
- Obstructive conditions

Symptoms
Hypertension

Dysuria

Flank pain

Increased frequency of urination

Treatment
Antibiotics for extended periods when reoccurring

Surgical reduction of obstruction

Glomerular Disorders

May be acute or chronic

Function of glomerulus is blood filtration

Glomerulonephritis
Inflammation of glomerulus

Cause
Drugs or toxins

Systemic disorder affecting many organs or idiopathic

May follow acute infections—most commonly streptococcal infections

Vascular pathology

Immune disorders

Treatment

Follows cause

Nephrotic Syndrome (Nephrosis)

Disease of kidneys that includes damage to membrane of the glomerulus causing excessive protein loss to urine

Accompanied by

- Hypoalbuminemia
- Hypercholesterolemia
- Hypercoagulability (excessive clotting)
- Prone to infections
- Edema
- Protein loss of >3.5 g

Damage to glomerulus results from

- Infection
- Immune response
  - Most predominant cause of dysfunction is exposure to toxins

May be a manifestation of an underlying condition, such as diabetes

Symptoms

Edema

Weight gain

Pallor

Proteinuria

Lipiduria

Treatment

Glucocorticoids, such as prednisone

- Reduces inflammation

Sodium and fat reduced diet

Protein supplements

Careful monitoring for continued inflammation

Acute Poststreptococcal Glomerulonephritis (APSGN)

Cause

Streptococcus infection

- With certain types of group A beta-hemolytic *Streptococcus*

Creates an antigen-antibody complex

- Infiltrates glomerular capillaries
- Results in inflammation in kidneys
- Inflammation interferes with normal kidney function
- Fluid and waste build-up
- Can lead to acute renal failure and scarring

Usually occurs in children 3 to 7 years of age

- Most often in boys

Symptoms
Back and flank pain

Cloudy, dark urine

Oliguria (decreased output)

Edema

Elevated blood pressure

Fatigue

Malaise

Headache

Nausea

Treatment
Sodium reduction

Antibiotics

Careful monitoring for continued inflammation

Urinary Tract Obstructions

Interference with urine flow

Causes urine backup behind obstruction of urinary system

Damage occurs to structures behind blockages

Increased urinary tract infection

Obstruction can be

- Functional

- Anatomic

  - Also known as obstructive uropathy

Kidney Stones (nephrolithiasis—renal calculi)
Formed of mineral salts (uric and calcuim)

Develop anywhere in urinary tract

Tend to form in presence of excess salt and decreased fluid intake

- Most stones are formed of calcium salts

- Staghorn calculus forms in renal pelvis

Symptoms
Asymptomatic until obstruction occurs

Obstruction results in renal colic

- Extremely intense pain in flank

- Nausea

- Vomiting

- Cold, clammy skin

- Increased pulse rate

Treatment
Stone usually passes spontaneously

May use extracorporeal ultrasound or laser lithotripsy to break up stone (also known as extracorporeal shock wave lithotripsy or ESWL)

Drugs may be used to dissolve stone

Preventative treatment to adjust pH level

- Increased fluid intake

Bladder Carcinoma
Malignant tumor
Most common site of malignancy in urinary system

Tumors originate in transitional epithelial lining

Tends to recur

Often metastatic to liver and bone

Tumor staging for renal cancer
Stage I tumor of kidney capsule only

Stage II tumor invading renal capsule/vein but within fascia

Stage III tumor extending to regional lymph/vena cava

Stage IV other organ metatasis

Symptoms
Often asymptomatic in early stage

Hematuria

Dysuria

Frequent urination

Infections common

Increased Risks
Cigarette smoking

Males age 50+

Working with industrial chemicals

Analgesics used in large amounts

Recurrent bladder infections

Treatment
Immunotherapy (bacillus Calmette-Guérin vaccine, BCG)

Excision

Chemotherapy

Radiation therapy

Hydronephrosis
Distention of kidney with urine

- Due to an obstruction

- Usually as a result of a kidney stone

- May also be due to scarring, tumor, edema from infection, or other obstruction

Symptoms
Usually asymptomatic

Mild flank pain

Infection may develop

May lead to chronic renal failure

Treatment
Treat underlying condition, such as removal of stone or antibiotics for infection

Dilation of stricture

Vascular Disorders

Nephrosclerosis
Excessive hardening and thickening of vascular structure of kidney

- Reduces blood supply

  - Increases blood pressure

  - Results in atrophy and ischemia of structures

  - May lead to chronic renal failure

Symptoms
Asymptomatic in early stages

Treatment
Diuretics

ACE (angiotensin-converting enzyme) inhibitors

Beta blockers that block release of resin

Antihypertensive drugs

Sodium intake reduction

Congenital Disorders

Polycystic Kidney (PKD)
Numerous kidney cysts

Genetic disease

Symptoms
Asymptomatic until 40s

Cysts progressive in development (both kidneys)

Nephromegaly, hematuria, URT, hypertension, uremia

Develops chronic renal failure

Cysts may spread to other organs, such as liver

Treatment
As for chronic renal failure

Wilms' Tumor—Nephroblastoma

Usually unilateral kidney tumors

Most common tumor in children

Usually advanced at time of diagnosis

- Metastasis to lungs at time of diagnosis is common

Symptoms

Asymptomatic until abdominal mass becomes apparent at age 1 to 5

Treatment

Excision

Radiation therapy

Chemotherapy

Usually a combination of above

URINARY SYSTEM PATHOPHYSIOLOGY QUIZ

1. Which of the following is NOT a type of acute renal failure?
   a. prerenal
   b. intrarenal
   c. interrenal
   d. postrenal

2. The loss of nephron function in end-stage renal disease is:
   a. 60%
   b. 70%
   c. 80%
   d. 90%

3. The cause of bacterial cystitis is usually:
   a. Proteus
   b. *Pseudomonas*
   c. *Staphylococci*
   d. *E. coli*

4. The primary treatment for acute pyelonephritis would be:
   a. prednisone
   b. sodium reduction
   c. antibiotics
   d. BCG

5. APSGN stands for:
   a. advanced poststaphylococcal glomerulonephritis
   b. acute poststreptococcal glomerulonephritis
   c. acute poststaphylococcal glomerulonephritis
   d. advanced poststreptococcal glomerulonephritis

6. Obstructive uropathy is also known as:
   a. pyelonephritis
   b. renal failure
   c. urinary tract obstruction
   d. nephrotic syndrome

7. A treatment for kidney stone may be:
   a. ESWL
   b. prednisone
   c. open surgical procedure
   d. diuretics

8. The treatment for hydronephrosis involves:
   a. an open surgical procedure
   b. use of diuretics
   c. treatment of the underlying condition
   d. BCG

9. This is a congential condition in which numerous cysts form in the kidney:
    a. Wilms' tumor
    b. polycystic kidney
    c. nephrosclerosis
    d. nephrotic syndrome

10. The treatment of Wilms' tumor would NOT include which of the following?
    a. excision
    b. chemotherapy
    c. diuretic
    d. radiation therapy

■ DIGESTIVE SYSTEM

DIGESTIVE SYSTEM—ANATOMY AND TERMINOLOGY

Function: digestion, absorption, and elimination

Includes gastrointestinal tract (alimentary canal) and accessory organs

Mouth (Fig. 1–35)

Roof: hard palate, soft palate, uvula (projection at back of mouth)

Floor: contains tongue (Fig. 1–36), muscles, taste buds, and lingual frenulum, which anchors tongue to floor of mouth

Teeth

Thirty-two teeth (permanent)

Names of teeth: incisor, cuspid, bicuspid, and tricuspid

Tooth has crown (outer portion), neck (narrow part below gum line), root (end section), and pulp cavity (core)

Salivary Glands (Fig. 1–37)

Surround mouth and produce saliva—1.5 liters daily

Parotid

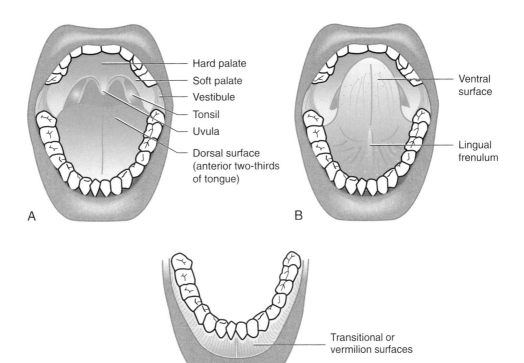

A

Hard palate
Soft palate
Vestibule
Tonsil
Uvula
Dorsal surface
(anterior two-thirds
of tongue)

B

Ventral
surface

Lingual
frenulum

C

Transitional or
vermilion surfaces

Lips are connected to
the gums by frenulum

Figure **1-35** Anatomic structures of the mouth.

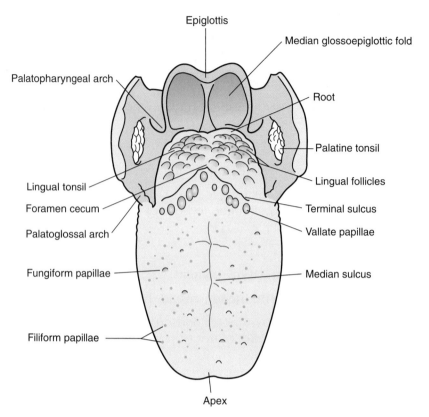

Figure **1-36** Dorsum of the tongue.

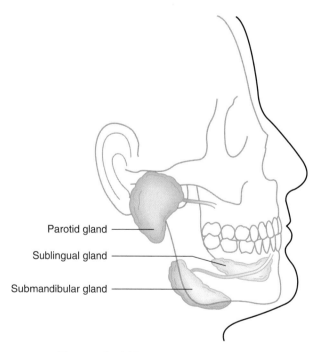

Figure **1-37** Major salivary glands.

Submandibular

Sublingual

Pharynx or Throat (Fig. 1–38)

Muscular tube (5 inches long) lined with mucus membrane through which air and food/water travel

Epiglottis covers larynx/esophagus when swallowing

Esophagus

Muscular tube (9-10 inches long) that carries food from pharynx to stomach by means of peristalsis (rhythmic contractions)

Stomach

Sphincter (ring of muscles) at entry into stomach (gastroesophageal or cardiac)

Three parts of stomach:

Fundus (upper part)

Body (middle part)

Antrum/pylorus (lower part)

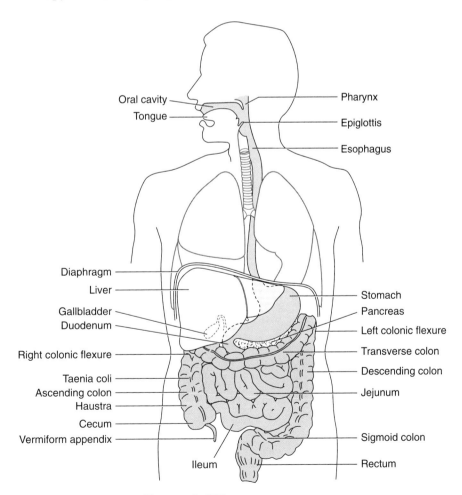

Figure **1-38** Digestive system.

Lined with rugae (folds of mucosal membrane)

Pyloric sphincter opens to allow chyme (thick liquid) to leave stomach and enter small intestine

Small Intestine

Duodenum (2 inches long): first portion beyond stomach—bile and pancreatic juice delivered here

Jejunum (96 inches long): connects duodenum to ileum

Ileum (132 inches long): attaches to large intestine

Large Intestine

Extends from ileum to anus

Cecum, from which appendix extends, connects ileum and colon

Colon (60 inches long), divided into:

    Ascending

    Transverse

    Descending

    Sigmoid

Sigmoid colon, connected to rectum, which terminates at anus

Accessory Organs

Liver produces bile, sent to gallbladder via hepatic duct and cystic duct

Gallbladder stores bile, sent to duodenum from cystic duct into common bile duct

Bile emulsifies fat (breaks up large globules)

Pancreas produces enzymes sent through pancreatic duct to hepatopancreatic ampulla (ampulla of Vater) then to duodenum

Pancreatic cells—Islets of Langerhans produce insulin and glucagon

Peritoneum

Serous membrane lines abdominal cavity and maintains organs in correct anatomic position

Food passes through digestive tract via:

    Mouth—including salivary glands

    Pharynx

    Esophagus

    Stomach

    Duodenum—pancreatic enzymes and bile produced in liver and stored in gallbladder enter

    Jejunum

Ileum

Cecum

Ascending colon

Transverse colon

Descending colon

Sigmoid colon

Rectum

Anus

COMBINING FORMS

1.	abdomin/o	abdomen
2.	an/o	anus
3.	appendic/o	appendix
4.	bil/i	bile
5.	bilirubin/o	bile pigment
6.	bucc/o	cheek
7.	cec/o	cecum
8.	celi/o	abdomen
9.	cheil/o	lip
10.	chol/e	gall/bile
11.	cholangio/o	bile duct
12.	cholecyst/o	gallbladder
13.	choledoch/o	common bile duct
14.	col/o	colon
15.	dent/i	tooth
16.	diverticul/o	diverticulum
17.	duoden/o	duodenum
18.	enter/o	small intestine
19.	esophag/o	esophagus
20.	faci/o	face
21.	gastr/o	stomach
22.	gingiv/o	gum
23.	gloss/o	tongue
24.	hepat/o	liver
25.	herni/o	hernia
26.	ile/o	ileum
27.	jejun/o	jejunum

28. labi/o	lip
29. lapar/o	abdomen
30. lingu/o	tongue
31. lip/o	fat
32. lith/o	stone
33. or/o	mouth
34. ordont/o	tooth
35. palat/o	palate
36. pancreat/o	pancreas
37. peritone/o	peritoneum
38. pharng/o	throat
39. polyp/o	polyp
40. proct/o	rectum
41. pylor/o	pylorus
42. rect/o	rectum
43. sial/o	saliva
44. sialaden/o	salivary gland
45. sigmoid/o	sigmoid colon
46. steat/o	fat
47. stomat/o	mouth
48. uvul/o	uvula

SUFFIXES

1. -ase	enzyme
2. -cele	hernia
3. -chezia	defecation
4. -iasis	abnormal condition
5. -phagia	eating
6. -prandial	meal

MEDICAL ABBREVIATIONS

1. EGD	esophagogastroduodenoscopy
2. EGJ	esophagogastric junction
3. ERCP	endoscopic retrograde cholangiopancreatography
4. GERD	gastroesophageal reflux disease
5. GI	gastrointestinal
6. HJR	hepatojugular reflux

7.	LLQ	left lower quadrant
8.	LUQ	left upper quadrant
9.	PEG	percutaneous endoscopic gastrostomy
10.	RLQ	right lower quadrant
11.	RUQ	right upper quadrant

MEDICAL TERMS

Anastomosis	Surgical connection of two tubular structures, such as two pieces of intestine
Biliary	Refers to gallbladder, bile, or bile duct
Cholangiography	Radiographic recording of bile ducts
Cholecystectomy	Surgical removal of gallbladder
Cholecystoenterostomy	Creation of a connection between gallbladder and intestine
Colonoscopy	Fiberscopic examination of entire colon that may include part of terminal ileum
Colostomy	Artificial opening between colon and abdominal wall
Diverticulum	Protrusion in wall of an organ
Dysphagia	Difficulty swallowing
Enterolysis	Releasing of adhesions of intestine
Eventration	Protrusion of bowel through an opening in abdomen
Evisceration	Pulling viscera outside of the body through an incision
Exstrophy	Condition in which an organ is turned inside out
Fulguration	Use of electric current to destroy tissue
Gastrointestinal	Pertaining to stomach and intestine
Gastroplasty	Operation on stomach for repair or reconfiguration
Gastrostomy	Artificial opening between stomach and abdominal wall
Hernia	Organ or tissue protruding through wall or cavity that usually contains it
Ileostomy	Artificial opening between ileum and abdominal wall
Imbrication	Overlapping
Incarcerated	Regarding hernias, a constricted, irreducible hernia that may cause obstruction of an intestine
Intussusception	Slipping of one part of intestine into another part
Jejunostomy	Artificial opening between jejunum and abdominal wall
Laparoscopy	Exploration of the abdomen and pelvic cavities using a scope placed through a small incision in abdominal wall
Lithotomy	Incision into an organ or a duct for the purpose of removing a stone
Lithotripsy	Crushing of a stone by sound wave or force

Paraesophageal or hiatal hernia	Protrusion of any structure through esophageal hiatus of diaphragm
Proctosigmoidoscopy	Fiberscopic examination of sigmoid colon and rectum
Sialolithotomy	Surgical removal of a stone of salivary gland or duct
Varices	Varicose veins
Volvulus	Twisted section of intestine

DIGESTIVE SYSTEM ANATOMY AND TERMINOLOGY QUIZ

1. This is NOT a part of the small intestine:
   a. ileum
   b. cecum
   c. duodenum
   d. jejunum

2. Term meaning a ring of muscles:
   a. pyloric
   b. parotid
   c. epiglottis
   d. sphincter

3. The throat is also known as the:
   a. larynx
   b. epiglottis
   c. esophagus
   d. pharynx

4. The three parts of the stomach:
   a. pyloric, rugae, fundus
   b. fundus, body, antrum
   c. antrum, pyloric, rugae
   d. ilium, fundus, pyloric

5. The projection at the back of the mouth:
   a. palate
   b. sublingual
   c. uvula
   d. parotid

6. Mucosal membrane that lines the stomach:
   a. cecum
   b. rugae
   c. frenulum
   d. fundus

7. The parts of the colon are:
   a. ascending, transverse, descending, sigmoid
   b. ascending, descending, sigmoid
   c. transverse, descending, sigmoid
   d. descending, sigmoid

8. Combining form meaning abdomen:
   a. an/o
   b. cec/o
   c. celi/o
   d. col/o

9. Term that means connecting two ends of a tube:
   a. anastomosis
   b. amylase
   c. aphthous stomatitis
   d. atresia

10. Abbreviation that means a scope placed through the esophagus, into the stomach, and to the duodenum:
    a. ERCP
    b. EGD
    c. GERD
    d. PEG

Disorders of Oral Cavity

Cleft Lip and Cleft Palate (Orofacial Cleft) (Fig. 1–39)

Congenital defect

Cleft lip and palate

Lip and palate do not properly join together

Causes feeding problems

- Infants cannot create sufficient suction for feeding

- Danger of aspirating food

- Results in speech defects

Treatment

Surgical repair of defects

Ulceration

Canker sore—caused by herpes simplex virus

- Ulceration of oral mucosa

Also known as

- Aphthous ulcer (aphtha: small ulcer)

- Aphthous stomatitis

Heals spontaneously

Infections

Candidiasis

Candida albicans is naturally found in mouth

Thrush (oral candidiasis) is overarching infection

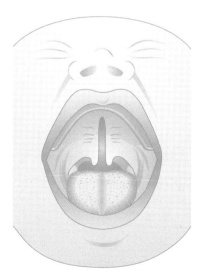

Figure **1-39** Cleft palate.

Causes

Antibiotic regimen

Chemotherapy

Glucocorticoids

Common in diabetics and AIDS patients

Treatment

Nystatin (topical fungal agent)

Herpes simplex type 1

Herpetic stomatitis

• Viral cold sores and blisters

• Associated with herpes simplex virus type 1 (HSV-1)

Treatment

No cure

May be alleviated somewhat by antiviral medications

Cancer of Oral Cavity

Most common type is squamous cell carcinoma

• Kaposi's sarcoma is type seen in AIDS patients

Increased in smokers

Lip cancer also increased in smokers, particularly pipe

Poor prognosis

Usually asymptomatic until later stages

Metastasis through lymph nodes

Esophageal Disorders

Scleroderma

Also known as progressive systemic sclerosis

Atrophy of smooth muscles of lower esophagus

Lower esophageal sphincter (LES) does not close properly

• Leads to esophageal reflux

• Strictures form

Symptom

Predominantly dysphagia

Esophagitis

Inflammation of esophagus

Types

Acute

Most common type is that caused by hiatal hernia

Infectious esophagitis is common in patients with AIDS

Ingestion of strong alkaline or acid substances

- Such as those in household cleaners

Inflammation leads to scarring

Chronic
Most common type is that caused by LES reflux

Cancer of Esophagus
Most common type is squamous cell or secondary adenocarcinoma

Usually caused by continued irritation

- Smoking

- Alcohol

- Hiatal hernia

- Chronic esophagitis/GERD

Poor prognosis

Hiatal Hernia (Diaphragmatic hernia)
Diaphragm goes over stomach

- Esophagus passes through diaphragm at natural opening (hiatus)

- Part of the stomach protrudes (herniates) through opening in diaphragm into thorax

Types (Fig. 1–40)
Sliding

- Stomach and gastroesophageal junction protrude through the hiatus

Paraesophageal/rolling hiatal

- Part of fundus protrudes

Symptoms
Heartburn

Reflux

Belching

Lying down causes discomfort

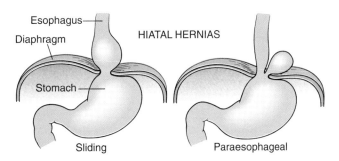

Figure **1-40** Sliding and paraesophageal hernias (hiatal hernias).

Dysphagia

Substernal pain after eating

Gastroesophageal Reflux Disease (GERD)
Associated with hiatal hernias

• Reflux of gastric contents

Lower esophageal sphincter does not constrict properly

Treatment
Reduce irritants, such as

- Smoking

- Spicy foods

- Alcohol

Antacids

Elevate head of bed

Avoid tight clothing

Stomach and Duodenum Disorders

Gastritis
Inflammation of stomach mucosa

Acute superficial gastritis
Mild, transient irritation

Causes
Excessive alcohol

Infection

Food allergies

Spicy foods

Aspirin

H. pylori (Helicobacter pylori)

Symptoms
Nausea

Vomiting

Anorexia

Bleeding in more severe cases

Epigastric pain

Treatment
Usually spontaneous remission in 2 to 3 days

Removal of underlying irritation

Antibiotics for infection

Chronic atrophic gastritis
Progressive atrophy of epithelium

Types

Type A, atrophic or fundal

- Involves fundus of stomach
- Autoimmune disease
  - Decreases acid secretion
  - Results in high gastrin levels

Type B, antral

- Involves antrum region of stomach
- Often associated with elderly
  - May be associated with pernicious anemia
- Low gastrin levels
- Usually caused by infection
- Irritated by alcohol, drugs, and tobacco

Symptom abatement

- Bland diet
- Alcohol avoidance
- ASA avoidance
- Antibiotics for *H. pylori*

Peptic Ulcers

Erosive area on mucosa

- Extends below epithelium
- Chronic ulcers have scar tissue at base of erosive area

Ulcers can occur anyplace on gastrointestinal tract but typically are found on the

- Lower esophagus
- Stomach
- Proximal duodenum

Some causes

Alcohol

Smoking

Aspirin

Severe stress

Bacterial infection caused by *Helicobacter pylori (H. pylori),* 90% of the time

Genetic factor

Constant use of anti-inflammatory drugs

Symptoms

Epigastric pain when stomach is empty

- Relieved by food or antacid

Burning

May include

- Vomiting blood
- Nausea
- Weight loss
- Anorexia

Severe cases may include

- Obstruction
- Hemorrhage
- Perforation

Treatment
Surgical intervention

Antacids

Dietary restrictions

Rest

Antibiotics

Gastric Cancer (malignant tumor of stomach)
Most often occurs in men over 40

Cause is unknown, but often associated with *Helicobacter pylori* (bacterial infection)

Predisposing Factors
Atrophic gastritis

Pernicious anemia

History of nonhealing gastric ulcer

Blood type A

Geographic factors

Environmental factors

Carcinogenic foods

- Smoked meats
- Nitrates
- Pickled foods

Symptoms
Usually asymptomatic in early stages

Treatment
Excision

Chemotherapy

Radiation (not good response)

Prognosis is poor

Pyloric Stenosis
Narrowing of the pyloric sphincter

Signs appear soon after birth

- Failure to thrive
- Projectile vomiting

Treatment
Surgery to relieve stenosis (pyloromyotomy)

Intestinal Disorders

■ Small Intestine

Malabsorption Conditions

Celiac disease
Most important malabsorption condition
Villi atrophy in response to food containing gluten and lose ability to absorb
- Gluten is a protein found in wheat, rye, oats, and barley

Symptoms
Malnutrition

Muscle wasting

Distended abdomen

Diarrhea

Fatigue

Weakness

Steatorrhea (excess fat in feces)

Treatment
Gluten-free diet

Steroids when necessary

Lactase deficiency
Enzyme deficiency
- Secondary to gastrointestinal damage, such as
  - Regional enteritis
  - Infection
- Common in blacks, occurring in adulthood

Symptoms
Intolerance to milk

Intestinal cramping

Diarrhea

Flatulence

Treatment
Elimination of milk products

Crohn's disease (regional enteritis)
Inflammatory bowel disease (IBD)—affects terminal ileum and colon

Cause
Unknown

Symptoms
Vary greatly/inflammatory disease of GI tract

Diarrhea

Gas

Fever

Abdominal pain

Malaise

Anorexia

Weight loss

Treatment
No specific treatment

Palliative medications to control symptoms

Resection of affected section of intestine with anastomosis

Diet modifications

Duodenal Ulcers
Most common ulcer

Develop in younger population

Common in type O blood types

Appendicitis
Inflammation of vermiform appendix that projects from cecum

Obstruction of lumen leads to infection

- Appendix becomes hypoxic (decreased oxygen levels)
- May cause gangrene
- May rupture, causing peritonitis

Symptoms
Periumbilical (around umbilicus) pain, initially

Right lower quadrant (RLQ) pain as inflammation progresses

Nausea

Vomiting

Possible diarrhea

Treatment
Appendectomy

Management of any perforation or abscess

Meckel's Diverticulum—an appendage of ileum near cecum derived from an unobliterated yolk stalk in fetal development. Symptoms can mimic appendicitis.

Peritonitis
Inflammation of peritoneum (membrane that lines abdominal cavity)

Usually a result of

- Spread of infection from abdominal organ
- Puncture wound to abdomen
- Rupture of gastrointestinal tract—appendicitis or Meckel's diverticulum

Abscesses form, resulting in adhesions

- May result in obstruction

Types
Acute

Chronic

Symptoms
    Abdominal pain

    Vomiting

    Rigid abdomen

    Fever

    Leukocytosis (increased white cells in blood)

Treatment
    Antibiotics

    Suction of stomach and intestines

    If possible, surgical removal of origin of infection, such as appendix

    Fluid replacement

    Bed rest

Obstruction
Any interference with passage of intestinal contents

May be

- Acute
- Chronic
- Partial
- Total

Types
    Nonmechanical

- Paralytic ileus
- Result of trauma or toxin

    Mechanical

- Result of tumors, adhesions, hernias
- Simple mechanical obstruction
  - One point of obstruction
- Closed-loop obstruction
  - At least two points of obstruction

    Diverticulosis

      Twisted bowel (volvulus)

      Telescoping bowel (intussception)

Symptoms
    Abdominal distention

    Pain

    Vomiting

    Total constipation

Treatment
    Surgical intervention

    Symptomatic treatment

■ Large Intestine

Diverticulosis

Herniation of intestinal mucosa

• Forms sacs in lining, called diverticula

Diverticulitis

Sacs fill and become inflamed

• Common in aged

Symptoms

    Diarrhea or constipation

    Gas

    Abdominal discomfort

Complications

    Perforation

    Bleeding

    Peritonitis

    Abscess

    Obstruction

Treatment

    Antimicrobials as necessary

    High-fiber diet (greater than 20 g daily)

    Stool softeners

    Dietary restrictions of solid foods

    Surgical intervention if necessary

Ulcerative Colitis (Fig. 1–41)

Inflammation of rectum that progresses to sigmoid colon

Intermittent exacerbations and remissions

May develop into toxic megacolon

• Leads to obstruction and dilation of colon

Increased risk of colorectal cancer

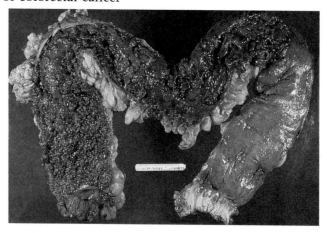

Figure **1-41** Ulcerative colitis. (From Damjanov I: *Pathology for the Health Professions,* ed 3, St. Louis, 2006, Saunders.)

Symptoms

Diarrhea

- Blood and mucus may be present

Cramping

Fever

Weight loss

Treatment

Remove physical or emotional stressors

Anti-inflammatory medications

Antimotility agents

Nutritional supplementation

Surgical intervention, if necessary

Colorectal Cancer

Usually develop from polyp

- In those 55 and older

Increased risks

Genetic factors

40 years of age and older

Diets high in

- Fat
- Sugar
- Red meat

Low-fiber diets

Symptoms

Asymptomatic until advanced

Some may experience

- Cramping
- Ribbon stools
- Feeling of incomplete evacuation
- Fatigue
- Weight loss
- Change in bowel habits
- Blood in stool

Treatment

Surgical excision

Radiation

Chemotherapy

Combination of above

Disorders of Liver, Gallbladder, and Pancreas

■ Disorders of Liver

Jaundice (Hyperbilirubinemia)

A symptom of biliary disease, not a disease itself

- Results in yellow eyes (sclera) and skin

Types

Prehepatic

- Excess destruction of red blood cells
- Result of hemolytic anemia or reaction to transfusion

Intrahepatic

- Impaired uptake of bilirubin and decreased blending of bilirubin by hepatic cells
- Result of liver disease, such as cirrhosis or hepatitis

Posthepatic

- Excess bile flows into blood
- Result of obstruction
  - Due to conditions such as inflammation of liver, tumors, cholelithiasis

Treatment

Removal of cause

Cancer of Liver

Most commonly a metastasis/primary CA rare

Risk for primary liver CA

- Hepatitis B, C, and D
- Cirrhosis
- Myotoxins
- Heavy smoking/alcohol use

Treatment

Surgical resection if localized

Survival typically 3 or 4 months

Viral Hepatitis

Liver cells are damaged

Results in inflammation and necrosis

Damage can be mild or severe

Scar tissue forms in liver

- Leads to ischemia

Hepatitis A (HAV)

Infectious hepatitis—caused by hepatitis A virus

Transmission

- Most commonly oral-fecal route—contaminated food or water

Does not have a chronic state

Slow onset—complete recovery characteristic

Vaccine available for those who are traveling

Gamma globulin may be administered to those just exposed

Hepatitis B (HBV)
Serum hepatitis

Carrier state is common

Caused by hepatitis B virus

- Asymptomatic but contagious

Long incubation period

Transmission

- Intravenous drug users
- Transfusion
- Exposure to blood and bodily fluids
- Sexual transmission
- Mother-to-fetus transmission
- Immune globulin is temporary prophylactic
- Vaccine is now routine for children and is given to those at risk

Severe forms cause liver cell destruction, cirrhosis, death

Hepatitis C (HCV)
Transmission of virus

- Most commonly by transfusion
- IV drug users

Half of cases develop into chronic hepatitis

Increases risk of hepatocellular cancer

Carrier state may develop

Hepatitis D (HDV)
Transmission of hepatitis D virus

- Blood
- Intravenous drug users

Hepatitis B is present for this type to develop

Hepatitis E (HEV)
Transmission of hepatitis E virus

- Oral-fecal route

Does not develop into chronic or carrier

Hepatitis G
Transmission of hepatitis G virus

- IV drug use
- Sexual transmission

Symptoms of hepatitis
Stages
Preicteric

- Anorexia

- Nausea and vomiting

Liver enzymes may be elevated—indication of liver cell damage

- Fatigue

- Malaise

- Generalized pain with low grade fever

- Cough

Icteric

- Jaundice

- Hepatomegaly (enlarged liver)

- Biliary obstruction

- Light-colored stools and dark urine

- Pruritus

- Abdominal pain

Posticteric (recovery)

- Reduction of symptoms

Treatment
None

In early stages gamma globulins may be used

Interferon may be used for cases of chronic hepatitis B and C

Nonviral hepatitis
Hepatitis that results from hepatotoxins

Symptoms

- Similar to viral hepatitis

Treatment

- Removal of hepatotoxin

Cirrhosis
Profuse liver damage

- Extensive fibrosis

  - Results in inflammation

Progressive disorder

Leads to liver failure

Types
Alcoholic liver

- Known as Laënnec's cirrhosis or portal

- Largest group

Biliary

- Associated with immune disorders

- Obstructions (intrahepatic or extrahepatic blood vessels) occur and disrupt normal function

Postnecrotic

- Associated with chronic hepatitis (A or C) and exposure to toxins

Symptoms
Asymptomatic in early stages

Nausea

Vomiting

Fatigue

Weight loss

Pruritus

Jaundice

Edema

Treatment
Symptomatic

Dietary restrictions

- Reduced protein and sodium

- Increased vitamins and carbohydrates

Diuretics

Antibiotics

Liver transplant

■ Disorders of Gallbladder

Cholecystitis
Inflammation of gallbladder and cystic duct

Cholangitis
Inflammation of bile duct

Cholelithiasis
Formation of gallstones (Fig. 1–42)

- Consists of cholesterol or bilirubin

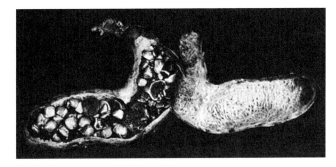

Figure **1-42** Resected gallbladder containing mixed gallstones. (From Kissane JM, editor: *Anderson's pathology,* ed 9, St Louis, 1990, Mosby.)

- Occurs most often in those with high levels of cholesterol, calcium, or bile salts

Stones cause irritation and inflammation

- May lead to infection
- Obstruction
  - May result in pancreatitis
  - Rupture is possible

Symptoms
Often asymptomatic

Dietary intolerance particularly to fat

Right upper quadrant (RUQ) pain

Pain in back and/or shoulder

Epigastric discomfort

Bloating heartburn, flatulence

Treatment
Surgical intervention (laparoscopic cholecystectomy)

Lithotripsy

Medical management by use of drugs that break down stone

■ Disorders of Pancreas

Pancreatitis
Inflammation of pancreas resulting from digestive enzyme attack to pancreas

Acute and chronic forms

Commonly associated with alcoholism/biliary tract obstruction, drug toxicity, gallstone obstruction of common bile duct and viral infections

Symptoms
Severe pain

Fever

Acute form is a medical emergency

Neurogenic shock

Septicemia

General sepsis

Complications
Adult respiratory distress syndrome (ARDS)

Renal failure

Treatment
No oral intake

- IV fluids given and carefully monitored

Analgesics

Stop process of autodigestion

Prevent systemic shutdown

Pancreatic Cancer
Increased risk
Cigarette smoking

Diet high in fat and protein

Symptoms
Weight loss

Jaundice

Anorexia

Most types of pancreatic cancer are asymptomatic until well advanced

Treatment
Palliative

Pain management

DIGESTIVE SYSTEM PATHOPHYSIOLOGY QUIZ

1. This type of hyperbilirubinemia is hallmarked by excess bile flow into the blood:
   a. intrahepatic
   b. prehepatic
   c. posthepatic
   d. jaundice

2. This type of hepatitis is transmitted by the oral-fecal route:
   a. A
   b. B
   c. C
   d. D

3. Which of the following is the recovery stage of hepatitis?
   a. prehepatic
   b. posthepatic
   c. preicteric
   d. posticteric

4. This type of cirrhosis is also known as portal cirrhosis:
   a. biliary
   b. alcoholic liver
   c. postnecrotic
   d. traumatic

5. This condition is the inflammation of the bile ducts:
   a. cholangitis
   b. cholecystitis
   c. cholelithiasis
   d. cholangioma

6. Formation of gallstones most often occurs with high levels of the following:
   a. bile salts and toxins
   b. cholesterol and toxins
   c. cholesterol and bile salts
   d. toxins

7. The primary factor that increases the risk of pancreatic cancer is:
   a. smoking
   b. alcohol
   c. intravenous drug use
   d. hepatitis

8. A potential complication of this condition is ARDS:
   a. hyperbilirubinemia
   b. hepatitis
   c. pancreatitis
   d. pancreatic cancer

9. The primary treatment for jaundice is:
   a. removal of cause
   b. antibiotics
   c. dialysis
   d. vaccine

10. This condition has as the largest group those that abuse alcohol:
    a. cirrhosis
    b. hepatitis
    c. pancreatitis
    d. pancreatic cancer

■ MEDIASTINUM AND DIAPHRAGM

MEDIASTINUM AND DIAPHRAGM—ANATOMY AND TERMINOLOGY

Not an organ system

Mediastinum

That area between lungs that a median (partition) divides (Fig. 1–43) into

- Superior
- Anterior
- Posterior
- Middle

Space that houses heart, thymus gland, trachea, esophagus, nerves, lymph and blood vessels and major blood vessels

- Aorta
- Inferior vena cava

Diaphragm

A dome-shaped muscular partition that separates abdominal cavity from thoracic cavity

- Assists in breathing
  - Expands to assist lungs in exhalation/relaxation of diaphragm
  - Flattens out during inspiration/contraction of diaphragm
- Diaphragmatic hernia: esophageal hernia

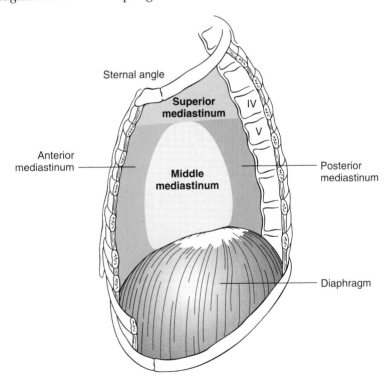

Figure **1-43** Mediastinum and diaphragm.

MEDIASTINUM AND DIAPHRAGM ANATOMY AND TERMINOLOGY QUIZ

1. The mediastinum is NOT an organ system.
   a. true
   b. false

2. The mediastinum is divided into:
   a. superior, anterior, posterior
   b. superior, anterior, posterior, middle
   c. anterior, posterior, middle
   d. middle, anterior, superior

3. During inspiration, the diaphragm:
   a. expands
   b. moves upward
   c. collapses
   d. flattens out

4. Term meaning partition:
   a. middle
   b. aspect
   c. median
   d. diaphragm

5. The diaphragm is said to be this shape:
   a. square
   b. flat
   c. dome
   d. round

6. This separates the abdominal cavity from the thoracic cavity:
   a. mediastinum
   b. diaphragm
   c. superior
   d. inferior

7. This is the area between the lungs:
   a. mediastinum
   b. diaphragm
   c. superior
   d. inferior

8. This is an esophageal hernia:
   a. mediastinal
   b. diaphragmatic
   c. paraesophageal
   d. hiatal

9. A diaphragmatic hernia is also known as:
    a. esophageal
    b. epiglottis
    c. partitional
    d. medial

10. The diaphragm assists in:
    a. percussion
    b. auscultation
    c. contraction
    d. breathing

■ HEMIC AND LYMPHATIC SYSTEM
HEMIC AND LYMPHATIC SYSTEM—ANATOMY AND TERMINOLOGY

Hemic refers to blood

Lymphatic system removes excess tissue fluid

- Lymph tissue is scattered throughout body
- Composed of lymph nodes, vessels, and organs

Lymph

Colorless fluid containing lymphocytes and monocytes

Originates from blood and after filtering, returns to blood

Transports interstitial fluids and proteins that have leaked from blood system into venous system

Absorbs and transports fats from villi of small intestine to venous system

Assists in immune function

Lymph Vessels

Similar to veins

Organized circulatory system throughout body

Lymph Organs

Lymph nodes, spleen, bone marrow, thymus, tonsils, and Peyer's patches (lymphoid tissue on mucosa of small intestine)

Lymph nodes, areas of concentrated tissue (Fig. 1–44)

Spleen, located in left upper quadrant (LUQ) of abdomen

- Composed of lymph tissue
  - Function is to filter blood; activates lymphocytes and B-cells to filter antigens
  - Stores blood

Thymus secretes thymosin causing T-cells to mature

- Larger in infants and shrinks with age

Tonsils

- Palatine tonsils
- Pharyngeal tonsils/adenoids

Hematopoietic Organ

Bone marrow, contains tissue that produces RBCs, WBCs, and platelets

- Produces stem cells

COMBINING FORMS

1.	aden/o	gland
2.	adenoid/o	adenoids

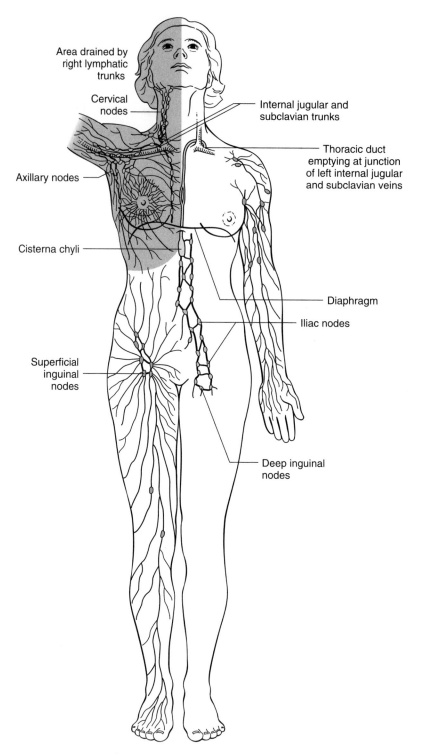

Area drained by
right lymphatic
trunks

Cervical
nodes

Internal jugular and
subclavian trunks

Thoracic duct
emptying at junction
of left internal jugular
and subclavian veins

Axillary nodes

Cisterna chyli

Diaphragm

Iliac nodes

Superficial
inguinal
nodes

Deep inguinal
nodes

Figure **1-44** Lymphatic system.

3.	axill/o	armpit
4.	cervic/o	neck/cervix
5.	immun/o	immune
6.	inguin/o	groin
7.	lymph/o	lymph
8.	lymphaden/o	lymph gland
9.	splen/o	spleen
10.	thym/o	thymus gland
11.	tonsill/o	tonsil
12.	tox/o	poison

PREFIXES

1.	hyper-	excess
2.	inter-	between
3.	retro-	behind

SUFFIXES

1.	-ectomy	removal
2.	-edema	swelling
3.	-itis	inflammation
4.	-megaly	enlargement
5.	-oid	resembling
6.	-oma	tumor
7.	-penia	deficient
8.	-pexy	fixation
9.	-phylaxis	protection
10.	-poiesis	production

MEDICAL TERMS

Axillary nodes	Lymph nodes located in armpit
Cloquet's node	Also called a gland; it is highest of deep groin lymph nodes
Inguinofemoral	Referring to groin and thigh
Jugular nodes	Lymph nodes located next to large vein in neck
Lymph node	Station along lymphatic system
Lymphadenectomy	Excision of a lymph node or nodes
Lymphadenitis	Inflammation of a lymph node
Lymphangiography	Radiographic recording of lymphatic vessels and nodes

Lymphangiotomy	Incision into a lymphatic vessel
Lymphangitis	Inflammation of lymphatic vessel or vessels
Parathyroid	Produces a hormone to mobilize calcium from bones to blood
Splenectomy	Excision of spleen
Splenography	Radiographic recording of spleen
Splenoportography	Radiographic procedure to allow visualization of splenic and portal veins of spleen
Stem cell	Immature blood cell
Thoracic duct	Largest lymph vessel which collects lymph from portions of body below diaphragm and from left side of body above diaphragm
Transplantation	Grafting of tissue from one source to another

HEMIC AND LYMPHATIC SYSTEM ANATOMY AND TERMINOLOGY QUIZ

1. The spleen is located in this quadrant of the abdomen:
   a. RUQ
   b. LUQ
   c. LLQ
   d. LRQ

2. Produces RBCs and platelets:
   a. thymus
   b. tonsils
   c. lymph node
   d. bone marrow

3. Which of the following is NOT a lymph organ?
   a. adrenal
   b. spleen
   c. thymus
   d. tonsil

4. Lymph transports fluids and _____ that have leaked from the blood system back to veins.
   a. stem cells
   b. lymphocytes
   c. B-cells
   d. proteins

5. This is largest in infants and shrinks with age:
   a. tonsils
   b. spleen
   c. thymus
   d. bone marrow

6. Combining form meaning gland:
   a. axill/o
   b. thym/o
   c. aden/o
   d. tox/o

7. Prefix meaning excess:
   a. hyper-
   b. hypo-
   c. inter-
   d. retro-

8. Suffix meaning enlargement:
   a. -edema
   b. -poiesis
   c. -penia
   d. -megaly

9. Lymph node located on neck:
   a. thoracic
   b. jugular
   c. Cloquet's
   d. axillary

10. These cells originate in the bone marrow:
    a. B-cells
    b. antigens
    c. erythrocytes
    d. stem cells

Anemia

Reduction in number of erythrocytes or decrease in quality of hemoglobin

- Less oxygen is transported in the blood

Aplastic Anemia

Diverse group of anemias

Characterized by bone marrow failure with reduced numbers of red and white cells and platelets

Causes

Genetic or acquired (primary or secondary)

Toxins/chemical agents

    Benzene and antibiotics such as chloramphenicol

Irradiation

Immunologic

Idiopathic (unknown)

Treatment

Blood transfusion

Bone marrow transplant

Iron Deficiency Anemia

Characterized by small erythrocytes and a reduced amount of hemoglobin

Caused by low or absent iron stores or serum iron concentrations

- Blood loss
- Decreased intake of iron
- Malabsorption of iron

Symptoms

Pallor

Headache

Stomatitis

Oral lesions

Gastrointestinal complaints

Retinal hemorrhages

Thinning, brittle nails and hair

Treatment

Iron supplement

Pernicious Anemia

Megaloblastic anemia (large stem cells)

Inability to absorb vitamin B_{12} due to a lack of intrinsic factor (found in gastric juices)

Usually in older adults

Caused by impaired intestinal absorption of vitamin B_{12}

Symptoms
Pallor

Weakness

Neurologic manifestations

Gastric discomfort

Treatment
Injections of vitamin B_{12}

Transfusions

Hemolytic Anemia
May be acute or chronic

Shortened survival of mature erythrocytes—excessive destruction of RBC

- Inability of bone marrow to compensate for decreased survival of erythrocytes

Treatment
Treat cause

Sickle Cell Anemia
Occurs primarily in those of West African descent

Abnormal sickle-shaped erythrocytes (sickle cell) caused by an abnormal type of hemoglobin (hemoglobin S)

Symptoms
Abdominal pain

Arthralgia

Ulceration of lower extremities

Fatigue

Dyspnea

Increased heart rate

Treatment
Symptomatic

Granulocytosis

Increase in granulocytes

- Neutrophils

- Eosinophils

- Basophils

Eosinophilia

Increase in number of eosinophilic granulocytes

Cause

Allergic disorders

Dermatologic disorders

Parasitic invasion

Drugs

Malignancies

Basophilia

Increase in basophilic granulocytes seen in leukemia

Monocytosis

Increased number of monocytes

Cause

Infection

Hematologic factors

Leukocytosis

Increased number of leukocytes

Cause

Acute viral infections, such as hepatitis

Chronic infections, such as syphilis

Leukocytopenia

Decreased number of leukocytes

Cause

Neoplasias

Immune deficiencies

Drugs

Virus

Radiation

Infectious Mononucleosis

Acute Infection of B Cells

Epstein-Barr virus most common cause

Symptoms

Fatigue

Fever

Weakness (asthenia)

Pharyngitis

Atypical lymphocytes in blood

Lymph node enlargement

Splenomegaly

Hepatomegaly

Transmission
Saliva

- Known as kissing disease

Treatment
Rest

Treatment of symptoms

Leukemia

Malignant disorder of blood and blood-forming organs

Leads to dysfunction of cells

- Primarily leads to proliferation of abnormal leukocytes—filling bone marrow and bloodstream

Acute Myelogenous Leukemia (AML)
Rapid onset

Short survival time

Symptoms
Abrupt onset

Fatigue

Lymphadenopathy

Bone pain and tenderness

Anemia

Bleeding

Fever

Infection

Anorexia

Splenomegaly

Hepatomegaly

Headache, vomiting, paralysis

Treatment
Chemotherapy

Bone marrow transplant following high-dose chemotherapy eradicating leukemic cells

Acute Lymphocytic Leukemia (ALL)
Immature lymphocytes (lymphoblasts)

Most cases occur in children and adolescents

Sudden onset

Treatment
Chemotherapy with drugs that suppress cell division/destroy rapid dividing cells

Remission

Relapse—leukemia cells in bone marrow and blood requiring treatment

Chronic Myelogenous Leukemia (CML)
Mature and immature granulocytes in bone marrow and blood

Slow progressive disease (those over 55 years live many years without life threat)

Cells are more differentiated

Gradual onset with milder symptoms

• Majority of cases are in adults

Symptoms
Extreme fatigue

Weight loss

Splenomegaly

Night sweats

Fever

Infections

Treatment
Chemotherapy—target abnormal proteins

Bone marrow transplant—following high-dose chemotherapy

Chronic Lymphocytic Leukemia (CLL)
Increased numbers of mature lymphocytes in marrow, lymph nodes, spleen

Most common form seen in elderly

Slowly progressive

Treatment
Chemotherapy

Lymphadenopathy

Lymphadenopathy
Any abnormality of lymph node

Enlargement of lymph node

Lymphangitis
Inflammation of lymphatic vessel

Lymphadenitis
Inflammation of lymph node

Localized inflammation associated with inflamed lesion

Generalized inflammation associated with disease

Inflammation can occur as result of

- Trauma

- Infection

- Drug reaction

- Autoimmune disease

- Immunologic disease

Malignant Lymphoma

Hodgkin's Disease
Initial sign is a painless mass commonly located on neck

Giant Reed-Sternberg cells are present in lymphatic tissue

Presentation
Enlarged spleen (splenomegaly)

Abdominal mass

Mediastinal mass

Localized node involvement

- Orderly spreading of node involvement

- Cervical, axillary, inguinal, and retroperitoneal lymph node involvement

Symptoms
Night sweats

Fever

Weight loss

Itching (pruritus)

Anorexia

Weakness

Treatment
If localized: radiation therapy and chemotherapy

If systemic: chemotherapy alone

High probability of cure with new treatments

Non-Hodgkin's Lymphoma
No giant Reed-Sternberg cells present

Involves multiple nodes scattered throughout body (follicular lymphoma)

Large cell lymphoma (large lymphocytes in diffuse nodes and lymph tissue)

- Noncontiguous spread of node involvement

- Not localized

Usually begins as a painless enlargement of node

Symptoms
Presents similar to Hodgkin's disease

Treatment
Chemotherapy cures or stops disease progression

Burkitt's Lymphoma
Type of non-Hodgkin's lymphoma

Usually found in Africa and New Guinea

Characterized by lesions in jaw and face

Epstein-Barr (herpes virus) has been found in Burkitt's lymphoma

Treatment
Radiation and chemotherapy for African type

Myeloma

Multiple Myeloma
B-cell cancer—lymphocytes that produce antibodies destroying bone tissue

• Also known as plasma cell myeloma

Increased plasma cells replace bone marrow

Overproduction of immunoglobulins—Bence Jones protein (found in urine)

Multiple tumor sites cause bone destruction

Results in weakened bone

Hypercalcemia

Anemia

Renal damage

Increased susceptibility to infections

Cause
Unknown

Treatment
Chemotherapy

Radiotherapy

Autologous bone marrow transplant (ABMT)—prolongs remission—may be a cure

Palliative treatments

HEMIC AND LYMPHATIC SYSTEM PATHOPHYSIOLOGY QUIZ

1. This condition involves a reduced number of erythrocytes and decreased quality of hemoglobin:
   a. monocytosis
   b. eosinophilia
   c. anemia
   d. leukocytosis

2. This condition is hallmarked by a shortened survival of mature erythrocytes and inability of bone marrow to compensate for decreased survival:
   a. hemolytic anemia
   b. granulocytosis
   c. eosinophilia
   d. monocytosis

3. The most common cause of this disease is Epstein-Barr virus:
   a. leukocytopenia
   b. infectious mononucleosis
   c. leukocytosis
   d. hemolytic anemia

4. Inflammation of the lymphatic vessels is:
   a. lymphadenitis
   b. lymphoma
   c. lymphadenopathy
   d. lymphangitis

5. What giant cell is present in Hodgkin's disease?
   a. B cell
   b. Reed-Sternberg
   c. T cell
   d. C cell

6. The average number of years of survival for multiple myeloma is:
   a. 5
   b. 10
   c. 3
   d. 20

7. Injection of vitamin B may be prescribed for this type of anemia:
   a. pernicious
   b. aplastic
   c. sideroblastic
   d. sickle cell

8. These are large stem cells:
   a. megaloblasts
   b. leukocytes
   c. erythrocytes
   d. granulocytes

9. This is known as the kissing disease:
   a. monocytosis
   b. leukocytopenia
   c. infectious mononucleosis
   d. granulocytosis

10. This lymphoma is usually found in Africa:
    a. multiple
    b. Burkitt's
    c. B-cell
    d. T-cell

■ ENDOCRINE SYSTEM

ENDOCRINE SYSTEM—ANATOMY AND TERMINOLOGY

Regulates body through hormones (chemical messengers)

Ductless endocrine glands secrete hormones directly to bloodstream

Affects growth, development, and metabolism

Endocrine Glands (Fig. 1–45)

Pituitary (Hypophysis): Master Gland
Located at base of brain in a depression in skull (sella turcica)

Anterior pituitary (adenohypophysis)

- Adrenocorticotropic hormone (ACTH)—stimulates adrenal cortex and increases production of cortisol

- Follicle-stimulating hormone (FSH)—males, stimulates sperm and testosterone production; females, with luteinizing hormone (LH) stimulates secretion of estrogen and follicle development and ovulation

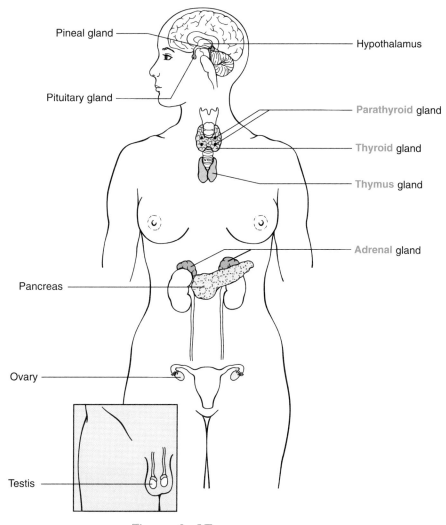

Figure **1-45** Endocrine system.

- Growth hormone (GH or somatotropin STH)—stimulates protein processing resulting in growth of bones, muscle, and fat metabolism, and maintains blood glucose levels

- Luteinizing hormone (LH)—males, stimulates testosterone production; females, stimulates secretion of progesterone and estrogen

- Melanocyte-stimulating hormone (MSH)—increases skin pigmentation

- Prolactin (PRL)—secreted by anterior pituitary, stimulates milk production and breast development

- Thyroid-stimulating hormone (TSH or thyrotropin)—stimulates thyroid gland

Posterior pituitary (neurohypophysis)—stores and releases hormones

- Antidiuretic hormone (ADH) or vasopressin—stimulates reabsorption of water by kidney tubules and increases blood pressure by constricting arterioles

- Oxytocin (OT)—stimulates contractions during childbirth, production and release of milk

Thyroid

Two lobes overlying trachea

Secretes two hormones that increase cell metabolism—thyroxine (T_4) and triiodothyronine (T_3)—synthesized from iodine

Secretes one hormone that decreases blood calcium—thyrocalcitonin (nasal spray used to treat osteoporosis)

Parathyroid Glands (4)

Located on posterior side of thyroid

Secretes PTH (parathyroid hormone) or parathoromone

Promotes calcium homeostasis in bloodstream

Adrenal Gland (Pair)

Located on top of each kidney

Adrenal cortex—outer region that secretes corticosteroids

- Cortisol—increases blood glucose

- Aldosterone—increases reabsorption of sodium (salt)

- Androgen, estrogen, progestin—sexual characteristics

Adrenal medulla—inner region that secretes catecholamines (epinephrine to dilate blood vessels to lower blood pressure, increase heart rate, dilate bronchial tubes, and release glycogen for energy and norepinephrine to constrict blood vessels to raise blood pressure)

Pancreas

Located behind stomach

Contains specialized cells (islets of Langerhans) that produce insulin and glycogen hormones

Insulin (decreases blood glucose), glucagon (converts glycogen to glucose, raising blood sugar), and somatostatin (regulates other cells of pancreas)

Thymus
Located behind sternum

Atrophies during adolescence

Produces thymosin—stimulates T-lymphocytes, effecting a positive immune response

Hypothalamus (Part of Brain)
Located below thalamus and above pituitary gland

Stimulates anterior pituitary to release hormones and posterior hypothalamus to store and release horomones

Pineal
Located between two cerebral hemispheres and above third ventricle

Secretes melatonin—more so at night, which affects sleep cycle

Also responsible for delaying sexual maturation in children

Also has neurotransmitters such as somatostatin, norepinephrine, seratonin, and histamine

Ovaries (Pair, Females)
Estrogen production stimulates ova production and secondary female sex characteristics

Progesterone—prepares the uterus for and maintains pregnancy

Placenta
Produces HCG (human chorionic gonadotropin) to sustain a pregnancy

Testes (Pair, Males)
Testosterone—male sex characteristics

COMBINING FORMS

1. aden/o — in relationship to a gland
2. adren/o — adrenal gland
3. adrenal/o — adrenal gland
4. andr/o — male
5. calc/o, calc/i — calcium
6. cortic/o — cortex
7. crin/o — secrete
8. dips/o — thirst
9. estr/o — female
10. gluc/o — sugar
11. glyc/o — sugar
12. gonad/o — ovaries and testes
13. home/o — same
14. hormon/o — hormone

15. kal/i	potassium
16. lact/o	milk
17. myx/o	mucus
18. natr/o	sodium
19. pancreat/o	pancreas
20. parathyroid/o	parathyroid gland
21. phys/o	growing
22. pituitar/o	pituitary gland
23. somat/o	body
24. ster/o, stere/o	solid, having three dimensions
25. thry/o	thyroid gland
26. thyroid/o	thyroid gland
27. toc/o	child birth
28. toxic/o	poison
29. ur/o	urine

PREFIXES

1. eu-	good/normal
2. oxy-	sharp, oxygen
3. pan-	all
4. tetra-	four
5. tri-	three
6. tropin-	act upon

SUFFIXES

1. -agon	assemble
2. -drome	run, relationship to conducting, to speed
3. -emia	blood condition
4. -in	a substance
5. -ine	a substance
6. -tropin	act upon
7. -uria	urine

MEDICAL TERMS

Adrenals	Glands, located at top of kidneys, that produce steroid hormones (cortex) and catecholamines (medulla)
Contralateral	Opposite side
Hormone	Chemical substance produced by body's endocrine glands

Isthmus	Connection of two regions or structures
Isthmus, thyroid	Tissue connection between right and left thyroid lobes
Isthmusectomy	Surgical removal of isthmus
Lobectomy	Removal of a lobe
Thymectomy	Surgical removal of thymus
Thymus	Gland that produces hormones important to immune response
Thyroglossal duct	A duct in embryo between thyroid and posterior tongue which occasionally persists into adult life and causes cysts, fistulas, or sinuses
Thyroid	Part of endocrine system that produces hormones that regulate metabolism
Thyroidectomy	Surgical removal of thyroid

ENDOCRINE SYSTEM ANATOMY AND TERMINOLOGY QUIZ

1. Which of the following is NOT affected by the endocrine system?
   a. digestion
   b. development
   c. progesterone
   d. metabolism

2. Gland that overlies the trachea:
   a. parathyroid
   b. adrenal
   c. pancreas
   d. thyroid

3. Gland that is located on the top of each kidney:
   a. parathyroid
   b. adrenal
   c. pancreas
   d. thyroid

4. The outer region of the adrenal gland that secretes corticosteroids:
   a. cortex
   b. medulla
   c. sternum
   d. medullary

5. Located on the thyroid:
   a. hypophysis
   b. thymus
   c. pineal
   d. parathyroid

6. Located at the base of the brain in a depression in the skull:
   a. pituitary
   b. thymus
   c. adrenal
   d. pineal

7. Stimulates contractions during childbirth:
   a. cortisol
   b. PTH
   c. ADH
   d. oxytocin

8. Produced only during pregnancy by the placenta:
   a. estrogen and progesterone
   b. melatonin
   c. thymosin
   d. adrenocorticotropic hormone

9. Combining form meaning secrete:
   a. dips/o
   b. crin/o
   c. gluc/o
   d. kal/i

10. Prefix meaning good:
    a. tri-
    b. tropin-
    c. pan-
    d. eu-

ENDOCRINE SYSTEM—PATHOPHYSIOLOGY

Diabetes Mellitus

Caused by a deficiency in insulin production or poor use of insulin by body cells

Islets of Langerhans (pancreatic cells) secrete glucagon and insulin to regulate fat, carbohydrate, and protein metabolism

Types of Diabetes Mellitus

Type 1, IDDM (insulin-dependent diabetes mellitus), immune mediated
Onset before age 30—peak onset age 12

Includes beta islet cell destruction, insulin deficiency

Acute onset

Positive family history

Requires insulin

Ketoacidosis (fats improperly burned leads to ketones and acids circulating)

Type 2, NIDDM (non–insulin-dependent diabetes mellitus)
Adult onset, after age 30, but it is now occurring earlier

Insidious onset/asymptomatic

Positive in immediate family

Dietary management and/or oral hypoglycemics and/or insulin

Most common type—85% are obese at onset

Insulin is present

Ketoacidosis does not occur

Symptoms
Polyuria

Polydipsia

Glycosuria

Hyperglycemia

Polyphagia

Unexplained weight loss

Acute complications
Hypoglycemia

Diabetic ketoacidosis

Chronic complications
Diabetic neuropathy (Fig. 1–46)

Retinopathy

Coronary artery disease (atherosclerosis)

Stroke

Peripheral vascular disease

Infection

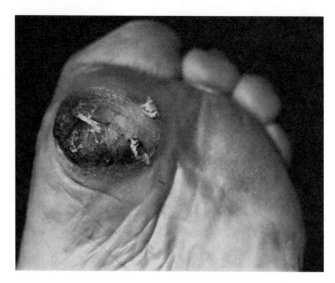

Figure **1-46** Patient with diabetes mellitus and neuropathy had severe claw toes, and shear forces across plantar surface of first metatarsal head caused recurrent ulceration. (From Canale ST, Beaty JH, *Campbell's Operative Orthopaedics*, ed 11, Philadelphia, 2008, Mosby.)

Gestational diabetes mellitus—predisposition to diabetes
Most often recognized in third trimester

Glucose intolerance may be temporary occurring only during pregnancy

Majority will develop diabetes mellitus within 15 years

Pituitary Disorders

Tumors

   Most common cause of pituitary disorders

   May secrete hormone

      Such as prolactin and ACTH

Anterior Pituitary
Dwarfism (hypopituitarism)
Can be caused by deficiency of somatotrophin (growth hormone)

Gigantism (Fig. 1–47) (hyperpituitarism)
Can be caused by excess of somatotrophin (growth hormone) in childhood

Treatment
Resection of tumor or irradiation of pituitary

Acromegaly (hyperpituitarism)
Increased GH in adulthood

Enlargement of facial bones, feet, and hands

Treatment
Pituitary adenoma is irradiated or removed

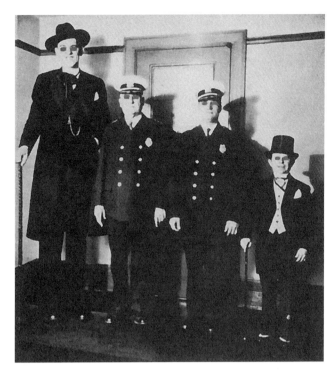

Figure **1-47** Gigantism. A pituitary giant and dwarf contrasted with normal-size men. (From Thibodeau GA, Patton KT: *Anatomy & physiology,* ed 5, St Louis, 2003, Mosby.)

Posterior Pituitary
Diabetes insipidus
Insufficient antidiuretic hormone—kidney tubules fail to retain needed water and salts

Causes polyuria, polydipsia, and dehydration

ADH or SIADH—syndrome of inadequate antidiuretic hormone

Excessive secretion of antidiuretic hormone

Causes excessive water retention

Treatment
Some types have no treatment

Others can be controlled with vasopressin (drugs)

Thyroid Disorders

Goiter (Fig. 1–48)
Enlargement of thyroid gland in the neck

Cause
Hypothyroid disorders

Hyperthyroid disorders

Hyperthyroidism—Thyrotoxicosis
Excessive thyroid hormone production

Most common form: Graves' disease (familial)—results of autoimmune process

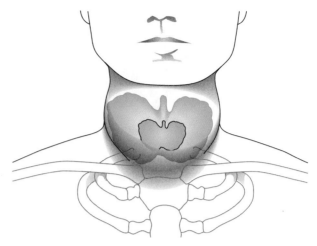

Figure **1-48** Goiter is an enlargement of thyroid gland.

Characterized by

Goiter

Tachycardia

Atrial fibrillation

Dyspnea

Palpitations

Fatigue

Tremor

Nervousness

Weight loss

Exophthalmos (protruding eyes)

• Decreased blinking

Treatment

Medication (antithyroid drugs)

Radioactive iodine

Surgical excision

Thyrotoxicosis storm/crisis

Thyroid storm/crisis is an acute life-threatening hypermetabolic state induced by excessive release of thyroid horomones

Most extreme state of thyrotoxicosis

Hypothyroidism

Primary: inadequate thyroid hormone production

Resulting in increasing levels of thyroid-stimulating hormone (TSH) production

Secondary: inadequate amounts of thyroid-stimulating hormone synthesized

Types

Cretinism

- Congenital
- Occurs in children
- If not treated, it will cause a severe delay in physical/mental development

Treatment
Thyroid hormone

Myxedema

- Severe form
- Occurs in adults
  - Atherosclerosis
- Symptoms
  - Cold intolerance
  - Weight gain
  - Mental sluggishness
  - Fatigue

Treatment
Thyroid hormone

Hashimoto's thyroiditis

- Autoimmune disorder

Treatment
Medication (levothyroxine synthetic hormone replacement)

Parathyroid Disorders

Hyperparathyroidism—Excessive Parathyroid Hormone (PTH)
Leads to hypercalcemia

- Affects heart and bones and damages kidneys

Symptoms
Brittle bones

Kidney stones

Cardiac disturbances

Treatment
Surgical excision

Hypoparathyroidism—Abnormally Low PTH
Leads to hypocalcemia

Symptoms
Nerve irritability—twitching or spasms

Muscle cramps

Tingling and burning (parathesias) fingertips, toes, and lips

Anxiety, nervousness

Tetany (constant muscle contraction)

Treatment
Calcium and vitamin D

Adrenal Gland Disorders

Cushing Syndrome—Hypercortisolism
Excess levels of adrenocorticotropic hormone (ACTH)

Cause
Hyperfunction of adrenal cortex

Long-term use of steroid medications

Symptoms
Weight gain

• Fat deposits on face (moonface) and trunk (buffalo hump)

Glucose intolerance

Hypernaturemia

Hypokalemia

Virilization

Hypertension

• Diabetes may develop (20%)

Muscle wasting

Osteoporosis

Change in mental status

Delayed healing

Treatment
Medication

Radiation therapy

Surgical intervention

Addison's Disease—Primary Adrenal Insufficiency
Deficiency of adrenocortical hormones resulting from destruction of adrenal glands
• Glucocorticoids

• Mineralocorticoids

Cause
Tumors

Autoimmune disorders

Viral

Tuberculosis

Infection

Symptoms
Decreased blood glucose levels

Elevated serum ACTH

Fatigue

Lack of ability to handle stress

Weight loss

Infections

Hypotension

Decreased body hair

Hyperpigmentation

Treatment
Hormone (glucocorticoid) replacement

Hyperaldosteronism
Excess aldosterone secreted by adrenal cortex

Types
Primary hyperaldosteronism (Conn's syndrome)

- Caused by an abnormality of adrenal cortex

  - Usually an adrenal adenoma

Secondary hyperaldosteronism

- Caused by other than adrenal stimuli

Symptoms
Hypertension

Hypokalemia

Neuromuscular disorders

Treatment
Treat the underlying condition that caused hyperaldosteronism

- Such as adrenal adenoma

Adrenal Medulla
Hypersecretion

Pheochromocytoma—benign tumor of medulla

Excessive production of epinephrine and norepinephrine

Symptoms
Severe headaches

Sweating

Flushing

Hypertension

Muscle spasms

Treatment
Antihypertensive drugs

Remove tumor

Androgen and Estrogen Hypersecretion
Androgen, male characteristic hormone

- Virilization, development of male characteristics

Feminization, hypersecretion of estrogen, female characteristic hormone

Cause
Underlying condition

- Adrenal tumor

- Cushing syndrome

- Adenomas or carcinomas

- Defects in steroid metabolism

Treatment
Surgical intervention for tumor

Underlying condition

ENDOCRINE SYSTEM PATHOPHYSIOLOGY QUIZ

1. This type of diabetes typically occurs before age 30:
   a. type 1
   b. type 2

2. The acronym that indicates that insulin is not required is:
   a. IDDM
   b. NIDDM
   c. PIDDM
   d. NDDMI

3. The most common cause of pituitary disorders is:
   a. hypersecretion
   b. hyposecretion
   c. tumor
   d. infection

4. In excess, this hormone can cause gigantism:
   a. somatotrophin
   b. thyroid
   c. mineralocorticoids
   d. adrenocortical

5. Goiter can be caused by which of the following:
   a. hypothyroidism
   b. parathyroidism
   c. hyperthyroidism
   d. both a and c

6. This type of hypothyroidism is an autoimmune disorder:
   a. myxedema
   b. Hashimoto's
   c. cretinism
   d. hypokalemia

7. Tetany can be caused by:
   a. hypoparathyroidism
   b. hyperthyroidism
   c. hyperparathyroidism
   d. hyperaldosteronism

8. Conn's syndrome is also known as:
   a. primary hypoparathyroidism
   b. primary hyperthyroidism
   c. primary hyperparathyroidism
   d. primary hyperaldosteronism

9. Development of male characteristics is known as:
    a. virilization
    b. feminization
    c. hypertrophy
    d. hyperaldosteronism

10. The treatment for Addison's disease is often:
    a. chemotherapy
    b. radiation
    c. hormone replacement
    d. all of the above

■ NERVOUS SYSTEM

NERVOUS SYSTEM—ANATOMY AND TERMINOLOGY

Controlling, regulating, and communicating system

Organization

- Central nervous system (CNS), brain and spinal cord
- Peripheral nervous system (PNS), cranial and spinal nerves
  - Autonomic nervous system—motor and sensory nerves of viscera (involuntary)
  - Somatic nervous system—motor and sensory nerves of skeletal muscles

Cells of the Nervous System (Fig. 1–49)

Neurons—Primary Cells of Nervous System

Classified according to function (afferent [sensory], efferent [motor], interneurons [associational])

- Dendrites (receive signals)
- Cell body (nucleus, within cell body)
- Axon (carries signals from cell body)
- Myelin sheath (insulation around axon)

Glia

Astrocytes

Star shaped—transport water and salts between capillaries and neurons

Microglia

Multiple branching processes—protect neurons from inflammation

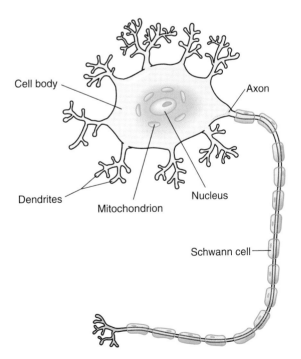

Figure **1-49** Myelinated axon.

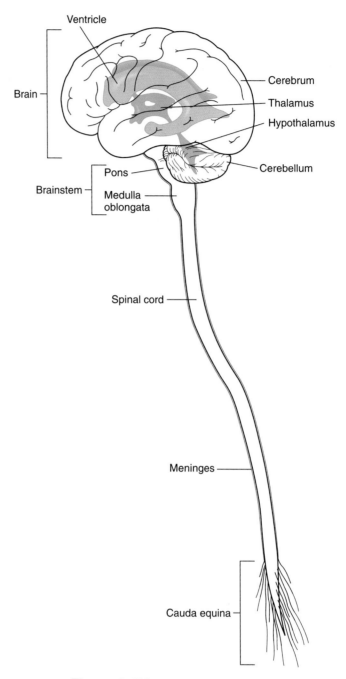

Figure **1-50** Brain and spinal cord.

Oligodendrocytes

Form myelin sheath

Ependymal

Lining membrane of brain and spinal cord where central spinal fluid circulates

Divisions of Central Nervous System (CNS) (Fig. 1–50)

Brain—Housed in Cranium (Box Comprised of 8 Bones)— Functioning to Enclose and Protect

Listing from inferior to superior

Brainstem

Medulla oblongata—cross over area left to right and center of respiratory and cardiovascular systems

Pons—connection of nerves (face and eyes)

Midbrain

Diencephalon

Hypothalamus controls autonomic nervous system, body temperature, sleep, apetite, and control of pituitary

Thalamus relays impulses to cerebral cortex for sensory system (pain)

Cerebellum

Controls voluntary movement and balance

Cerebrum

Largest part of brain

Functions

Mental processes, personality, sensory interpretation, movements, and memory

Two hemispheres

Right controls left side of body

Left controls right side of body

Divided into five lobes

- Frontal

- Parietal

- Temporal

- Occipital

- Insula

Vertebral Column—33 Vertebrae

7 cervical

12 thoracic

5 lumbar

5 sacrum (fused)

4 coccygeal (fused)—tailbone

Spinal Cord—housed within vertebrae from medulla oblongata to second lumbar

Spinal and brain meninges (coverings—dura mater [external], archnoid, pia mater [internal])

Spine and brain spaces bathed by cerebrospinal fluid (CSF) (subarachnoid space)

Cavities within brain contain cerebrospinal fluid (ventricles)

Peripheral Nervous System (PNS)

Cranial nerves, 12 pair

Spinal nerves, 31 pair

Autonomic Nervous System (ANS)—Housed within Both PNS and CNS

Two divisions

- Sympathetic system—functions in fight and flight (stress)

- Parasympathetic system—functions to restore and conserve energy

COMBINING FORMS

1.	cephal/o	head
2.	cerebell/o	cerebellum
3.	cerebr/o	cerebrum
4.	crani/o	cranium
5.	dur/o	dura mater
6.	encephal/o	brain
7.	gangli/o	ganglion
8.	ganglion/o	ganglion
9.	gli/o	glial cells
10.	lept/o	slender
11.	mening/o	meninges
12.	meningi/o	meninges
13.	ment/o	mind
14.	mon/o	one
15.	myel/o	bone marrow, spinal cord
16.	neur/o	nerve
17.	phas/o	speech
18.	phren/o	mind
19.	poli/o	gray matter
20.	pont/o	pons
21.	psych/o	mind
22.	quadr/i	four
23.	radic/o	nerve root
24.	radicul/o	nerve root
25.	rhiz/o	nerve root
26.	vag/o	vagus nerve

PREFIXES

1.	hemi-	half
2.	per-	through

232

3. quadri-   four

4. tetra-   four

SUFFIXES

1. -algesia   pain sensation

2. -algia   pain

3. -cele   hernia

4. -esthesia   feeling

5. -iatry   medical treatment

6. -ictal   pertaining to

7. -kines/o   movement

8. -paresis   incomplete paralysis

9. -plegia   paralysis

MEDICAL ABBREVIATIONS

1. ANS   autonomic nervous system

2. CNS   central nervous system

3. CSF   cerebrospinal fluid

4. CVA   stroke/cerebrovascular accident

5. EEG   electroencephalogram

6. LP   lumbar puncture

7. PNS   peripheral nervous system

8. TENS   transcutaneous electrical nerve stimulation

9. TIA   transient ischemic attack

MEDICAL TERMS

Burr	Drill used to create an entry into the cranium
Central nervous system	Brain and spinal cord
Craniectomy	Permanent, partial removal of skull
Craniotomy	Opening of the skull
Cranium	That part of the skeleton that encloses the brain
Diskectomy	Removal of a vertebral disk
Electroencephalography	Recording of the electric currents of the brain by means of electrodes attached to the scalp
Laminectomy	Surgical excision of posterior arch of vertebra—includes spinal process
Peripheral nerves	12 pairs of cranial nerves, 31 pairs of spinal nerves, and autonomic nervous system; connects peripheral receptors to the brain and spinal cord

Shunt	An artificial passage
Skull	Entire skeletal framework of the head
Somatic nerve	Sensory or motor nerve
Stereotaxis	Method of identifying a specific area or point in the brain
Sympathetic nerve	Part of the peripheral nervous system that controls automatic body function and sympathetic nerves activated under stress
Trephination	Surgical removal of a disk of bone
Vertebrectomy	Removal of vertebra

NERVOUS SYSTEM ANATOMY AND TERMINOLOGY QUIZ

1. Portion of nervous system that contains cranial and spinal nerves:
   a. central
   b. peripheral
   c. autonomic
   d. parasympathetic

2. Part of neuron that receives signals:
   a. dendrites
   b. cell body
   c. axon
   d. myelin sheath

3. NOT associated with glia:
   a. monocytes
   b. astrocytes
   c. microglia
   d. oligodendrocytes

4. Largest part of brain:
   a. cerebellum
   b. cerebrum
   c. cortex
   d. pons

5. Divided into two hemispheres:
   a. cerebellum
   b. cerebrum
   c. cortex
   d. pons

6. Number of pairs of cranial nerves:
   a. 10
   b. 11
   c. 12
   d. 13

7. Controls right side of body:
   a. left cerebrum
   b. right cerebrum
   c. right cortex
   d. left cortex

8. Combining form that means brain:
   a. mening/o
   b. mon/o
   c. esthesi/o
   d. encephal/o

9. Prefix that means four:
   a. per-
   b. tetra-
   c. para-
   d. bi-

10. Combining form that means speech:
    a. phas/o
    b. rhiz/o
    c. poli/o
    d. myel/o

Dementias—Classified by Causative Factor

Cognitive deficiencies

Causes

Alzheimer's disease

Vascular disease

Head trauma

Tumors

Infection

Toxins

Substance abuse

AIDS

Alzheimer's Disease

Most common type of dementia

Progressive intellectual impairment

- Results in damage to neurons (neurofibrillary tangles)

- Fatal within 3 to 20 years

Causes

Mostly unknown

Perhaps genetic defect, autoimmune reaction, or virus

Symptoms

Behavior change

Memory loss

Confusion

Disorientation

Restlessness

Speech disturbances

Personality change—anxiety, depression

Irritability

Inability to complete activities of daily living

Treatment

- No cure

- Aricept (drug has modest effect in early stages)

- Symptomatic treatment

- Support for family

Vascular Dementia

Result of brain infarctions (vascular occlusion resulting in loss of brain function)

Nutritional Degenerative Disease
Deficiency

- B vitamins

- Niacin

- Pantothenic acid

Associated with alcoholism

Amyotrophic Lateral Sclerosis (ALS)
Motor neuron disease (MND)

Also known as Lou Gehrig's disease

- Baseball player who died of ALS

Deterioration of neurons of spinal cord and brain

Results in atrophy of muscles and loss of fine motor skills

Difficulty walking, talking, and breathing

Mental functioning remains normal

Survival is 2 to 5 years after diagnosis

Genetic cause/familial chromosome 21 aberration

- Death usually results from respiratory failure

Treatment
Symptomatic only

Emotional support

No cure

Huntington's Disease—Chorea
Inherited progressive atrophy of cerebrum

Symptoms
Restlessness

Rapid, jerky movements in arms and face (uncontrollable jerking and facial grimacing)

Rigidity

Intellectual impairment/bradyphrenia/apathy

Treatment
Genetic defect of chromosome 4

No cure

Symptomatic

Parkinson's Disease (Parkinsonism)
Decreased secretion of dopamine

Typically occurs after age 40

Cause

Unknown

Symptoms

Muscle rigidity and weakness

Bradykinesia—slow voluntary movements

Postural instability, stooped

Shuffling gait

Tremors at rest

Masklike facial appearance

Depression

Treatment

Medications to reduce symptoms

Dopamine replacement

Multiple Sclerosis (MS)

Common neurologic condition

- Demyelination of central nervous system—replaced by sclerotic tissue

Affects young adults 20–40 years old

Results in myelin destruction and gliosis of white matter of central nervous system

Speculation that it is an autoimmune condition or result of a virus

Exacerbations and remission patterns

Symptoms

Precipitated by "an event," i.e., infection, pregnancy, stress

Loss of feeling (paresthesias)

Vision problems

Bladder disorder

Mood disorders

Weakness of limbs—unsteady gait and paralysis

Treatment

Symptomatic

Management of relapses

Reducing relapses and disease progression—disease-modifying drugs (DMDs)

Myasthenia Gravis (MG)

Means grave muscle weakness

Autoimmune neuromuscular condition—antibodies block neurotransmission to muscle cells

Most have pathologic changes of thymus

Symptoms

Insidious

Muscle weakness and fatigability

May be localized or generalized

Often affects

- Swallowing

- Breathing

- Compromised swallowing and breathing may lead to crisis

Treatment
Anticholinesterase drugs

- Restores normal muscle strength and recoverability after fatigue

Corticosteroids (prednisone) and immunosuppressive drugs

Thymectomy

Tourette syndrome

Symptoms

Spasmodic, twitching movements, uncontrollable vocal sounds, inappropriate words

Begins with twitching eyelids and facial muscles (tics)

Verbal outbursts

Cause

Unknown

Excess dopamine or hypersensitivity to dopamine

Treatment

Antipsychotic drugs

Antidepressant drugs

Mood-elevating drugs

Poliomyelitis
Contagious viral disease

Affects motor neurons

Causes paralysis and respiratory failure

Prevent with vaccination

Postpolio Syndrome (PPS)
Also known as postpoliomyelitis neuromuscular atrophy

Progressive muscle weakness

- Past history of paralytic polio

Symptoms
Muscle weakness and fatigability

- May include atrophy and muscle twitching

Treatment
Symptomatic

Maintenance of respiratory function

Guillain-Barré Syndrome

Also known as

- Idiopathic polyneuritis
- Acute inflammatory polyneuropathy
- Landry's ascending paralysis

Demyelination of peripheral nerves—acquired disease

Symptoms

Primary ascending motor paralysis

Variable sensory disturbances

Treatment

Supportive

Congenital Neurologic Disorders

Hydrocephalus

Excessive amounts circulating of cerebrospinal fluid in ventricles of brain

Circulation is impaired in brain or spinal cord

Compresses brain

Treatment

Surgical placement of a shunt

Spina Bifida (Fig. 1–51)

Developmental birth defect which causes incomplete development of spinal cord and its coverings.

Vertebrae overlying open portions of spinal cord do not fully form and remain unfused and open.

- Spina bifida occulta—may not be noticed, no protrusion through defect
- Spina bifida manifesta which includes:
  - Myelomeningocele (spina bifida cystical)
    - Meninges and spinal cord protrude through defect
  - Meningocele
    - Meninges herniated through defect

Results in neurologic deficiencies

Treatment

Surgical repair

Mental Disorders

Schizophrenia

Variety of syndromes

Results in changes in brain

Hereditary factors are considered a cause

- Also, fetal brain damage is caused by viral infections, complications of pregnancy, nutritional deficiences

Stress usually precipitates onset

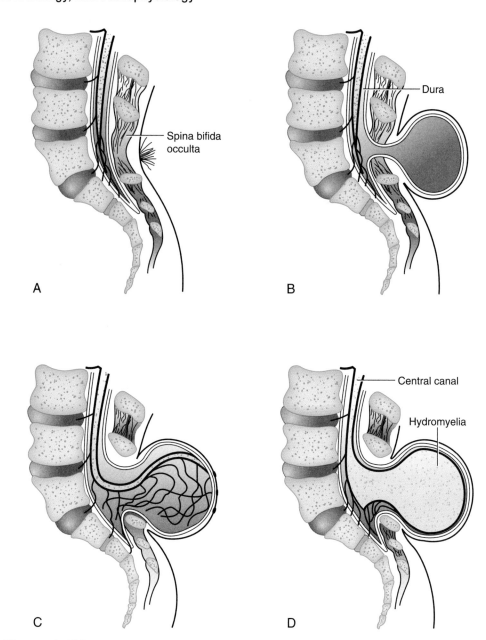

Figure **1-51** **A,** Spina bifida occulta. **B,** Meningocele. **C,** Myelomeningocele. **D,** Myelocystocele or hydromyelia.

Symptoms

Delusions of persecution and/or grandeur

Disorganized thought

Repetitive behaviors

Behavior issues

Decreased speech

Decreased ability to solve problems

Loss of emotions/flat affect

Hallucinations

Types are based on characteristics

Treatment
Antipsychotic drugs

Drugs have very unpleasant side effects such as tardive dyskinesia, with symptoms as follows:

- Excessive movement
- Grimacing
- Jerking
- Tremors
- Shuffling gait
- Dry mouth
- Blurred vision

Depression
Mood (sustained emotional state) disorder

Exact cause is unknown

Symptoms
Sadness

Hopelessness

Lethargy

Insomnia

Anorexia

Treatment
Antidepressant drugs

Electroconvulsive therapy

Central Nervous System (CNS) Disorders

■ Vascular Disorder

Transient Ischemic Attack (TIA)
Temporary reduction of blood flow to brain which produces strokelike symptoms but no lasting damage

Often a warning sign of cerebrovascular accident

Symptoms
Depend on location of ischemia

- Usual recovery in 24 hours

No loss of consciousness

Slurred, indiscernible speech

May display muscle weakness in legs/arms

Paresthesia (numbness) of face

Mental confusion may be present

Repeated attacks common in the presence of atherosclerotic disease

Cerebrovascular Accident (CVA) or Stroke
Infarction of brain due to lack of blood/oxygen flow

Necrosis of tissue with total occlusion of vessel

Causes
Atherosclerotic disease—thrombus formation

Embolus

Hemorrhage—arterial aneurysm

Symptoms
Depend on location of obstruction

- Thrombus
  - Gradual onset
  - Often occurs at rest
  - Intracranial pressure (ICP) minimal
  - Localized damage
- Embolus
  - Sudden onset
  - Occurs anytime
  - ICP minimal
  - Localized damage unless multiple emboli
- Hemorrhage
  - Sudden onset
  - Occurs most often with activity
  - ICP high
  - Widespread damage
  - May be fatal

Treatment
Anticoagulant drugs (clot dissolving) if caused by thrombus or embolus—tissue plasminogen activator (tPA)

Carotid endarterectomy (removes artherosclerotic plaque)

Oxygen treatment

Underlying condition treated, such as

- Hypertension
- Atherosclerosis
- Thrombus

Aneurysm—Cerebral
Dilation of artery

- May be localized or multiple

Rupture possible, often on exertion

- Fatal if rupture is massive

Symptoms
May display visual effects, such as

- Loss of visual fields

- Photophobia

- Diplopia

Headache

Confusion

Slurred speech

Weakness

Stiff neck (nuchal rigidity)

Treatment
Dependent on diagnosis prior to rupture

Surgical intervention

Encephalitis
Infection of parenchymal tissue of brain or spinal cord

- Often viral

Accompanying inflammation

Usually results in some permanent damage

Symptoms
Stiff neck

Headaches

Vomiting

Fever

May have seizure

Lethargy

Some types of encephalitis
Herpes simplex

Lyme disease

West Nile fever

Western equine

Treatment
Symptomatic

Supportive

Reye's Syndrome
Associated with viral infection

- Especially when aspirin has been administered

Changes occur in brain and liver

- Leads to increased intracranial pressure

Symptoms
Headaches

Vomiting

Lethargy

Seizures

Treatment
Symptomatic treatment

Brain Abscess
Localized infection

Necrosis of tissue

Usually spread from infection elsewhere, such as ears or sinus

Symptoms
Neurologic deficiencies

Increased intracranial pressure

Treatment
Antibiotics for bacterial infections

Surgical drainage

■ Epilepsies
Chronic seizure disorder

Types
Partial seizures (focal)
State of altered focus but conscious—simple

Impaired consciousness—complex

Specialized epileptic seizures

Aura

• Auditory or visual sign that precedes a seizure

Generalized seizures
Absence seizures—petit mal

• Brief loss of awareness

• Most common in children (febrile causation)

Tonic-clonic—grand mal or ictal event

• Loss of consciousness

• Alternate contraction and relaxation

• Incontinence

• No memory of seizure

Causes
Tumor

Hemorrhage

Trauma

Edema

Infection

Excessive cerebrospinal fluid

High fever

Treatment

Correct cause

Anticonvulsant drugs

Neurosurgery

Postictal event—after seizure—neurologic symptoms (weakness, etc.)

■ Trauma

Head Injury—Traumatic Brain Injury (TBI)
Concussion
Mild blow to head

Temporary axonal disturbances

Grade 1: temporary confusion and amnesia (brief)

Grade 2: memory loss for very recent events and confusion

Grade 3: amnesia for recent events and disorientation (longer duration)

Results in reversible interference with brain function

• Recover in 24 hours with no residual damage

Contusion
Bruising of brain

Force of blow determines outcome

Hematomas—blood accumulation (clot)
Compresses surrounding structures

Classified based on location

• Epidural
  • Develops between dura and skull
• Subdural
  • Develops between dura and arachnoid
    · Development within 24 hours is acute
    · Development within a week is subacute
  • ICP increases with enlargement of hematoma
• Subarachnoid
  • Develops between pia and arachnoid
  • Blood mixes with cerebrospinal fluid
    · No localized hematoma forms

- Intracerebral
  - As a result of a contusion

Symptoms
Increased ICP

Others dependent on location and severity of injury

Treatment
Identification of the location of hematoma

Medications to decrease edema

Antibiotics

Surgical intervention—Burr hole if necessary to decrease the ICP

Spinal Cord Injury
Result of trauma to vertebra, cord, ligaments, intervertebral disc

Vertebra injuries classified as
- Simple—affects spinous or transverse process

- Compression—anterior fracture of vertebrae

- Comminuted—vertebral body is shattered

- Dislocation—vertebrae are out of alignment

- Flexion injury in which hyperflexion compresses vertebra

Dislocation

Rotation

Symptoms
Depend on vertebral level and severity

Paralysis

Loss of sensation

Drop in blood pressure

Loss of bladder and rectal control

Decreased venous circulation

Treatment
Identification of area of injury

Immobilization

Corticosteroids to decrease edema

Bladder and bowel management

Rehabilitation

■ Tumors of Brain and Spinal Cord

Increases ICP

Life threatening

Rarely metastasize outside of central nervous system

Secondary brain tumors are common

Metastasis from lung or breast

Gliomas Common Type

Primary malignant tumor—encapsulated and invasive

Types based on cell from which tumor arises and location of tumor

Glioblastoma
Located in cerebral hemispheres (deep in white matter)

Highly aggressive

Oligodendrocytoma
Usually located in frontal lobes

Oligodendroblastoma, more aggressive form

Ependymoma
Located in ventricles

Most often occurs in children

Ependymoblastoma, more aggressive form

Astrocytoma
Located anywhere in brain and spinal cord

Invasive but slow growing

Pineal Region
Germ cell tumors
Usually in adolescents

Rare

Variable growth rate

Several other pineal tumors
Pineocytoma

Teratoma

Germinoma

Blood Vessel
Angioma
Usually located in posterior cerebral hemispheres

Slow growing

Hemangioblastoma
Located in cerebellum

Slow growing

Medulloblastoma
Aggressive tumor

Located in posterior cerebellar vermis (fourth ventricle roof)

Meningioma
Originates in arachnoid

Slow growing

Pituitary Tumor
Related to aging

Slow growing

• Such as macroadenomas

Cranial Nerve Tumors
Neurilemmomas most common location: cranial nerve VIII

Slow growing

Metastatic

Spinal Cord Tumors

Symptoms are based on location of spinal compression

Intramedullary

• Originates in neural tissue

Extramedullary

• Originates outside the spinal cord

Metastatic tumors of spinal cord are more common

• Myeloma—marrow

• Lymphoma—lymph

• Carcinomas—lung, breast, prostate

Most common type of primary extramedullary tumor

• Meningiomas—anyplace in spine

• Neurofibromas—common in thoracic and lumbar

NERVOUS SYSTEM PATHOPHYSIOLOGY QUIZ

1. Most common dementia is:
   a. Alzheimer's disease
   b. secondary
   c. nutritional degenerative disease
   d. Lou Gehrig's disease

2. MND stands for:
   a. maximal neuron disorder
   b. migrating niacin disorder
   c. motor neuron disease
   d. motor neuropathic disorder

3. Dopamine replacement is useful in treating:
   a. multiple sclerosis
   b. Parkinson's disease
   c. Huntington's disease
   d. CVA

4. Condition in which primary symptoms are muscle weakness and fatigability:
   a. amyotrophic lateral sclerosis
   b. multiple sclerosis
   c. dyskinesis
   d. myasthenia gravis

5. Another name for idiopathic polyneuritis is:
   a. Guillain-Barré syndrome
   b. multiple sclerosis
   c. amyotrophic lateral sclerosis
   d. postpolio syndrome

6. This condition is thought to be caused by genetic factors and possibly fetal brain damage:
   a. Parkinson's
   b. schizophrenia
   c. spina bifida
   d. Guillain-Barré syndrome

7. This condition is associated with viral infection, especially when aspirin has been administered:
   a. Reye's syndrome
   b. Guillain-Barré syndrome
   c. Lou Gehrig's disease
   d. Conn's syndrome

8. Concussion is a mild blow to the head in which recovery is expected within _____ hours.
   a. 12
   b. 24
   c. 48
   d. 1 week

9. ICP means:
   a. intercranial pressure
   b. intracranial pressure
   c. interior cranial pressure
   d. intensive cranial pressure

10. In this type of hematoma, blood mixes with cerebrospinal fluid:
    a. epidural
    b. subdural
    c. subarachnoid
    d. intracerebral

■ SENSES

SENSES—ANATOMY AND TERMINOLOGY

Sight	Eyes
Hearing	Ears
Smell	Nose
Taste	Tongue
Touch	Skin

Sight: Three Layers of Eye (Fig. 1–52)

Cornea (Outer Layer)
Fibrous, transparent layer that extends over dome of eye

Refracts (bends) light to focus on receptor cells (posterior eye)

Avascular (nourished by sclera)

Sclera (Extension of Outer Layer)
White of eye

Extends from cornea (anterior or surface) to optic nerve (posterior surface)

- Lies over iris

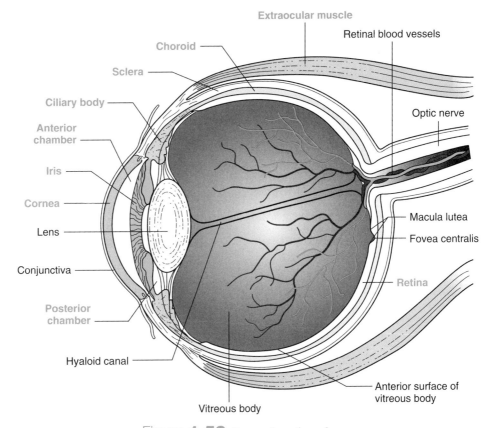

Figure **1-52** Eye and ocular adnexa.

Choroid (Middle Layer)
Pigment layer

Ciliary muscle and iris on front portion of layer

- Contracts

Retina (Inner Layer)
Contains rods and cones

- Rods provide night and peripheral vision

- Cones provide day and color vision and are stimulated by primary colors of red, green, and blue

Conjunctiva
Covers front of sclera and lines eyelid (contiguous layer)

Lens
Behind pupil

Lens is connected by zonules to ciliary body

Ciliary body muscles cause lens to change shape to refract light rays (accommodation)

Fluids
Aqueous humor (front of lens)—watery substance secreted by ciliary body

    Maintains shape of front portion of eye

    Refracts light

Vitreous humor (behind lens)—gel-like substance (not readily reformed) filling large space behind lens

    Maintains shape of eyeball

    Refracts light

Optic Nerve
Light rays from rods and cones travel from eye to brain via optic nerve

Optic nerve meets retina in optic disc (no light receptors)—blind spot

Pathway of light ray

    Cornea—refraction site

    Anterior chamber (aqueous humor)—refraction site

    Pupil

    Lens—refraction site

    Posterior chamber (vitreous humor)—refraction site

    Retina (rods and cones)

    Optic nerve fibers—first portion of brain that light is transmitted

    Optic chiasm

    Thalamus

    Cerebral cortex (occipital lobe)—light is interpreted

Hearing, Three Divisions of Ear

External Ear

Auricle (pinna)—sound waves enter ear

External auditory canal—tunnel from auricle to middle ear

Middle Ear

Begins with tympanic membrane (eardrum)

Ossicles—small bones conducting sound waves from middle to inner ear

- Malleus

- Incus

- Stapes

Eustachian tube—leads to pharynx

Inner Ear (Labyrinth)

Vestibule

Semicircular canals/vestibular apparatus

Cochlea contains perilymph and endolymph (liquids through which sound waves are conducted)

Organ of Corti—auditory receptor area

Auditory nerve—electrical impulse is conducted to cerebral cortex for interpretation (hearing)

Pathway of sound vibration (exterior to brain)

Pinna

External auditory canal

Tympanic membrane

Malleus

Incus

Stapes

Oval window

Cochlea

Auditory fluid/receptors in organ of Corti

Auditory nerve

Cerebral cortex

Smell

Olfactory Sense Receptors

Located in nasal cavity

Closely related to sense of taste

Cranial nerve I

Taste

Gustatory sense—sweet, salt, and sour differentiated

Taste buds located on anterior portion of tongue

Cranial nerves VII and IX

Touch

Mechanoreceptors
Widely distributed throughout body

Reacts to touch and pressure

- Meissner corpuscles (touch)

- Pacinian corpuscles (pressure)

Proprioceptors
Position and orientation

Dysfunctions

- Vestibular nystagmus—involuntary movement of eyes

- Vertigo—sense of spinning/dizziness

Thermoreceptors
Under skin

Sense temperature changes

Nociceptors
Pain sensors

In skin and internal organs

COMBINING FORMS

1. ambly/o	dim, dullness
2. aque/o	water
3. audi/o	hearing
4. blephar/o	eyelid
5. conjunctiv/o	conjunctiva
6. cor/o, core/o	pupil
7. corne/o	cornea
8. cycl/o	ciliary body
9. dacry/o	tear
10. essi/o, esthesi/o	sensation
11. glauc/o	gray
12. ir/o	iris
13. irid/o	iris

14. kerat/o — cornea
15. lacrim/o — tear
16. mi/o — smaller
17. myring/o — eardrum
18. ocul/o — eye
19. ophthalm/o — eye
20. opt/o — eye, vision
21. optic/o — eye
22. ot/o — ear
23. palpebr/o — eyelid
24. papill/o — optic nerve
25. phac/o — eye lens
26. phak/o — eye lens
27. phot/o — light
28. presby/o — old age
29. pupill/o — pupil
30. retin/o — retina
31. scler/o — sclera
32. scot/o — darkness
33. staped/o — stapes
34. tympan/o — eardrum
35. uve/o — uvea
36. vitre/o — glassy
37. xer/o — dry

PREFIXES

1. audi- — hearing
2. eso- — inward
3. exo- — outward

SUFFIXES

1. -opia — vision
2. -omia — smell
3. -tropia — to turn

MEDICAL ABBREVIATIONS

1. AD — right ear
2. AS — left ear
3. AU — both ears

257

4.	H or E	hemorrhage or exudate
5.	IO	intraocular
6.	IOL	intraocular lens
7.	OD	right eye
8.	OS	left eye
9.	OU	each eye
10.	PERL	pupils equal and reactive to light
11.	PERRL	pupils equal, round, and reactive to light
12.	PERRLA	pupils equal, round, and reactive to light and accommodation
13.	REM	rapid eye movement
14.	TM	tympanic membrane

MEDICAL TERMS

Anterior segment	Those parts of eye in the front of and including lens, orbit, extraocular muscles, and eyelid
Apicectomy	Excision of a portion of temporal bone
Astigmatism	Condition in which refractive surfaces of eye are unequal
Aural atresia	Congenital absence of external auditory canal
Blepharitis	Inflammation of eyelid
Cataract	Opaque covering on or in lens
Chalazion	Granuloma around sebaceous gland
Cholesteatoma	Tumor that forms in middle ear
Conjunctiva	The lining of eyelids and covering of sclera
Dacryocystitis	Blocked, inflamed infection of nasolacrimal duct
Dacryostenosis	Narrowing of lacrimal duct
Ectropion	Eversion (outward sagging) of eyelid
Entropion	Inversion of eyelid (lashes rubbing cornea)
Enucleation	Removal of an organ or organs from a body cavity
Episclera	Connective covering of sclera
Exenteration	Removal of an organ all in one piece, commonly used to describe radical excision
Exophthalmos	Protrusion of eyeball
Exostosis	Bony growth
Fenestration	Creation of a new opening in inner wall of middle ear
Glaucoma	Eye diseases that are characterized by an increase of intraocular pressure
Hordeolum	Stye—infection of sebaceous gland (nodule on lid margin)
Hyperopia	Farsightedness, eyeball is too short from front to back
Keratomalacia	Softening of cornea associated with a deficiency of vitamin A

Keratoplasty	Surgical repair of the cornea
Labyrinth	Inner connecting cavities, such as internal ear
Labyrinthitis	Inner ear inflammation
Lacrimal	Related to tears
Mastoidectomy	Removal of mastoid bone
Ménière's disease	Condition that causes dizziness, ringing in ears, and deafness
Myopia	Nearsightedness, eyeball too long from front to back
Myringotomy	Incision into tympanic membrane
Ocular adnexa	Orbit, extraocular muscles, and eyelid
Ophthalmoscopy	Examination of the interior of eye by means of a scope, also known as funduscopy
Otitis media	Noninfectious inflammation of middle ear; serous otitis media produces liquid drainage (not purulent), and suppurative otitis media produces purulent (pus) matter
Otoscope	Instrument used to examine ear
Papilledema	Swelling of optic disk (papilla)
Posterior segment	Those parts of eye behind lens
Ptosis	Drooping of upper eyelid
Sclera	Outer covering of eye
Strabismus	Extraocular muscle deviation resulting in unequal visual axes
Tarsorrhaphy	Suturing together of eyelids
Tinnitus	Ringing in the ears
Transmastoid	Creates an opening in mastoid for drainage antrostomy
Tympanolysis	Freeing of adhesions of the tympanic membrane
Tympanometry	Test of the inner ear using air pressure
Tympanostomy	Insertion of ventilation tube into tympanum
Uveal	Vascular tissue of the choroid, ciliary body, and iris
Vertigo	Dizziness
Xanthelasma	Yellow plaque on eyelid (lipid disorder)

SENSES ANATOMY AND TERMINOLOGY QUIZ

1. The middle layer of the eye:
   a. sclera
   b. retina
   c. episclera
   d. choroid

2. The covering of the front of sclera and lining of eyelid:
   a. aqueous humor
   b. ossicles
   c. vitreous
   d. conjunctiva

3. Which of the following is NOT a bone of the middle ear?
   a. cochlea
   b. stapes
   c. malleus
   d. incus

4. This cranial nerve controls the sense of smell:
   a. I
   b. II
   c. III
   d. IV

5. Which of the following is NOT part of the inner ear?
   a. pinna
   b. vestibule
   c. semicircular canals
   d. cochlea

6. These receptors react to touch:
   a. nociceptors
   b. mechanoreceptors
   c. proprioceptors
   d. thermoreceptors

7. These react to position and orientation:
   a. nociceptors
   b. mechanoreceptors
   c. proprioceptors
   d. thermoreceptors

8. Combining form meaning eyelid:
   a. aque/o
   b. blephar/o
   c. optic/o
   d. uve/o

9. Combining form meaning eye lens:
   a. cor/o
   b. irid/o
   c. ocul/o
   d. phak/o

10. Abbreviation meaning the pupils are equal, round, and reactive to light and accommodation:
    a. PERRLA
    b. PERRL
    c. PERL
    d. PURL

Eye

Visual Disturbances

Astigmatism

Irregular curvature of refractive surfaces (cornea or lens) of eye

Can be congenital or acquired (as a result of disease or trauma)

Image is distorted

Treatment

Corrected with cylindrical lens

Diplopia

Double vision

Amblyopia

Dimness of vision—impairment of vision without detectable organic lesion of eye

Hyperopia

Farsightedness

Shortened eyeball

- Can see objects in distance, not close up

Treatment

Corrected with convex lens

Presbyopia

Age-related farsightedness

Treatment

Magnification (reading glasses or bifocals)

Myopia

Nearsightedness

Elongated eyeball

- Can see objects up close, not in distance

Treatment

Corrected with concave lens thicker at periphery

Nystagmus—unilateral or bilateral

Rapid, involuntary eye movements

Movements can be

- Vertical
- Horizontal
- Rotational
- Combination of above

Cause

  Brain tumor or inner ear disease

Normal in newborns

Due to underlying condition or adverse effect of drug

Various types, such as

- Vestibular nystagmus
- Rhythmic eye movements

Strabismus
Cross-eyed

Due to muscle weakness or neurologic defect

Forms of strabismus

- Hypotropia (downward deviation of one eye)
- Hypertropia (upward deviation of one eye)
- Estropia (one eye turns inward)
- Exotropia (one eye turns outward)

Treatment
- Eye exercises/patching of normal eye
- Surgery to establish muscle balance

Infections
Conjunctivitis (pink eye)
Inflammation of conjunctival lining of eyelid or covering of sclera

Due to

- Infection
- Allergy
- Irritation

Treatment

- Varies with cause
- Antibiotic eye drops

Hordeolum (stye)
Bacterial infection of eyelid hair follicle

- Usually *Staphylococci*

Results in mass on eyelid

Treatment

- Antibiotics
- Incision and drainage may be necessary

Keratitis
Corneal inflammation

Caused by herpes simplex virus

Causes tearing and photophobia

Macular Degeneration

Destruction of fovea centralis

- Fovea centralis is small pit in center of retina (fovea centralis retinae)

Usually age related—leading cause of blindness in elderly

Results from exposure to ultraviolet rays or drugs

- Also may have a genetic component

Central vision is lost

Two types of macular degeneration

- Wet—development of new vascularization and leaking blood vessels near macula

- Dry (85% of cases)—atrophy and degeneration of retinal cells and deposits of drusen (clumps of extracellular waste)

Treatment

None for "dry" macular degeneration

Surgical intervention with laser for "net" macular degeneration to coagulate leaking vessels; success is limited

Medications

Detached Retina

Retinal tear—two layers of retina separate from each other

- Vitreous humor then leaks behind retina

- Retina then pulls away from choroid

Results in increasing blind spot in visual field

Condition is painless

Pressure continues to build if left unattended

Final result is blindness

Treatment

Surgical intervention with laser to repair tear (emergency/urgency)— photocoagulation for small tears

Scleral buckle for large retinal detachments

Pneumatic retinopexy for medium to large retinal detachment. Gas bubble is injected to vitreous cavity; pressure to tear resulting in retinal reattachment.

Cataracts

Lens becomes opaque with protein aggregates

Classified by morphology

Size

Shape

Location

Also may be classified by etiology (cause) or time cataract occurs

Examples of classification
Congenital cataract

- Bilateral opacity present at birth

- Also known as developmental cataract

Heat cataract

- Also known as glassblowers' cataract

- Caused by exposure to radiation

Traumatic cataract (Fig. 1–53)

- Result of injury to eye

Senile cataract

- Age related

- Usually forms on corneal area of lens

Symptoms
Blurring of vision

Halos around lights

Treatment
Removal of cataract with intraocular lens implantation

If no intraocular lens implant, then glasses or contact lenses for refraction

Glaucoma
Excess accumulation of intraocular aqueous humor

- Results in decreased blood flow and edema

- Damages retinal cells and optic nerve

Narrow angle glaucoma
Acute type of glaucoma

Chronic glaucoma
Also known as

- Wide angle glaucoma

- Open angle glaucoma

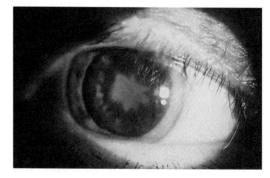

Figure **1-53** A concussion injury that resulted in a traumatic cataract. (From Yanoff M, Duker J: *Ophthalmology*, ed 2, St Louis, 2004, Mosby.)

Asymptomatic

Diagnosed in eye examination using tonometry to test anterior chamber pressure

Treatment

Medications that decrease output of aqueous humor and decreased intraocular pressure (IOP)

Laser treatment to provide drainage

Ear

■ Infections

Otitis Media

Infection or inflammation of middle ear cavity

Chronic infection produces adhesions

Results in loss of hearing

Often occurs in children in combination with URI (upper respiratory infection)

Causes severe ear pain (otalgia)

Treatment

Antibiotics

Surgical intervention with placement of tubes to allow for drainage

- Useful in patients with recurrent infection

Otitis Externa

Also known as swimmer's ear

Infection of external auditory canal and pinna (exterior ear)

Caused by bacteria or fungus

Results in pain and discharge

Treatment

Antibiotic

Encouraged to keep ear dry

■ Hearing Loss

Conductive Hearing Loss

Due to a defect of sound-conducting apparatus

- Accumulation of wax
- Scar tissue on tympanic membrane

Also known as:

- Transmission hearing loss
- Conduction deafness

Treatment

- Hearing aids

Sensorineural

Due to a lesion of cochlea or central neural pathways

Also known as

- Perceptive deafness

May be divided into

- Cochlear hearing loss
  - Due to a defect in receptor or transducing mechanisms of cochlea
- Retrocochlear hearing loss
  - Due to defect located proximal to cochlea (vestibulocochlear nerve or auditory area of brain)

Presbycusis is age-related sensorineural hearing loss

Treatment
- Unknown

Ototoxic Hearing Loss

Due to ingestion of toxic substance

Also known as toxic deafness

Ménière's Disease

Inner ear disturbance

Also known as idiopathic endolymphatic hydrops

Cause unknown

Most common cause of vertigo (dizziness) of inner ear

Other symptoms include vertigo, hearing loss, and tinnitus

SENSES PATHOPHYSIOLOGY QUIZ

1. This condition can be acquired or congenital and results in an irregular curvature of the refractive surfaces of the eye:
   a. diplopia
   b. hyperopia
   c. nystagmus
   d. astigmatism

2. In this condition the eyeball is shorter than normal and results in being able to see objects in the distance but not close up:
   a. diplopia
   b. hyperopia
   c. nystagmus
   d. astigmatism

3. Rapid, involuntary eye movement is the predominant symptom of this condition:
   a. diplopia
   b. hyperopia
   c. nystagmus
   d. astigmatism

4. Age-related farsightedness is:
   a. presbyopia
   b. hyperopia
   c. diplopia
   d. myopia

5. Another name for a stye is:
   a. keratitis
   b. hordeolum
   c. hyperopia
   d. strabismus

6. An inflammation of the cornea that is caused by herpes simplex virus is:
   a. keratitis
   b. hordeolum
   c. hyperopia
   d. strabismus

7. In this condition there is destruction of the fovea centralis:
   a. macular degeneration
   b. detached retina
   c. glaucoma
   d. cataract

8. This is an infection that occurs in the middle ear cavity:
   a. otitis media
   b. otitis externa
   c. ototoxic
   d. retrocochlear

9. The hearing loss that can be due to a lesion on the cochlea is:
   a. conductive
   b. sensorineural
   c. ototoxic
   d. transmission

10. This condition is also known as perceptive deafness:
    a. conductive
    b. sensorineural
    c. otitis media
    d. transmission

Integumentary System

Anatomy and Terminology Quiz

1. c	6. c
2. d	7. d
3. a	8. b
4. b	9. c
5. d	10. c

Pathophysiology Quiz

1. c	6. c
2. c	7. d
3. a	8. b
4. d	9. d
5. b	10. a

Musculoskeletal System

Anatomy and Terminology Quiz

1. b	6. d
2. c	7. b
3. a	8. d
4. c	9. a
5. a	10. c

Pathophysiology Quiz

1. d	6. d
2. c	7. a
3. b	8. c
4. a	9. b
5. d	10. d

Respiratory System

Anatomy and Terminology Quiz

1. b	6. c
2. d	7. c
3. c	8. b
4. a	9. d
5. a	10. d

Pathophysiology Quiz

1. b	6. a
2. a	7. c
3. d	8. b
4. d	9. a
5. d	10. c

Cardiovascular System

Anatomy and Terminology Quiz

1. d	7. d
2. a	8. a
3. c	9. d
4. a	10. d
5. d	11. b
6. b	12. c

Pathophysiology Quiz

1. b	6. a
2. c	7. c
3. d	8. c
4. c	9. a
5. d	10. d

Female Genital System and Pregnancy

Anatomy and Terminology Quiz

1. d   6. a
2. a   7. b
3. a   8. b
4. b   9. c
5. c   10. d

Pathophysiology Quiz

1. b   6. a
2. d   7. a
3. a   8. c
4. c   9. b
5. b   10. c

Male Genital System

Anatomy and Terminology Quiz

1. c   6. a
2. a   7. a
3. d   8. d
4. b   9. d
5. a   10. b

Pathophysiology Quiz

1. a   6. b
2. b   7. d
3. d   8. b
4. a   9. a
5. c   10. b

Urinary System

Anatomy and Terminology Quiz

1. c   6. d

2. d   7. c

3. a   8. b

4. c   9. d

5. b   10. a

Pathophysiology Quiz

1. c   6. c

2. d   7. a or c

3. d   8. c

4. c   9. b

5. b   10. c

Digestive System

Anatomy and Terminology Quiz

1. b   6. b

2. d   7. a

3. d   8. c

4. b   9. a

5. c   10. b

Pathophysiology Quiz

1. c   6. c

2. a   7. a

3. d   8. c

4. b   9. a

5. a   10. a

Mediastinum and Diaphragm

Anatomy and Terminology Quiz

1. a   6. b

2. b   7. a

3. d   8. b

4. c   9. a

5. c   10. d

Hemic and Lymphatic System

Anatomy and Terminology Quiz

1. b	6. c
2. d	7. a
3. a	8. d
4. d	9. b
5. c	10. d

Pathophysiology Quiz

1. c	6. c
2. a	7. a
3. b	8. a
4. d	9. c
5. b	10. b

Endocrine System

Anatomy and Terminology Quiz

1. c	6. a
2. d	7. d
3. b	8. a
4. a	9. b
5. d	10. d

Pathophysiology Quiz

1. a	6. b
2. b	7. a
3. c	8. d
4. a	9. a
5. d	10. c

Nervous System

Anatomy and Terminology Quiz

1. b	6. c
2. a	7. a
3. a	8. d
4. b	9. b
5. b	10. a

Pathophysiology Quiz

1. a	6. b
2. c	7. a
3. b	8. b
4. d	9. b
5. a	10. c

Senses

Anatomy and Terminology Quiz

1. d	6. b
2. d	7. c
3. a	8. b
4. a	9. d
5. a	10. a

Pathophysiology Quiz

1. d	6. a
2. b	7. a
3. c	8. a
4. a	9. b
5. b	10. b

Reimbursement Issues and Data Quality

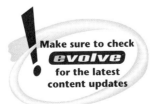

Make sure to check **evolve** for the latest content updates

REIMBURSEMENT ISSUES

Your Responsibility

Accurately code services that are provided and supported by documentation

Submit complete, accurate, and compliantly coded claims to obtain correct reimbursement for services rendered

Upcoding (maximizing) or downcoding is never appropriate

Stay abreast of continuing changes

- Reimbursement and coverage policies, i.e., Local Medical Review Policies, Local Coverage Determinations, or National Coverage Decisions

- Coding guidelines from authoritative sources, i.e., AHA's *Coding Clinic for ICD-9-CM*; AHA's *Coding Clinic for HCPCS*; *UHDDS (Uniform Hospital Discharge Data) Guidelines*; and AMA's *CPT Assistant*

- Stay current with regulatory and Medicare Requirements. The CMS website (http://www.cms.hhs.gov/) offers links to many regulations for specific settings, including hospitals and physician practices. Some examples are:

Regulations such as the Health Insurance Portability and Accountability Act (HIPAA)

  - Centers for Medicare and Medicaid Policy Manuals

  National Correct Coding Guidelines

  MedLearn Matters Alerts and Educational Material

- Health Information Management Professionals are bound by the AHIMA Code of Ethics and Standards of Ethical Coding (www.ahima.org)

For the certification examination:
   You need a working knowledge of national reimbursement and regulatory guidelines.

Population Change = Reimbursement Change

Elderly patients are the fastest growing patient segment due to "Baby Boomers"

By 2030, there will be one elderly person for each person younger than 19 years

Medicare is the primary insurance for the elderly

Medicare

Getting bigger all the time!
Over the next ten years, Medicare spending will total more than $3 trillion (http://www.cbo.gov/ftpdoc.cfm?index=308&type=0)

Health care will continue to expand to meet enormous future demands

- Job security for coders!

Those covered—beneficiaries
Originally established in 1965 for those 65 and older

Added coverage for disabled and End Stage Renal Disease (ESRD) in 1972

Basic Structure

■ Part A: Hospital and Institutional Care Coverage

> For the certification examination:
>   You need to know what is covered and not covered under Part A and what can be reported outside the MS-DRG payment.

Covered inpatient expenses include

Room
Semiprivate room rate

- Pays the same amount whether the patient has a private room that is or is not medically necessary

Semiprivate room

Ward accommodations

- Accommodations must meet program standards

Patient pays the difference between private and semiprivate room when
Private room is not medically necessary or

Patient has requested the private room

- Provider must inform patient of the additional charge for private room

Patient does not pay the difference between private and semiprivate room when isolation is required to avoid jeopardizing the health or recovery of the patient or others

Example:

- Communicable diseases
- Heart attacks
- Cerebrovascular accidents
- Psychotic episodes
- Hospital has no semiprivate or ward accommodations available at the time of admission and
    - Patient requires immediate hospitalization

Patients may be assigned to ward accommodations if
All semiprivate accommodations are occupied

Facility has no semiprivate accommodations

- Patient must be moved to semiprivate room when one is available
    - Accommodations must meet program standards

Nursing services and other related services
Defined as use of hospital facilities and medical social services ordinarily furnished by the hospital for the care/treatment of inpatients

Drugs, biologicals, supplies, appliances, and equipment
FDA-approved drugs and biologicals for use in the hospital

- Must usually be furnished by the hospital for the care/treatment of inpatients

Supplies, appliances, and equipment

• Must be used for care/treatment solely during the inpatient hospital stay

OR

When unreasonable or impossible to limit the use to the inpatient period

Example:

• Items permanently installed in/attached to the patient's body while an inpatient, such as cardiac valves, cardiac pacemakers, and artificial limbs
• Items which are temporarily installed in/attached to the patient's body while an inpatient and are necessary to permit the patient's release from the hospital, such as tracheotomy or drainage tubes

Hospital must have purchased the item

• A cost was incurred by the hospital for the item
  • Excluded are items given to the hospital

  Example: Free pharmaceutical samples

Certain other covered diagnostic or therapeutic services

Diagnostic or therapeutic items/services ordinarily furnished to inpatients by hospital

• This includes the supply by others under arrangements made by the hospital

Example:

• Diagnostic or therapeutic services of an audiologist provided off the hospital premises but billed for by the hospital
• Surgical dressings and splints, casts, and other devices used for the reduction of fractures and dislocations

Prosthetic devices are covered that replace all/part of an organ

• The function of a permanently inoperative or malfunctioning internal body organ

Example:

• Braces, trusses, artificial replacements, such as legs, arms, and eyes

Diagnostic/therapeutic inpatient services of a psychologist/physical therapist

• Must be a salaried member of the staff of a hospital

Inpatient diagnostic services furnished by an independent, certified clinical lab under arrangements with the hospital

• Lab certified under CLIA
  • CLIA = Clinical Laboratories Improvement Act

Reasonable cost of medical/surgical services of medical/osteopathic interns or residents under an approved teaching program

Transportation services

Includes transport by ambulance

Additionally covered expenses when they meet certain criteria

Inpatient rehabilitation

Skilled nursing

Some personal convenience items for long-term illness/disability

Home health visit

Hospice care

Noncovered inpatient-hospital expenses
Non-medically necessary services or supplies

Private-duty nurse or other private-duty attendant

Deluxe or non-medically necessary private room

Personal convenience items

- Those not routinely furnished to patients

Non-physician inpatient services that have not been provided directly or arranged for by hospital staff

Coverage under Part A is compulsory
Paid for by Social Security tax

Eligibility is determined by the Social Security Administration (SSA)

Reimbursement is for all covered and medically necessary services

- Once annual deductible is met

ICD-9-CM diagnosis and procedure codes are basis for Part A payment

Charges are submitted on UB-04

- UB = Uniform Billing
- Also known as CMS-1450

■ Part B: Supplemental
Provides coverage for non-hospital charges
Physician services

Outpatient hospital services

Home health care

Medically necessary supplies and equipment

Those services and supplies not covered under Part A that are medically necessary

Payment for the hospital stay if the patient has exhausted all Part A benefits prior to admission

Beneficiaries purchase coverage with monthly premiums

Three coding systems used to report Part B services and supplies that are medical necessity for services
HCPCS Level I = CPT—services

HCPCS Level II (also known as National Codes)—supplies, services, and drugs not included or covered by CPT coding system

ICD-9-CM—diagnoses

Charges submitted on CMS-1500 (Figure 2-1)
Also known as Universal Health Care form

■ Part C: Medicare Advantage
Variety of health care options are available

- Such as managed care

Added after Part A and B

1500

HEALTH INSURANCE CLAIM FORM

APPROVED BY NATIONAL UNIFORM CLAIM COMMITTEE 08/05

PICA | PICA

CARRIER

1. MEDICARE (Medicare #) | MEDICAID (Medicaid #) | TRICARE CHAMPUS (Sponsor's SSN) | CHAMPVA (Member ID#) | GROUP HEALTH PLAN (SSN or ID) | FECA BLK LUNG (SSN) | OTHER (ID)

1a. INSURED'S I.D. NUMBER (For Program in Item 1)

2. PATIENT'S NAME (Last Name, First Name, Middle Initial)

3. PATIENT'S BIRTH DATE MM DD YY SEX M F

4. INSURED'S NAME (Last Name, First Name, Middle Initial)

5. PATIENT'S ADDRESS (No., Street)

6. PATIENT RELATIONSHIP TO INSURED Self Spouse Child Other

7. INSURED'S ADDRESS (No., Street)

CITY STATE

8. PATIENT STATUS Single Married Other

CITY STATE

ZIP CODE TELEPHONE (Include Area Code) ( )

Employed Full-Time Student Part-Time Student

ZIP CODE TELEPHONE (Include Area Code) ( )

9. OTHER INSURED'S NAME (Last Name, First Name, Middle Initial)

10. IS PATIENT'S CONDITION RELATED TO:

11. INSURED'S POLICY GROUP OR FECA NUMBER

a. OTHER INSURED'S POLICY OR GROUP NUMBER

a. EMPLOYMENT? (Current or Previous) YES NO

a. INSURED'S DATE OF BIRTH MM DD YY SEX M F

b. OTHER INSURED'S DATE OF BIRTH MM DD YY SEX M F

b. AUTO ACCIDENT? YES NO PLACE (State)

b. EMPLOYER'S NAME OR SCHOOL NAME

c. EMPLOYER'S NAME OR SCHOOL NAME

c. OTHER ACCIDENT? YES NO

c. INSURANCE PLAN NAME OR PROGRAM NAME

d. INSURANCE PLAN NAME OR PROGRAM NAME

10d. RESERVED FOR LOCAL USE

d. IS THERE ANOTHER HEALTH BENEFIT PLAN? YES NO ***If yes,*** return to and complete item 9 a-d.

READ BACK OF FORM BEFORE COMPLETING & SIGNING THIS FORM.

12. PATIENT'S OR AUTHORIZED PERSON'S SIGNATURE I authorize the release of any medical or other information necessary to process this claim. I also request payment of government benefits either to myself or to the party who accepts assignment below.

SIGNED ______ DATE ______

13. INSURED'S OR AUTHORIZED PERSON'S SIGNATURE I authorize payment of medical benefits to the undersigned physician or supplier for services described below.

SIGNED ______

PATIENT AND INSURED INFORMATION

14. DATE OF CURRENT: MM DD YY ILLNESS (First symptom) OR INJURY (Accident) OR PREGNANCY(LMP)

15. IF PATIENT HAS HAD SAME OR SIMILAR ILLNESS. GIVE FIRST DATE MM DD YY

16. DATES PATIENT UNABLE TO WORK IN CURRENT OCCUPATION FROM MM DD YY TO MM DD YY

17. NAME OF REFERRING PROVIDER OR OTHER SOURCE 17a. 17b. NPI

18. HOSPITALIZATION DATES RELATED TO CURRENT SERVICES FROM MM DD YY TO MM DD YY

19. RESERVED FOR LOCAL USE

20. OUTSIDE LAB? YES NO $ CHARGES

21. DIAGNOSIS OR NATURE OF ILLNESS OR INJURY (Relate Items 1, 2, 3 or 4 to Item 24E by Line)

1. ___ . ___ 3. ___ . ___

2. ___ . ___ 4. ___ . ___

22. MEDICAID RESUBMISSION CODE ORIGINAL REF. NO.

23. PRIOR AUTHORIZATION NUMBER

	24. A. DATE(S) OF SERVICE From MM DD YY	To MM DD YY	B. PLACE OF SERVICE	C. EMG	D. PROCEDURES, SERVICES, OR SUPPLIES (Explain Unusual Circumstances) CPT/HCPCS	MODIFIER	E. DIAGNOSIS POINTER	F. $ CHARGES	G. DAYS OR UNITS	H. EPSDT Family Plan	I. ID. QUAL.	J. RENDERING PROVIDER ID. #
1												
2												
3												
4												
5												
6												

PHYSICIAN OR SUPPLIER INFORMATION

25. FEDERAL TAX I.D. NUMBER SSN EIN

26. PATIENT'S ACCOUNT NO.

27. ACCEPT ASSIGNMENT? (For govt. claims, see back) YES NO

28. TOTAL CHARGE $

29. AMOUNT PAID $

30. BALANCE DUE $

31. SIGNATURE OF PHYSICIAN OR SUPPLIER INCLUDING DEGREES OR CREDENTIALS (I certify that the statements on the reverse apply to this bill and are made a part thereof.)

SIGNED DATE

32. SERVICE FACILITY LOCATION INFORMATION

a. b.

33. BILLING PROVIDER INFO & PH # ( )

a. b.

NUCC Instruction Manual available at: www.nucc.org

OMB APPROVAL PENDING

Figure **2-1** The CMS-1500 (08-05) Health Insurance Claim Form. This form was revised in 2007 to accommodate the National Provider Identifier (NPI) number. (Courtesy U.S. Department of Health and Human Services, Centers for Medicare and Medicaid Services.)

■ Part D: Prescription Drug, Improvement, and Modernization Act of 2003

Prescription drug plan

Piloted through 2005

Open enrollment began January 1, 2006

Premium paid by beneficiary

Officiating Office

Department of Health and Human Services (DHHS)

Delegated to Centers for Medicare and Medicaid Services (CMS)

CMS runs Medicare and Medicaid

CMS delegates daily operation for Part A and Part B to companies that have contracted to adjudicate Medicare claims

- The Medicare Prescription Drug Improvement and Modernization Act of 2003 allowed CMS to reduce the current 48 FIs to 19* Medicare Administrative Contractors (MACs)

  - Phased in with the final 19* MACs in place by 2011

Funding for Medicare

Social security taxes

Equal match from government

CMS sends money to MACs

MACs handle paperwork and pay claims

Government publishes updates, revisions, deletions (changes) in *Federal Register* (Figure 2-2)

Updates to payment systems occur throughout the year

Part A hospital inpatient payment changes are effective October 1

Hospital outpatient facility payment changes and physician payment system changes are effective January 1

Quarterly revisions to HCPCS are published by CMS

AMA publishes changes to CPT Category III codes effective January 1 and July 1

*http://www.cms.hhs.gov/MedicareContractingReform/07_PartA_PartBMedicareAdministrativeContractor.asp

9. Supplementary information

5342   **Federal Register** / Vol. 73, No. 19 / Tuesday, January 29, 2008 / Proposed Rules

1. Issuing office

DEPARTMENT OF HEALTH AND HUMAN SERVICES

Centers for Medicare & Medicaid Services

42 CFR Part 412

[CMS–1393–P]

RIN 0938–AO94

2. Subject

Medicare Program; Prospective Payment System for Long-Term Care Hospitals RY 2009: Proposed Annual Payment Rate Updates, Policy Changes, and Clarification

3. Agency

AGENCY: Centers for Medicare & Medicaid Services (CMS), HHS.

4. Action

ACTION: Proposed rule.

5. Summary

SUMMARY: This proposed rule would update the annual payment rates for the Medicare prospective payment system (PPS) for inpatient hospital services provided by long-term care hospitals (LTCHs). In addition, we are proposing to consolidate the annual July 1 update for payment rates and the October 1 update for Medicare severity long-term care diagnosis related group (MS–LTC–DRG) weights to a single fiscal year (FY) update.

In this proposed rule, we are also clarifying various policy issues.

This proposed rule would also describe our evaluation of the possible one-time adjustment to the Federal payment rate.

6. Dates

DATES: To be assured consideration, comments must be received at one of the addresses provided below, no later than 5 p.m. on March 24, 2008.

7. Address

ADDRESSES: In commenting, please refer to file code CMS–1393–P. Because of staff and resource limitations, we cannot accept comments by facsimile (FAX) transmission.

8. Further information

You may submit comments in one of four ways (please choose only one of the ways listed):

1. *Electronically.* You may submit electronic comments on specific issues in this regulation to *http://www.regulations.gov/.* Follow the instructions for "Comment or Submission" and enter the filecode to find the document accepting comment.

2. *By regular mail.* You may mail written comments (one original and two copies) to the following address ONLY:

Centers for Medicare & Medicaid Services, Department of Health and Human Services, *Attention:* CMS–1393–P, P.O. Box 8013, Baltimore, MD 21244–8013.
Please allow sufficient time for mailed comments to be received before the close of the comment period.

3. *By express or overnight mail.* You

may send written comments (one original and two copies) to the following address ONLY:

Centers for Medicare & Medicaid Services, Department of Health and Human Services, Attention: CMS–1393–P, Mail Stop C4–26–05, 7500 Security Boulevard, Baltimore, MD 21244–1850.

4. *By hand or courier.* If you prefer, you may deliver (by hand or courier) your written comments (one original and two copies) before the close of the comment period to one of the following addresses. If you intend to deliver your comments to the Baltimore address, please call telephone number (410) 786–7195 in advance to schedule your arrival with one of our staff members.

Room 445–G, Hubert H. Humphrey Building, 200 Independence Avenue, SW., Washington, DC 20201; or 7500 Security Boulevard, Baltimore, MD 21244–1850.

(Because access to the interior of the HHH Building is not readily available to persons without Federal Government identification, commenters are encouraged to leave their comments in the CMS drop slots located in the main lobby of the building. A stamp-in clock is available for persons wishing to retain a proof of filing by stamping in and retaining an extra copy of the comments being filed.)

Comments mailed to the addresses indicated as appropriate for hand or courier delivery may be delayed and received after the comment period.

Submission of comments on paperwork requirements. You may submit comments on this document's paperwork requirements by mailing your comments to the addresses provided at the end of the "Collection of Information Requirements" section in this document.

For information on viewing public comments, see the beginning of the **SUPPLEMENTARYINFORMATION** section.

FOR FURTHER INFORMATION CONTACT:

Tzvi Hefter, (410) 786–4487 (General information).

Judy Richter, (410) 786–2590 (General information, payment adjustments for special cases, onsite discharges and readmissions, interrupted stays, co-located providers, and short-stay outliers).

Michele Hudson, (410) 786–5490 (Calculation of the payment rates, MS–LTC–DRGs, relative weights and case-mix index, market basket, wage index, budget neutrality, and other payment adjustments).

Ann Fagan, (410) 786–5662 (Patient classification system).

Linda McKenna, (410) 786–4537 (Payment adjustments and interrupted stay).

Elizabeth Truong, (410) 786–6005 (Federal rate update, budget neutrality, other adjustments, and calculation of the payment rates).

Michael Treitel, (410) 786–4552 (High cost outliers and cost-to-charge ratios).

Table of Contents

I. Background
  A. Legislative and Regulatory Authority
  B. Criteria for Classification as a LTCH
  1. Classification as a LTCH
  2. Hospitals Excluded From the LTCH PPS
  C. Transition Period for Implementation of the LTCH PPS
  D. Limitation on Charges to Beneficiaries
  E. Administrative Simplification Compliance Act (ASCA) and Health Insurance Portability and Accountability Act (HIPAA) Compliance
II. Summary of the Provisions of This Proposed Rule
III. Medicare Severity Long-Term Care Diagnosis-Related Group (LTC–DRG) Classifications and Relative Weights
  A. Background
  B. Patient Classifications into MS–LTC–DRGs
  C. Organization of MS–LTC–DRGs
  D. Method for Updating the MS–LTC–DRG Classifications and Relative Weights
  1. Background
  2. FY 2008 MS–LTC–DRG Relative Weights
IV. Proposed Changes to the LTCH PPS Payment Rates and other Proposed Changes for the 2009 LTCH PPS Rate Year
  A. Overview of the Development of the Payment Rates
  B. Proposed Consolidation of the Annual Updates for Payment and MS–LTC–DRG weights to One Annual Update
  C. LTCH PPS Market Basket
  1. Overview of the RPL Market Basket
  2. Market Basket Estimate for the 2009 LTCH PPS Rate Year
  D. Discussion of a One-time Prospective Adjustment to the Standard Federal Rate
  E. Proposed Standard Federal Rate for the 2009 LTCH PPS Rate Year
  1. Background
  2. Proposed Standard Federal Rate for the 2009 LTCH PPS Rate Year
  F. Calculation of Proposed LTCH Prospective Payments for the 2009 LTCH PPS Rate Year
  1. Proposed Adjustment for Area Wage Levels
  a. Background
  b. Proposed Updates to the Geographic Classifications/Labor Market Area Definitions
  (1) Background
  (2) Proposed Update to the CBSA-based Labor Market Area Definitions
  (3) New England Deemed Counties
  (4) Proposed Codification of the Definitions of urban and rural under 42 CFR Part 412, subpart O
  c. Proposed Labor-Related Share
  d. Proposed Wage Index Data
  2. Proposed Adjustment for Cost-of-Living in Alaska and Hawaii

Figure **2-2** Example of page from the *Federal Register.* (From *Federal Register*, January 29, 2008, vol. 73, no. 19, Proposed Rules.)

NATIONAL CORRECT CODING INITIATIVE (NCCI)

Developed by the Centers for Medicare and Medicaid Services to

- Promote national correct coding methods, to reduce/alleviate separate reporting of bundled services
- Control improper multiple procedure coding that leads to inappropriate payment of Part B physician claims and hospital outpatient claims
- Complete list may be found at http://www.cms.hhs.gov/NationalCorrectCodInitEd/02_hoppscciedits.asp

Unbundling

CMS defines unbundling as

- Billing separately each component of an all-inclusive procedure

Example:

Billing 15260, Full thickness graft, free, including direct closure of donor site; nose, ears, eyelids and/or lips PLUS 12016, Simple repair of superficial wounds of face, ears, eyelids, nose lips . . . when code 15260 states "including direct closure of donor site"

AMBULATORY PAYMENT CLASSIFICATIONS (APCs)

Omnibus Budget Reconciliation Act of 1986 (OBRA)

Prior to OBRA, Medicare hospital outpatient services paid on a cost-based system

- Also known as a retrospective system

Act mandated

Replacement of cost-based system with a PPS (prospective payment system)

Hospitals to report services and some supplies/drugs on claims using CMS Healthcare Common Procedure Coding System (HCPCS), which includes CPT codes

CMS uses claims data to determine payment rates and coverage policies for future years

- Data were used to develop Outpatient Prospective Payment System (OPPS)

Developed Ambulatory Patient Groups (APGs)

Grouped outpatient services

Differ from MS-DRGs because an outpatient can be assigned multiple APGs

Outpatient claims may have multiple APGs on any given day, but only one MS-DRG is paid for the entire inpatient encounter

Final version of the classification system was Ambulatory Payment Classifications (APCs)

Implementation on August 1, 2000

APCs mandatory for

Most Medicare hospital outpatient services

Some exceptions are lab and therapy services that are paid by a separate fee schedule

Inpatient services covered under Part B

- If beneficiary has exhausted Part A benefits

Inpatient services not covered by Part A

Partial hospitalization services

- Furnished by community mental health centers and some hospitals

APCs are used for reimbursement for hospital-based outpatient services
Such as

- Outpatient surgery
- Hospital-based outpatient clinics
- Emergency departments
- Outpatient ancillary services

   Example: Radiology (Laboratory is paid on a separate fee schedule)

APC Structure

Consists of over 500 groups of services

- Each HCPCS code is assigned to an APC and has a status indicator defining how and whether separate payment is made (Figure 2-3)

Services in each APC are alike:

- Clinically
- In resources required to provide the services

APC includes some items/services that contribute to cost of the service but

Medicare does not usually reimburse separately

- These incidentals are packaged into the APC payment

APC	HCPCS	APC Description	HCPCS Description	SI	Rel. Wt.	Pay Rate	Natl. Coin.	Min. Coin.
0006		**Level I Incision & Drainage**		T	1.4066	$89.59	$	$17.92
0006	10060		Drainage of skin abscess					
0006	10061		Drainage of skin abscess					
0006	10080		Drainage of pilonidal cyst					
0006	10120		Remove foreign body					
0006	20000		Incision of abscess					
0006	20950		Fluid pressure, muscle					
0006	21725		Revision of neck muscle					
0006	26010		Drainage of finger abscess					
0006	69000		Drain external ear lesion					
0006	69020		Drain outer ear canal lesion					
0007		**Level II Incision & Drainage**		T	11.5594	$736.26		$147.25
0007	10081		Drainage of pilonidal cyst					
0007	10140		Drainage of hematoma/fluid					
0007	26011		Drainage of finger abscess					
0007	38300		Drainage lymph node lesion					
0007	55100		Drainage of scrotum abscess					
0007	57022		I & D vaginal hematoma					

Figure **2-3** APC grouping of HCPCS codes.

Example:

- Supplies
- Observation services (limited exceptions)
- Many drugs
- Medical visits on the same day of service or procedure unless separately identifiable and modified

Medicare does reimburse separately for some items and services that are not packaged, such as casting, splinting, and strapping services

Further APC information available
http://www.cms.hhs.gov/HospitalOutpatientPPS/

Pass-through codes

Services, procedures, and/or supplies not included in APC package

Paid an additional pass-through APC payment

Payment rate and co-insurance

Co-insurance amount is 20% of the median charge for all services in the APC

- This means the payment rate and co-insurance will not change until the co-insurance amount becomes 20% of the individual APC payment

APC Payment Status Indicators (SI) (Figure 2-4)

One letter designating a status indicator is assigned to each HCPCS/CPT code

Indicates if service, procedure, or supply is reimbursable under the Outpatient Prospective Payment System (OPPS) or other fee schedule

Also identifies if the reimbursement is bundled or separately payable and/or discounted

Example:

- HCPCS/CPT codes under SI "A" are not paid under OPPS but are paid under a fee schedule or another payment method
- Such as: 77057, mammogram screening (SI "A")
- Routine Dialysis Services
- Ambulance Services

Each APC is assigned a co-insurance amount and payment rate

- Adjusted by hospital's wage index (labor costs)

Figure 2-5 illustrates the payment rate and co-insurance amounts

Example:

- Drainage of skin abscess (10060) is paid at $89.59, co-insurance amount of 20% ($17.92)
- Red blood cell irradiation (P9038) is paid at $195.18, co-insurance amount of 20% ($39.04)

Can receive payment for multiple services provided on the same day

Multiple procedures that have the status indicator of S are reimbursed at 100%

Multiple significant surgical procedures performed on the same day that have a status indicator of T are discounted

- Full payment made for the highest reimbursed procedure APC
- 50% reimbursed for each additional surgical procedure APC

ADDENDUM D1. — OPPS PAYMENT STATUS INDICATORS		
Indicator	**Item/Code/Service**	**OPPS Payment Status**
A	Services furnished to a hospital outpatient that are paid under a fee schedule or payment system other than OPPS, for example: • Ambulance Services. • Clinical Diagnostic Laboratory Services .... • Non-Implantable Prosthetic and Orthotic Devices. • EPO for ESRD Patients. • Physical, Occupational, and Speech Therapy. • Routine Dialysis Services for ESRD Patients Provided in a Certified Dialysis Unit of a Hospital. • Diagnostic Mammography. • Screening Mammography	Not paid under OPPS. Paid by fiscal intermediaries/MACs under a fee schedule or payment system other than OPPS. Not subject to deductible or coinsurance. Not subject to deductible.
B	Codes that are not recognized by OPPS when submitted on an outpatient hospital Part B bill type (12x and 13x).	Not paid under OPPS. • May be paid by fiscal intermediaries/MACs when submitted on a different bill type, for example, 75x (CORF), but not paid under OPPS. • An alternate code that is recognized by OPPS when submitted on an outpatient hospital Part B bill type (12x and 13x) may be available.
C	Inpatient Procedures	Not paid under OPPS. Admit patient. Bill as inpatient.
D	Discontinued Codes	Not paid under OPPS or any other Medicare payment system.
E	Items, Codes, and Services: • That are not covered by Medicare based on statutory exclusion. • That are not covered by Medicare for reasons other than statutory exclusion. • That are not recognized by Medicare but for which an alternate code for the same item or service may be available. • For which separate payment is not provided by Medicare.	Not paid under OPPS or any other Medicare payment system.
F	Corneal Tissue Acquisition; Certain CRNA Services and Hepatitis B Vaccines.	Not paid under OPPS. Paid at reasonable cost.
G	Pass-Through Drugs and Biologicals	Paid under OPPS; separate APC payment includes pass-through amount.
H	Pass-Through Device Categories	Separate cost-based pass-through payment; not subject to copayment.
K	(1) Nonpass-Through Drugs and Biologicals .... (2) Therapeutic Radiopharmaceuticals .... (3) Brachytherapy Sources .... (4) Blood and Blood Products	(1) Paid under OPPS; separate APC payment. (2) Paid under OPPS; separate APC payment. (3) Paid under OPPS; separate APC payment. (4) Paid under OPPS; separate APC payment.
L	Influenza Vaccine; Pneumococcal Pneumonia Vaccine	Not paid under OPPS. Paid at reasonable cost; not subject to deductible or coinsurance.
M	Items and Services Not Billable to the Fiscal Intermediary/MAC.	Not paid under OPPS.
N	Items and Services Packaged into APC Rates	Paid under OPPS; payment is packaged into payment for other services, including outliers. Therefore, there is no separate APC payment.
P	Partial Hospitalization	Not paid under OPPS; per diem APC payment.
Q	Packaged Services Subject to Separate Payment under OPPS Payment Criteria.	Paid under OPPS; Addendum B displays APC assignments when services are separately payable. (1) Separate APC payment based on OPPS payment criteria. (2) If criteria are not met, payment is packaged into payment for other services, including outliers. Therefore, there is no separate APC payment.
S	Significant Procedure, Not Discounted when Multiple	Paid under OPPS; separate APC payment.
T	Significant Procedure, Multiple Reduction Applies	Paid under OPPS; separate APC payment.
V	Clinic or Emergency Department Visit	Paid under OPPS; separate APC payment.
X	Ancillary Services	Paid under OPPS; separate APC payment.
Y	Non-Implantable Durable Medical Equipment	Not paid under OPPS. All institutional providers other than home health agencies bill to DMERC.

Figure **2-4** Payment Status Indicators for the Hospital Outpatient Prospective Payment System Addendum D1. (From *Federal Register,* vol. 72, Tuesday, November 27, 2007.)

CPT/ HCPCS	Description	Status Indicator	APC	Relative Weight	Payment Rate	Minimum Unadjusted Copayment
10060	Drainage of skin abscess	T	0006	1.4066	$89.59	$17.92
10061	Drainage of skin abscess	T	0006	1.4066	$89.59	$17.92
1006F	Osteoarthritis assess	M				
1007F	Anti-inflm/anlgsc otc assess	M				
10080	Drainage of pilonidal cyst	T	0006	1.4066	$89.59	$17.92
10081	Drainage of pilonidal cyst	T	0007	11.5594	$736.26	$147.25
1008F	Gi/renal risk assess	M				
P9038	RBC irradiated	K	9505	3.0643	$195.18	$39.04
P9039	RBC deglycerolized	K	9504	5.4516	$347.23	$69.45
P9040	RBC leukoreduced irradiated	K	0969	3.7722	$240.27	$48.05

Figure 2-5 APC payment rate and co-insurance amount.

-CA Modifier

Used with status indicator "C" services, these are inpatient procedures provided on an emergency basis in the outpatient setting

- Patient expires before admission to the hospital

- Patient is transferred to hospital as inpatient
  - Transfer due to an unexpected occurrence during a scheduled outpatient procedure necessitating an inpatient procedure

-CA is assigned to inpatient-only procedure

Payment is allowed for only one procedure

All other services on same day are packaged into APC for services identified with -CA

Transitional pass-through payments for certain devices and items

Payments made for certain innovative devices, drugs, and biologicals

Paid as an additional APC payment

Such as

- Chemotherapeutic agents
  - Including supportive and adjunctive drugs used
- Implantable devices
- Immunosuppressive drugs
- Orphan drugs
- Some new drugs
- Certain drugs given in the emergency room for heart attacks

Have co-insurance amounts that can be less than 20% of the Average Wholesale Price (AWP)

Payments for pass-throughs made for at least 2 years but not more than 3 years

Reported devices and drugs with HCPCS C or J codes and SI "G"

When a pass-through transitional payment has expired

289

- C code removed from HCPCS and is usually given an applicable "J" code
- Payment is no longer made for item

Current HCPCS codes, including C codes, can be viewed and/or downloaded from the CMS website at http://www.cms.hhs.gov/HCPCSReleaseCodeSets/ANHCPCS/list.asp#/TopOfPage

Pass-through items for which separate payment expires should be reported on the claim to identify the cost to CMS

HCPCS codes for drugs, biologicals, devices, and radiopharmaceuticals that have a separate APC payment are listed in HOPPS Manual Addendum B

Currently, very few devices are paid separately

Most devices have no separate APC payment because the item is packaged into the APC payment for the procedure. Although hospitals do not receive additional payment for these devices, they are encouraged to report the HCPCS codes on the claim

> In some cases, hospitals are required to report the device HCPCS code. See the following section "Device Dependent Procedures"

Most recent information concerning applications and requirements for APC payments for new technologies, additional device categories, and pass-through payments for drugs and biologicals is located on the CMS website at http://www.cms.hhs.gov/HospitalOutpatientPPS/04_passthrough_payment.asp#/TopOfPage

Device Dependent Procedures

Effective January 1, 2005, when hospitals report certain procedure codes that require the use of devices

> Must also report the applicable HCPCS codes and charges for all devices used to perform the procedures. This information is used in calculating future OPPS payment amounts

If such a procedure is reported without at least one device HCPCS code, the OCE will return the claim to the provider

The procedures that require device HCPCS codes are listed in the Device to Procedure Edits document

Download from CMS the device edits:

> http://www.cms.hhs.gov/hospitaloutpatientpps/01_overview.asp?

Discounting

Multiple surgical procedures during the same operative procedure

- Status indicator "T" indicates multiple procedure payment reduction applied

Highest weighted procedure APC paid in full (after applicable co-pay and deductible)

- 50% discount for the other status "T" procedural APCs

Terminated surgical procedures before the induction of anesthesia paid at 50%

- Indicated by use of modifier -73 added to surgical procedure code

Outlier adjustments

Some costs that exceed 2.5 times the payment rate receive an adjusted higher reimbursement

Inpatient-only procedures with status indicator "C"

CMS publishes a list of procedures that are "inpatient-only" procedures

Procedures that are life-threatening and require substantial mortality risks as an outpatient

http://www.cms.hhs.gov/HospitalOutpatientPPS/ and go to Hospital Outpatient Regulations and Notices

- Example of Status Indicator "C" procedures
  - 27258 Treat hip dislocation
  - 32900 Removal of rib(s)
  - 33535 CABG, arterial, three

CMS publishes a list of procedures approved for ASC procedures

http://www.cms.hhs.gov/ASCPayment/

- Example of approved ASC procedures
  - 10121 Removal of foreign body
  - 19340 Immediate breast prosthesis
  - 23155 Removal of humerus lesion

Observation status
Paid only for the three clinical conditions

1. Congestive heart failure

2. Chest pain

3. Asthma

The complete OPPS program for 2008 is in the *Federal Register*, August 2, 2007, Volume 72, Number 148.

There are other circumstances that a patient can be admitted for observation, such as post-op care, severe epileptic attack, TIA, etc.

Observation status (G0378, G0379)
Beginning January 1, 2006, observation services are to be reported with:

- HCPCS codes:
  - G0378—Hospital observation services, per hour
  - G0379—Direct admission of patient for hospital observation care (APC604)
- Revenue code:
  - 0762, observation room

The claims processing logic will determine if the observation services are separately payable or if they will be packaged into the payment to the hospital for other services in the same encounter

Hospitals should bill HCPCS code G0378 for observation services regardless of the patient's condition

The units of service should equal the number of hours the patient is in observation status

G0379 is reported when patient is directly admitted to "observation status" without an associated emergency room visit, hospital outpatient clinic visit, or critical care service on the day of initiation of observation services

CMS states that all hospital observation services, regardless of the duration of the observation care, that are medically reasonable and necessary are covered by Medicare, and hospitals receive either packaged or separate OPPS payment for these covered observation services

Claim must include one of the following in addition to the reported observation services. The additional services must have a line item date of service on the same day or the day before the observation service date:

- An emergency department visit, or

- A clinic visit, or

- Critical care, or

- Direct admission to observation reported with HCPCS code G0379

No procedure with status indicator of "T" can be reported on the same day or day before observation services.

Separate Payment for Direct Admission to Observation:
- Both HCPCS codes G0378 (Hourly Observation) and G0379 (Direct Admit to Observation) with the same date of service;

- No services with a status indicator "T" or "V" or critical care were provided on the same day of service as HCPCS code G0379; and

- The observation care does not qualify for separate payment under APC 0339

Packaged Payment for Direct Admission to Observation;
- Payment is not allowed when billed with the same date of service as a hospital clinic visit, emergency room visit, critical care service, or "T" status procedure

- If the requirements are not met, then payment for the direct admission to observation service will be packaged into payments for other separately payable services during the same encounter

Outpatient Code Edit (OCE)
General functions of the OCE system

- Edits claims data to identify errors and returns an edit flag(s)

- Edits are based upon HCPCS and ICD-9-CM codes

Assigns an APC number to each service covered under OPPS

PROSPECTIVE PAYMENT SYSTEMS (PPS)

Established by TEFRA of 1982

For services provided in

- Acute care hospitals

- Skilled nursing facilities

- Inpatient rehabilitation facilities

- Long-term care hospital settings
  - Psychiatric hospitals or exempt psychiatric units

Hospital/facility paid fixed amount for patient discharged in a treatment category

Excludes hospitals:

- Children's
- Rehabilitation
- Cancer

MEDICARE SEVERITY DIAGNOSIS RELATED GROUPS (MS-DRG)

System of Classifying Patients Into Groups by Related Diagnoses

For payment of operating costs based on prospectively set rates

For acute care hospital inpatient stays under Medicare Part A

Each diagnosis code is categorized into an MS-DRG

MS-DRGs have payment weights assigned based on the average resources used to treat patients in that MS-DRG

- Similar types of patients
- Similar types of illnesses or injuries
- Severity of illness
- Treatments provided
  - Similar use of resources

System Based On

Principal diagnosis

Medical or surgical service

Any qualifying complication(s) or comorbidity(ies)

Structure of MS-DRGs

Divides all principal diagnoses into 25 major diagnostic categories (MDCs) (Figure 2-6)

16 MDCs correspond to major organ systems

Example:

- Respiratory
- Gastrointestinal
- Cardiology

9 MDCs correspond to an etiology (cause)

Example:

Lung cancer

MS-DRG Index

1 - Diseases and Disorders of the Nervous System
2 - Diseases and Disorders of the Eye
3 - Diseases and Disorders of the Ear, Nose, Mouth and Throat
4 - Diseases and Disorders of the Respiratory System
5 - Diseases and Disorders of the Circulatory System
6 - Diseases and Disorders of the Digestive System
7 - Diseases and Disorders of the Hepatobiliary System and Pancreas
8 - Diseases and Disorders of the Musculoskeletal System and Connective Tissue
9 - Diseases and Disorders of the Skin, Subcutaneous Tissue and Breast
10 - Endocrine, Nutritional and Metabolic Diseases and Disorders
11 - Diseases and Disorders of the Kidney and Urinary Tract
12 - Diseases and Disorders of the Male Reproductive System
13 - Diseases and Disorders of the Female Reproductive System
14 - Pregnancy, Childbirth and the Puerperium
15 - Newborns and Other Neonates with Conditions Originating in the Perinatal Period
16 - Diseases and Disorders of the Blood and Blood Forming Organs and Immunological Disorders
17 - Myeloproliferative Diseases and Disorders, and Poorly Differentiated Neoplasms
18 - Infectious and Parasitic Diseases (Systemic or Unspecified Sites)
19 - Mental Diseases and Disorders
20 - Alcohol/Drug Use and Alcohol/Drug Induced Organic Mental Disorders
21 - Injuries, Poisonings and Toxic Effects of Drugs
22 - Burns
23 - Factors Influencing Health Status and Other Contacts with Health Services
24 - Multiple Significant Trauma
25 - Human Immunodeficiency Virus Infections

Figure 2-6 Major Diagnostic Categories of the Diagnosis-Related Groups. (From *Diagnosis Related Groups,* Version 25.0, Definitions Manual, 3M Health Information Systems.)

MS-DRGs are then further defined by a particular set of patient attributes defined in the Uniform Hospital Discharge Data Set (UHDDS)

By diagnosis

Principal diagnosis — Defined as "that condition established after study to be chiefly responsible for occasioning the admission of the patient to the hospital for care"

Secondary diagnosis — Conditions that co-exist at the time of admission, that develop subsequently to the admission, or that affect the treatment received and/or length of stay

By procedure

Principal procedure — A procedure that is performed for definitive treatment rather than for diagnostic or exploratory purposes or that is necessary in order to take care of a complication

Significant procedure — Medicare defines a significant procedure as one that is

- Surgical in nature
- Carries an anesthetic/procedural risk, and
- Requires specialized training

By patient

Sex   Male/Female

Discharge status   Condition and/or place to which the patient is being
                          discharged, such as to home, skilled nursing facility,
                          rehabilitation, home health care, long-term care

MS-DRGs are not affected by age.

Surgical classes in each MDC are defined in a hierarchical (least-to-most resource intense) order

Multiple procedures related to principal diagnosis during hospital stay are
assigned to only the highest surgical class in the hierarchy

- MS-DRG Grouper performs assignment

  - Computer program

Case Study

The principal diagnosis is congestive heart failure (428.0). Additional diagnoses are
morbid obesity (278.01), diabetes (250.00), coronary atherosclerosis (414.01), psoriasis
(696.1), depressive disorder (311), unspecified personality disorder (301.9), hypercholesterolemia (272.0), cardiomegaly (429.3), and initial episode of subendocardial infarction
(410.71). If 410.71 had been listed within the top nine diagnoses, the reimbursement
would have been based on MS-DRG 293 (0.876) compared to 282 (1.0617) if the complication of subendocardial infarction has been correctly listed. Review the principal
reason for admission and the principal diagnosis assignment after study for correct
MS-DRG assignment.

MS-DRGs

Medicare Payment Advisory Commission (MedPAC) recommended DRG system
be revised to recognize severity of illness (SOI)

- Changes were proposed and published in the *Federal Register*, April 13, 2007

- Most drastic change to the inpatient prospective payment system since
  inception in 1983

New reimbursement system will be effective for discharges occurring on or after
October 1, 2007

- Termed Medicare severity DRGs or MS-DRGs (version 25.0)

- Replaced the 538 DRGs with 745 new MS-DRGs

- During conversion some DRGs eliminated

  - Example:

    · Pediatric DRGs

    · Low-volume DRGs

    · DRGs determined by diagnosis complexity, such as complex cardiac
      diagnoses

Change due to the determination that current CC listing had lost ability to
distinguish the differences in resource consumption

- All diagnoses were reviewed to determine if they qualify as a CC or non-CC

  - Key criterion being the increase in hospital resources

- All diagnoses were divided into three severity levels:

- Major complications or comorbidities (MCC)

- Complications or comorbidities (CC)

- Non-CCs—do not affect MS-DRG assignment

The MS-DRG system is 1-999 with allowances for future changes and are listed in Figure 2-7

Chronic conditions may have to be decompensated or in exacerbation to qualify as a CC for MS-DRGs

According to 2006 statistical claims data from Medicare Provider Analysis and Review File (MedPAR), about 78% of claims had at least 1 CC under the DRG system

- Under the MS-DRG system and with the revised CC list, the percentage of claims with a CC is expected to drop to about 40%

A hospital's income will depend even more on complete documentation and accurate coding

MS-DRGs are affected by the CC exclusions list

- Also revised

- Lists certain diagnoses that would not be considered CCs when coded as a secondary diagnosis with a certain principal diagnosis

- Example: 518.3 (pulmonary infiltrates) is excluded as a CC when most of the pneumonia codes are assigned as principal diagnosis

The changes that will affect coders the most are the creation of three different levels of complication/comorbidity (CC) severity and the revision of the CC listing

- Good documentation and accurate coding will be even more important to obtain the optimum reimbursement for the hospital

The challenges for coding staff include:

- It may take more time to review and code a record resulting in decreased productivity

- Greater specificity in code assignment will be necessary with MS-DRGs

- There will be an increase in physician queries and communications

MS-DRGs	# of MS-DRGs
No severity levels	73
Three levels of severity (MCC/CC/non-CC)	456
Two levels: With CC/MCC or Without CC/MCC	88
Two levels: With MCC or Without MCC	126
Error MS-DRGs	2
Total	**745**

Figure **2-7** MS-DRG system.

- Assigning POA (present on admission) indicators will require extra attention and may decrease productivity

- A coder's knowledge base about clinical conditions and disease will have to expand

MS-DRG Classification

Begins with diagnosis and pre-MDC (Figure 2-8)

Pre-Major Diagnostic Categories (Pre-MDCs)

Pre-MDC MS-DRGs are very resource intensive

Services for these MS-DRGs may be performed for diagnoses in many different MDCs

Assigned independently of the MDC to indicate the procedure performed

For year 2008, there were 13 MS-DRGs to which cases were directly assigned based on ICD-9-CM procedure codes

Cases are assigned to these MS-DRGs before they are assigned a MDC

MS-DRG	MS-DRG Title
001	Heart transplant or implant of heart assist system w MCC
002	Heart transplant or implant of heart assist system w/o MCC
003	ECMO or trach w MV 96+ hrs or PDX exc face, mouth & neck w maj O.R.
004	Trach w MV 96+ hrs or PDX exc face, mouth & neck w/o maj O.R.
005	Liver transplant w MCC or intestinal transplant
006	Liver transplant w/o MCC
007	Lung transplant
008	Simultaneous pancreas/kidney transplant
009	Bone marrow transplant
010	Pancreas transplant
011	Tracheostomy for face, mouth & neck diagnoses w MCC
012	Tracheostomy for face, mouth & neck diagnoses w CC
013	Tracheostomy for face, mouth & neck diagnoses w/o CC/MCC

If care involves a procedure/principal diagnosis contained within the pre-MDCs, the patient is assigned to both:

- Pre-MDC

- MDC of the principal diagnosis

  Example: HIV patient admitted for chronic respiratory failure on ventilator. An open bronchial biopsy procedure was performed, assigned to both MDC 25 and 6

- 25 HIV

- 6 Diseases and disorders of the respiratory system

If admitting principal diagnosis/procedure is not one contained within the pre-MDCs flow chart, the remaining 25 MDCs are reviewed

Use surgical procedure MS-DRG if surgery was performed (Figure 2-9)

- Surgical procedures pay more than nonsurgical MDCs

Use principal diagnosis to select MS-DRG if no surgery was performed

ALL PATIENTS

Heart Transplant or Implant of Heart Assist System

MCC			DRG
Yes			001
No			002

ECMO or Tracheostomy with MV 96+ Hours or PDX Except Face, Mouth and Neck

ECMO	Tracheostomy	Major O.R. Procedure	DRG
Yes			003
No	Yes	Yes	003
No	Yes	No	004

Liver or Intestinal Transplant

Instestinal Transplant	MCC		DRG
Yes			005
No	Yes		005
No	No		006

Lung Transplant

	DRG
	007

Simultaneous Pancreas/Kidney Transplant

	DRG
	008

Bone Marrow Transplant

	DRG
	009

Pancreas Transplant

	DRG
	010

Tracheostomy for Face, Mouth and Neck Diagnoses

MCC	CC		DRG
Yes			011
No	Yes		012
No	No		013

PDX of Trauma and At Least Two Significant Diagnoses of Different Body Site Categories

	MDC
	24

PDX of HIV Infection OR PDX of HIV Significant Related Condition and SDX of HIV Infection

	MDC
	25

Figure **2-8** Pre-MDC flow chart, DRG Grouper Version 25.0. (From *Diagnosis Related Groups*, Version 25.0, Definitions Manual, 3M Health Information Systems.)

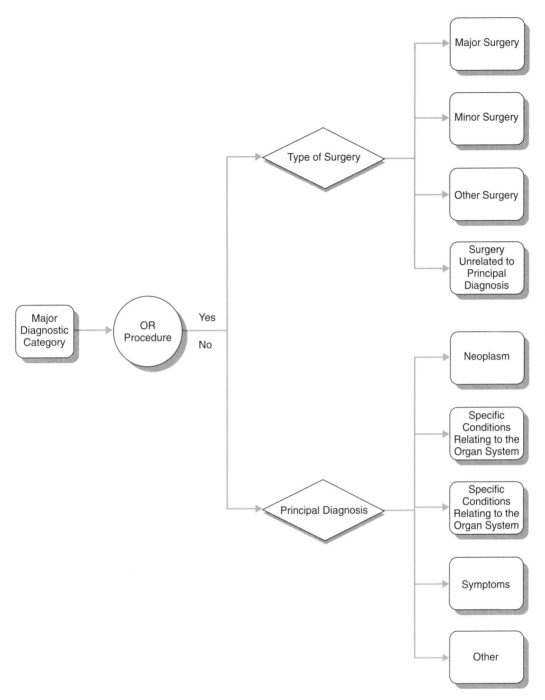

Figure **2-9** Typical DRG structure for a Major Diagnostic Category. The Medical and Surgical Classes are further divided according to the age of the patient or the presence of complications or co-morbidities. (From *Diagnosis Related Groups*, Version 25.0, Definitions Manual, 3M Health Information Systems.)

MS-DRG selection if no surgical procedure is performed is based on:
- Qualifying MCC/CC

- Discharge disposition

- **Must be significant**

  - An MCC/CC is likely to result in increased use of hospital resources

Example:

- Pneumonia (486) is an MCC; benign hypertension (401.1) is not an MCC or a CC

- **May be excluded if MCC/CC**

  - Chronic and acute manifestations of the same disease (not CCs for one another)

  - Is closely related to the principal diagnosis

Example:

- Cardiomyopathy is not considered a CC with congestive heart failure

- Dehydration is considered a CC with congestive heart failure

Separate MS-DRGs for

Burn patients

Newborns transferred to another acute care facility

Drug or alcoholism abuse patients leaving against medical advice

Myocardial infarction patients and newborns who die

MS-DRGs for patients whose medical records contain inconsistency or invalid information are classified to

MS-DRG	MS-DRG Title
981	Extensive O.R. procedure unrelated to principal diagnosis w MCC
982	Extensive O.R. procedure unrelated to principal diagnosis w CC
983	Extensive O.R. procedure unrelated to principal diagnosis w/o CC/MCC
984	Prostatic O.R. procedure unrelated to principal diagnosis w MCC
985	Prostatic O.R. procedure unrelated to principal diagnosis w CC
986	Prostatic O.R. procedure unrelated to principal diagnosis w/o CC/MCC
987	Non-extensive O.R. proc unrelated to principal diagnosis w MCC
988	Non-extensive O.R. proc unrelated to principal diagnosis w CC
989	Non-extensive O.R. proc unrelated to principal diagnosis w/o CC/MCC
998	Principal diagnosis invalid as discharge diagnosis
999	Ungroupable

Hospital charges are reported on CMS-1450 (UB-04) (Figure 2-10)

See Table 2-1 for UB-04 information for each field locator

Calculating MS-DRG Payment

2008 MS-DRG weights are available in Table S of 2008 Final Rule

According to the list, MS-DRG 185, Major Chest Trauma w/o CC, is assigned the following weights and means

Relative Weight   0.7298

Geometric mean LOS (GMLOS)   2.7

Arithmetic mean LOS (AMLOS)   3.3

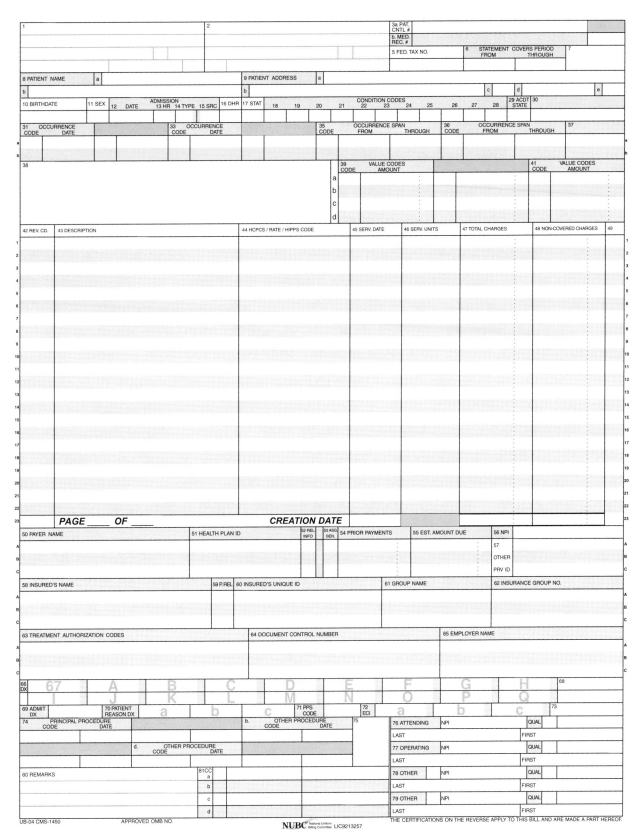

Figure **2-10** CMS-1450/UB-04.

2007 is a year of transition from the DRG to MS-DRG and as such these calculations are based on the current system.

The following is an example of how the MS-DRG payment is calculated:

A Medicare patient was admitted with a principal dx of closed fracture of three ribs (807.03) or MS-DRG 185. No surgical procedures were performed. The patient was discharged on day 3 with no complications or comorbidities indicated in the documentation. The patient has not paid any of the Part A deductible for the year ($912 for 2007). If the Hospital Specific Rate is $2,000, calculation of the amount the hospital would receive from Medicare would be:

Relative Weight × Hospital Specific Rate − Medicare deductible = Amount Due from Medicare

$$0.7298 \times \$2,000 = \$1,459.60 - \$912 = \textbf{\$547.60} \text{ amount due from Medicare}$$

If the same patient developed pneumonia (486), which is a complication (MS-DRG 183), the following would be the weights and means:

Relative Weight   1.2664
Geometric mean LOS   5.7
Arithmetic mean LOS   7.2

Calculation would be:

Relative Weight × Hospital Specific Rate − Medicare deductible = Amount Due from Medicare

$$1.2664 \times \$2,000 = \$2,532.80 - \$912 = \textbf{\$1,620.80} \text{ amount due from Medicare}$$

CMS publishes a list of ICD-9-CM codes that are complications and comorbidities

Analyzing Case Mix

Refer to Figure 2-11, which illustrates six hospital admissions with relative weights

Relative Weight × Number of Cases = Total Value of Service

MS-DRG	MDC	TYPE	MS-DRG TITLE	Relative Weight	Number of Cases	Total Value of Service
025	01	SURG	Craniotomy & endovascular intracranial procedures w MCC	4.2362	5	21.1810
026	01	SURG	Craniotomy & endovascular intracranial procedures w CC	3.1582	9	28.4235
027	01	SURG	Craniotomy & endovascular intracranial procedures w/o CC/MCC	2.3259	12	27.9105
031	01	SURG	Ventricular shunt procedures w MCC	3.2226	3	9.6677
032	01	SURG	Ventricular shunt procedures w CC	1.9342	4	7.7370
033	01	SURG	Ventricular shunt procedures w/o CC/MCC	1.4281	10	14.2811
052	01	MED	Spinal disorders & injuries w CC/MCC	1.4329	9	12.8960
053	01	MED	Spinal disorders & injuries w/o CC/MCC	1.1172	15	16.7578
054	01	MED	Nervous system neoplasms w MCC	1.4228	3	4.2683
055	01	MED	Nervous system neoplasms w/o MCC	1.1213	8	8.9703
					78	152.0932

Figure **2-11** Ten hospital admissions with relative weights.

Table 2-1   UB-04 Field Locators

UB-04		UB-04	
FL	**Description**	**FL**	**Description**
FL01	Provider Name	FL35	Occurrence Span Code/From/Through
FL01	Provider Street Address	FL35	Occurrence Span Code/From/Through
FL01	Provider City, State, Zip	FL36	Occurrence Span Code/From/Through
FL01	Provider Telephone, Fax, Country Code	FL36	Occurrence Span Code/From/Through
FL02	Pay-to Name	FL37	Unlabeled
FL02	Pay-to Address	FL37	Unlabeled
FL02	Pay-to City, State		*Moved to FL64*
FL02	Pay-to ID		*Moved to FL64*
FL03a	Patient Control Number		*Moved to FL64*
FL03b	Medical Record Number	FL38	Responsible Party Name/Address
FL04	Type of Bill	FL38	Responsible Party Name/Address
FL05	Federal Tax Number	FL38	Responsible Party Name/Address
FL05	Federal Tax Number	FL38	Responsible Party Name/Address
FL06	Statement Covers Period – From/Through	FL38	Responsible Party Name/Address
FL07	Unlabeled	FL39	Value Code – Code
FL08	Patient Name – ID	FL39	Value Code – Amount
FL08	Patient Name	FL39	Value Code – Code
FL09	Patient Address – Street	FL39	Value Code – Amount
FL09	Patient Address – City	FL39	Value Code – Code
FL09	Patient Address – State	FL39	Value Code – Amount
FL09	Patient Address – ZIP	FL39	Value Code – Code
FL09	Patient Address – Country Code	FL39	Value Code – Amount
FL10	Patient Birthdate	FL40	Value Code – Code
FL11	Patient Sex	FL40	Value Code – Amount
	Eliminated	FL40	Value Code – Code
FL12	Admission Date	FL40	Value Code – Amount
FL13	Admission Hour	FL40	Value Code – Code
FL14	Type of Admission/Visit	FL40	Value Code – Amount
FL15	Source of Admission	FL40	Value Code – Code
FL16	Discharge Hour	FL40	Value Code – Amount
FL17	Patient Discharge Status	FL40	Value Code – Code
	Moved to FL3b	FL40	Value Code – Amount
FL18	Condition Codes	FL41	Value Code – Code
FL19	Condition Codes	FL41	Value Code – Amount
FL20	Condition Codes	FL41	Value Code – Code
FL21	Condition Codes	FL41	Value Code – Amount
FL22	Condition Codes	FL41	Value Code – Code
FL23	Condition Codes	FL41	Value Code – Amount
FL24	Condition Codes	FL41	Value Code – Code
FL25	Condition Codes	FL41	Value Code – Amount
FL26	Condition Codes	FL41	Value Code – Code
FL27	Condition Codes	FL41	Value Code – Amount
FL28	Condition Codes	FL42	Revenue Code
FL29	Accident State	FL43	Revenue Code Description
FL30	Unlabeled	FL44	HCPCS/Rates/HIPPS Rate Codes
FL30	Unlabeled	FL45	Service Date
FL31	Occurrence Code/Date	FL45	Creation Date
FL31	Occurrence Code/Date	FL46	Units of Service
FL32	Occurrence Code/Date	FL47	Total Charges
FL32	Occurrence Code/Date	FL48	Non-Covered Charges
FL33	Occurrence Code/Date	FL49	Unlabeled
FL33	Occurrence Code/Date	FL50	Payer Name – Primary
FL34	Occurrence Code/Date	FL50	Payer Name – Secondary
FL34	Occurrence Code/Date	FL50	Payer Name – Tertiary
		FL51	Health Plan ID
		FL51	Health Plan ID
		FL51	Health Plan ID
		FL52	Release of Information – Primary

Table 2-1 UB-04 Field Locators—cont'd

UB-04		UB-04	
FL	Description	FL	Description
FL52	Release of Information – Secondary	FL67E	Other Diagnosis
FL52	Release of Information – Tertiary	FL67F	Other Diagnosis
FL53	Assignment of Benefits – Primary	FL67G	Other Diagnosis
FL53	Assignment of Benefits – Secondary	FL67H	Other Diagnosis
FL53	Assignment of Benefits – Tertiary	FL67I	Other Diagnosis
FL54	Prior Payments – Primary	FL67J	Other Diagnosis
FL54	Prior Payments – Secondary	FL67K	Other Diagnosis
FL54	Prior Payments – Tertiary	FL67L	Other Diagnosis
	Eliminated Patient Prior Payments	FL67M	Other Diagnosis
FL55	Estimated Amount Due – Primary	FL67N	Other Diagnosis
FL55	Estimated Amount Due – Secondary	FL67O	Other Diagnosis
FL55	Estimated Amount Due – Tertiary	FL67P	Other Diagnosis
	Eliminated Due from Patient	FL67Q	Other Diagnosis
FL56	NPI	FL68	Unlabeled
FL57	Other Provider ID – Primary	FL68	Unlabeled
FL57	Other Provider ID – Secondary	FL69	Admitting Diagnosis Code
FL57	Other Provider ID – Tertiary	FL70	Patient's Reason for Visit Code
	Deleted from UB-04	FL70	Patient's Reason for Visit Code
FL58	Insured's Name – Primary	FL70	Patient's Reason for Visit Code
FL58	Insured's Name – Secondary	FL71	PPS Code
FL58	Insured's Name – Tertiary	FL72	External Cause of Injury Code
FL59	Patient's Relationship – Primary	FL72	External Cause of Injury Code
FL59	Patient's Relationship – Secondary	FL72	External Cause of Injury Code
FL59	Patient's Relationship – Tertiary	FL73	Unlabeled
FL60	Insured's Unique ID – Primary		*Deleted from UB-04*
FL60	Insured's Unique ID – Secondary	FL74	Principal Procedure Code/Date
FL60	Insured's Unique ID – Tertiary	FL74a	Other Procedure Code/Date
FL61	Insurance Group Name – Primary	FL74b	Other Procedure Code/Date
FL61	Insurance Group Name – Secondary	FL74c	Other Procedure Code/Date
FL61	Insurance Group Name – Tertiary	FL74d	Other Procedure Code/Date
FL62	Insurance Group Number – Primary	FL74e	Other Procedure Code/Date
FL62	Insurance Group Number – Secondary	FL75	Unlabeled
FL62	Insurance Group Number – Tertiary	FL75	Unlabeled
FL63	Treatment Authorization Code – Primary	FL75	Unlabeled
FL63	Treatment Authorization Code – Secondary	FL75	Unlabeled
FL63	Treatment Authorization Code – Tertiary	FL76	Attending – NPI/QUAL/ID
FL64	Document Control Number	FL76	Attending – Last/First
FL64	Document Control Number	FL77	Operating – NPI/QUAL/ID
FL64	Document Control Number	FL77	Operating – Last/First
	Deleted from UB-04	FL78	Other ID – QUAL/NPI/QUAL/ID
	Deleted from UB-04	FL78	Other ID – Last/First
	Deleted from UB-04	FL79	Other ID – QUAL/NPI/QUAL/ID
FL65	Employer Name – Primary	FL79	Other ID – Last/First
FL65	Employer Name – Secondary	FL80	Remarks
FL65	Employer Name – Tertiary	FL80	Remarks
	Deleted from UB-04	FL80	Remarks
	Deleted from UB-04	FL80	Remarks
	Deleted from UB-04	FL81	Code-Code – QUAL/CODE/VALUE
FL66	DX Version Qualifier	FL81	Code-Code – QUAL/CODE/VALUE
FL67	Principal Diagnosis Code	FL81	Code-Code – QUAL/CODE/VALUE
FL67A	Other Diagnosis	FL81	Code-Code – QUAL/CODE/VALUE
FL67B	Other Diagnosis		*Deleted from UB-04*
FL67C	Other Diagnosis		*Deleted from UB-04; See FL45, line 23*
FL67D	Other Diagnosis		

Example:

- MS-DRG 025: **4.2362** (Relative Weight) × **5** (number of cases) = **21.1810** (Total Value of Services)

- Total Value of Services / Number of cases = Case Mix Index (CMI)

Example:

- **152.0932** (Total Value of Services) / **78** (Total Number of Cases) = **1.9499** (CMI)

Highest total reimbursement is MS-DRG 10, Nervous system neoplasm w CC (28.1543)

Highest relative weight is MS-DRG 025, Craniotomy and endovascular intracranial procedures with MCC (4.2362)

POST ACUTE TRANSFER

CMS thought it was overpaying the acute care hospital for these patients at the full MS-DRG rate so a reduction in payment formula was implemented.

- Medicare developed special rules that apply to particular MS-DRGs in which patients are frequently discharged immediately to a rehab hospital, skilled nursing facility, a long-term care hospital or home health care

- Termed transfer MS-DRGs

- Part of the Balance Budget Act of 1997

- Initially there were 10 DRGs that were identified in 1999 as "transfer DRGs."

- This number has grown significantly over the years with 209 for FY07.

Payment is adjusted when the covered days preceding the "transfer" are less than the Geometric Mean Length of Stay (GMLOS) of the assigned MS-DRG

- The facility is reimbursed on a per diem rate that is calculated by taking the Hospital's normal reimbursement for the MS-DRG divided by the GMLOS.

There are three types of transfers that are affected:

- Transfers to another acute care hospital
  - The transferring hospital receives double the per diem rate for the first day plus the per diem rate for each subsequent day prior to the transfer
  - Not to exceed the total MS-DRG payment
- Designated MS-DRGs transferred to a post acute care setting
  - The same formula as a transfer to another acute care hospital
- Designated special pay MS-DRGs transferred to a post acute care setting
  - The transferring hospital receives the per diem rate for the first day plus one-half the per diem rate for each subsequent day prior to the transfer.

PRESENT ON ADMISSION INDICATOR (POA)

Effective October 1, 2007, hospital to submit Medicare inpatient claims with a Present On Admission (POA) indicator for every diagnosis

Exempt are:

- Critical access hospital
- Maryland waiver hospitals
- Long-term care hospitals
- Cancer and psychiatric hospitals
- Inpatient rehabilitation facilities
- Children's inpatient facilities

Beginning on April 1, 2008, Medicare will return claims without POA codes Hospital will have to correct and resubmit a claim

POA guidelines are provided in Appendix I of the *ICD-9-CM Official Guidelines for Coding and Reporting*

POA defined as present at the time the order for inpatient admission occurs

- Conditions that develop during an outpatient encounter are considered as present on admission
    - Example: Emergency room, observation, outpatient surgery

The reporting options are:

Y Yes, this diagnosis was present at the time of admission

N No, this diagnosis was not present at the time of admission

U Unknown, documentation is insufficient to determine if condition is present at time of inpatient admission

W Clinically undetermined, provider is unable to clinically determine whether the condition was present at the time of admission or not

1 Unreported/Not used, exempt from POA reporting

72-Hour rule
Also known as the "3-day window"

Part of Medicare's Prospective Payment System (PPS)

States that reimbursement for any hospital outpatient diagnostic or other services provided for the same diagnosis occasioning the admission 3 days prior to admission is included in the DRG payment for that hospital stay

Monitoring MS-DRG Reimbursement

Accounts receivable (AR)
List of all cases not paid yet because codes are not available

Bills have not yet been sent on these accounts

Monitor AR amounts

Remittance advice
Sent by MACs listing amounts paid to hospital

Always verify correct MS-DRG was paid based on MS-DRG initially submitted

Audit for underpayments of transfer MS-DRGs

All Patient Refined Diagnosis Related Groups (APR-DRG)

CMS did not utilize the APR-DRG because it is a proprietary system and instead they developed their own system of MS-DRGs

CMS contracted with a consulting firm to review available severity of illness systems and make recommendations on the most appropriate system to use

- Classification related type of patient treated to resources consumed

APR-DRG developed by National Association of Children's Hospitals and Related Institutions (NACHRI) and 3M

- Expansion of basic DRG (measures/compares consumption of resources) to better reflect non-Medicare patient attributes with severity of illness and risk of mortality

- Four subclassifications for severity of illness and risk of mortality for each APR-DRG

  - Minor, moderate, major, and extreme
  - Severity levels are not comparable from one APR-DRG to another. For example, a level 3 severity for one APR-DRG is not comparable to a level 3 severity of another APR-DRG
  - Severity levels are based on variables that include secondary diagnoses, age, procedure, and birth weight

Resource Utilization Groups (RUGs)

Reimbursement system used in long-term skilled health care settings

- Long-term care hospitals (LTCH) are defined as those with average stays greater than 10 days

Based on resources

Utilizes information from the minimum data set (MDS)

- Rehabilitation services
- Special care needs
- Clinical requirements
- Activity of daily living
- Cognitive function
- Behavioral symptoms and resident's distressed mood

Assessment of patient must be on days 5, 14, 30, 60, and 90

- Defined by federal law

Home Health Prospective Payment System (HHPPS)

Reimbursement system used in home care agencies

Based on information in Outcome and Assessment Information Set (OASIS)

Payment based on the visit

Home Assessment Validation and Entry (HAVEN) is the CMS free data entry software utilized by most Home Health Agencies (HHA)

Inpatient Rehabilitation Facility (IRF) Prospective Payment System

Paid on a per-discharge basis

Utilizes information from an Inpatient Rehabilitation Facility Patient Assessment Instrument (IRF PAI)

- Classifies patients into distinct groups based on clinical characteristics and expected resource needs

Inpatient Psychiatric Facility (IPF) Prospective Payment System

- Originally excluded from PPS
- Also excluded were rehabilitation, children's, cancer, and long-term care hospitals, rehabilitation and hospitals located outside the 50 states and Puerto Rico
- Referred to as TEFRA (Tax Equity and Fiscal Responsibility Act) facilities and paid on a per diem amount

As of January 1, 2005, payment made under IPF prospective payment system

Paid per diem rate

- Adjusted based on:
    1. Diagnosis Related Group classification
    2. Patient age
    3. Length of stay
    4. Any co-morbidities

REVENUE CODES

Four digit classification system that

- Identifies services or procedures
- Identifies location where services were rendered

Three Main Categories

1. Billing revenue codes

    Example:

    - *0137, replacement of a prior claim for a hospital outpatient charge*

2. Accommodation revenue codes

    Example:

    - *0120, semiprivate room and board for obstetrical patient*

3. Ancillary revenue codes

    Example:

    - *0314, laboratory pathological services for a biopsy*

The digits and their placement further define elements of the revenue code (Figure 2-12)

Example:

Revenue code for laboratory pathological service is 031X

				RVU Category
0	3	1	X	Laboratory Pathological
				Subcategory
			0	General Classification
			1	Cytology
			2	Histology
			4	Biopsy
			9	Other

Figure **2-12** Chart of Laboratory Pathological Revenue code category breakdown.

The fourth digit (X) is assigned from one of five subcategory digits

• Subcategory identifies type of service/procedure within category

Example:

• *Fourth digit (4) identifies biopsy services (0314)*

Medicare determines included and excluded services based on
Revenue codes

HCPCS codes (FL44)

Principal and other diagnoses

• FL 67 = PDx

• FLs 68-75 = Other Dx

Under the OPPS, Medicare requires use of HCPCS codes by hospital outpatient departments when a code for that service is available

Example of services that require HCPCS codes

Revenue Code	Description	HCPCS Codes
0274	Prosthetic and orthotic devices	L9900, Orthotic
0331	Injected chemotherapy	96401, Chemotherapy administration
0481	Cardiac catheterization laboratory	93526, Combined heart cath
0623	Surgical dressing	G0168, Wound closure
0636	Pharmacy	J1645, Dalteparin
0901	Electroshock therapy	90870, Electroconvulsion

DATA QUALITY

Charge Description Master

Data base used by hospitals

Includes all services, procedures, supplies, and drugs with a

• Corresponding internal numbered description of everything utilized by the patient

• Revenue code

- CPT/HCPCS codes
- Charge (Figure 2-13)

Elements of a charge description master
- Unique department code number
- Description number (charge code) that is internally assigned to identify each procedure, supply, drug, and service. The charge code is a unique alpha or alphanumeric code that remains constant year after year
- Procedure/service description
- CPT/HCPCS codes—HCPCS code may change from time to time based on CPT/HCPCS code changes and changes in payer requirements
- Revenue code—may change from time to time based on payer requirements
- Cost/Charge—generally this is evaluated and changed annually
- Hard-coded modifiers when applicable

Should be reviewed annually and updated as needed to assist in
Reduction of claim denials

Accurate reimbursement

Compliance

Better data management and quality

- Such as tracking of services and supplies

Review for
Invalid/inaccurate codes

- Unclear/incorrect descriptions
- Omitted procedures or supplies
- Correct service/supply and revenue code linkage
- Appropriate fees

MEDICARE FRAUD AND ABUSE

Program established by Medicare

- To decrease and eliminate fraud and abuse

HCPCS	Description	Active Date	Revenue Code	Charge
Q0171	Chlorpromazine Tablet 10 mg	11/02/2001	635	$2.23
96413	Chemotherapy Admin Infusion up to one hour	01/01/2007	261	$152.75
P9016	Red blood cells, leukocytes reduced, each unit	02/10/2003	380	$295.00
L3810	WHFO, addition to short and long opponens, thumb abduction bar	05/14/2003	274	$403.23
96360	Infusion therapy, not chemotherapy drugs, per visit	01/01/2007	450	$153.00
J9370	Vincristine Sulfate, 1 mg	09/30/2003	636	$202.02

Figure **2-13** Example of basic "Charge Description Master."

Beneficiary signatures on file

- Service, charges submitted without need for patient signature

Presents opportunity for fraud

Fraud

Intentional deception to benefit

Example: Submitting for services not provided

Anyone who submits for Medicare services can be violator

- Physicians
- Hospitals
- Laboratories
- Billing services
- YOU

Fraud Can Be

Billing for services not provided

Misrepresenting diagnosis, CPT, or HCPCS code(s)

Kickbacks

Unbundling services

Falsifying medical necessity

Systematic waiver of co-payment

Fraud Examples

Patient presents with chest pain and is treated.
  Progress note indicates myocardial infarction (MI) is to be ruled out.
  Laboratory tests do not suggest or indicate MI.
  Coder assigns MI as PDx as the reason for encounter/admission.
Chest pain pays less than MI.
This is fraud!

Other examples of fraud

Upcoding is using a higher-level code for a lower-level service

Misrepresenting the diagnosis for a patient to justify the service or equipment furnished

Unbundling or exploding charge

Example: Reporting multichannel lab tests (many tests in one process) to appear as if the individual tests were performed

Billing noncovered services

Example: Routine foot care reported as more involved form of foot care that is paid under the Medicare program

Applying for duplicate payment

> ***Example:*** Patient has Medicare and another insurance and both are billed without indicating that there is another third-party payer

OFFICE OF THE INSPECTOR GENERAL (OIG)

Develops and publishes work plan annually

Outlines Medicare monitoring program

MACs monitor those areas identified in plan

Complaints of Fraud or Abuse

Submitted orally or in writing to MACs

Allegations made by anyone against anyone

Allegations followed up by MACs

Abuse

Generally involves

- Impropriety

- Lack of medical necessity for services reported

Review takes place after claim is submitted

- MACs go back and do historical review of claims

Kickbacks

Bribe or rebate for referring patient for any service covered by Medicare

Any personal gain kickback

A felony

- $25,000 fine or

- 5 years in jail or

- Both

Protect Yourself

Use your common sense

Submit only truthful and accurate claims

If you are unsure about charges, services, or procedures check with physician or supervisor

MANAGED HEALTH CARE

Network health care providers and facilities that offer health care services under one organization

Group hospitals, physicians, or other providers

90% of people with health care coverage are covered by an organization (e.g., HMO, PPO, POS)

Managed Care Organizations

Responsible for health care services to an enrolled group or person

Coordinate various health care services

Negotiate with facilities and providers

Capitation method common in managed care

- Prepaid, fixed amount for each person in the plan
  - Regardless of resource use

Preferred Provider Organization (PPO)

Providers and facilities form network to offer health care services as group

Enrollees who seek health care outside PPO pay more

Point of service (POS)

In-network or out-of-network providers may be used

Benefits are paid at a higher rate to in-network providers

Subscribers are not limited to providers, but to amount covered by plan

Health Maintenance Organization (HMO)

Total package health care

Out-of-pocket expenses minimal

Assigned physician acts as gatekeeper to refer patient outside organization

ABBREVIATIONS

AMLOS	Arithmetic Mean Length of Stay
APCs	Ambulatory Patient Classifications
APGs	Ambulatory Patient Groups
APR-DRG	All Payer Diagnosis Related Groups
AWP	Average Wholesale Price
CC	Complications and Co-morbidities
CLIA	Clinical Laboratories Improvement Act
DCN	Document Control Number
DME	Durable Medical Equipment
DRG	Diagnosis Related Groups
EDI	Electronic Data Interchange
EIN	Employer Identification Number
EOB	Explanation of Benefits
ESRD	End Stage Renal Disease
FL	Field Locators
FUD	Follow-up Days
GMLOS	Geometric Mean Length of Stay
GPN	Group Provider Number
HAVEN	Home Assessment Validation and Entry
HCPCS	Healthcare Common Procedural Coding System
HHA	Home Health Agencies
HHPPS	Home Health Prospective Payment System
HICN	Health Insurance Claim/Identification Number
HIPAA	Health Insurance Portability and Accountability Act
HMO	Health Maintenance Organization
HOPPS	Hospital Outpatient Prospective Payment System
HPMP	Hospital Payment Monitoring Program
ICN	Internal Control Number
IPF	Inpatient Psychiatric Facility
IRF	Inpatient Rehabilitation Facility
IRF PAI	Inpatient Rehabilitation Facility Patient Assessment Instrument
LCD	Local Coverage Determination
LMRP	Local Medical Review Policies, replaced by LCD, Local Coverage Determination
MDCs	Major Diagnostic Categories
NCCI	National Correct Coding Initiative
NCD	National Coverage Decisions
NCHS	National Centers for Health Statistics
NPI	National Provider Identifier
OASIS	Outcome and Assessment Information Set
OBRA	Omnibus Budget Reconciliation Act of 1986
OCE	Outpatient Code Edit
OIG	Office of the Inspector General
OR	Operating Room
PDx	Principal Diagnosis
PIN	Provider Identification Number
PPO	Preferred Provider Organization
PPS	Prospective Payment System
PRO	Peer Review Organizations, now QIO
QIO	Quality Improvement Organizations
RBRVS	Resource-Based Relative Value Scale
RUGs	Resource Utilization Groups
SDRG	Severity Diagnosis Related Groups
SI	Status Indicators
UCR	Usual, Customary, and Reasonable
UHDDS	Uniform Hospital Discharge Data Set
WHO	World Health Organization

REIMBURSEMENT TERMINOLOGY

Advance Beneficiary Notice	ABN, notification in advance of services that Medicare may not pay for them, including the estimated cost to the patient
Ancillary Service	A service that is supportive of care of a patient, such as laboratory services
APC	A classification system used to group like services based upon clinical similarities and resources utilized
Assignment	A legal agreement that allows the provider to receive direct payment from a payer and the provider to accept payment as payment in full for covered services
Attending Physician	The physician legally responsible for oversight of an inpatient's care
Beneficiary	The person who benefits from insurance coverage; also known as subscriber, dependent, enrollee, member, or participant
Birthday Rule	When both parents have insurance coverage, the parent with the birthday earliest in the year is the primary coverage for a dependent
Certified Registered Nurse Anesthetist	CRNA, an individual with specialized training and certification in nursing and anesthesia
Charge Description Master	Record of services, procedures, supplies, and drugs with corresponding codes, descriptions, and charges billed
Co-insurance	Cost-sharing of covered services
Compliance Plan	Written strategy developed by medical facilities to ensure appropriate, consistent documentation within the medical record and ensure compliance with third-party payer guidelines
Concurrent Care	More than one physician providing care to a patient at the same time
Coordination of Benefits	COB, management of multiple third-party payments to ensure overpayment does not occur
Co-payment	Cost-sharing between beneficiary and payer
Correct Coding Initiative	CCI, developed by CMS to control improper unbundling of CPT codes leading to inappropriate payment
Deductible	That portion of covered services paid by the beneficiary before third-party payment begins
Denial	Statement from the payer that reimbursement is denied
Documentation	Detailed chronology of facts and observations regarding a patient's health
Diagnosis Related Groups	DRGs, A case mix classification system established by CMS consisting of classes of patients who are similar clinically and in consumption of hospital resources; replaced with MS-DRGs
Durable Medical Equipment	DME, medically related equipment that is not disposable, such as wheelchairs, crutches, and vaporizers
Electronic Data Interchange	EDI, computerized submission of health care insurance information exchange
Employer Identification Number	EIN, an Internal Revenue Service (IRS)–issued identification number used on tax documents

316

Encounter Form	Medical document that contains information regarding a patient visit for health care services
Explanation of Benefits	EOB, written, detailed listing of medical service payments by third-party payer to inform beneficiary and provider of payment
Fee Schedule	Established list of payments for medical services, i.e., lab, physician services
Follow-up Days	FUD, established by third-party payers and listing the number of days after a procedure for which a provider must provide normal uncomplicated related services to a patient for no fee (also known as global days, global package, or global period)
Group Provider Number	GPN, numeric designation for a group of providers that is used instead of the individual provider number
Hospital Payment Monitoring System	HPMS, an inpatient PPS audit system used by CMS to reduce improper payments
Invalid Claim	Claim that is missing necessary information and cannot be processed or paid
Inpatient	CMS defines an inpatient as a person who has been formally admitted to a hospital with the expectation that he or she will remain at least overnight and occupy a bed even if it later develops that the patient can be discharged or transferred to another hospital and not actually use a hospital bed overnight
Medical Record	Documentation about the health care of a patient
Medicare Administrative Contractors	MACs, will replace Fiscal Intermediaries (FIs) by 2011
Medicare Severity Diagnosis Related Groups	MS-DRG, classification system implemented October 2007 that is based on the principal diagnosis and the medical or surgical service provided to the Medicare inpatient in which the hospital/facility is paid a fixed amount for each patient discharged in a treatment category
Noncovered Services	Any service not included by a third-party payer in the list of services for which payment is made
National Provider Identifier	NPI, 10-digit number assigned to provider and used for identification purposes when submitting services to third-party payers
Hospital Outpatient	An individual who is not an inpatient of a hospital but who is registered as an outpatient at the hospital
Prior Authorization	Also known as preauthorization, which is a requirement by the payer to receive written permission prior to patient services if the service is to be considered for payment by the payer
Provider Identification Number	PIN, or UPIN, assigned by the third-party payer to providers to be used for identification purposes when submitting services to third-party payers
Rejection	A claim that does not pass edits and is returned to the provider as rejected
Reimbursement	Payment from a third-party payer for services rendered to a patient covered by the payer's health care plan

State License Number

Identification number issued by a state to a physician who has been granted the right to practice in that state

Usual, Customary, and Reasonable

UCR, used by third-party payers to establish a payment rate for a service in an area with the usual (standard fee in area), customary (standard fee by the physician), and reasonable (as determined by payer) rate

REIMBURSEMENT QUIZ

1. Any person who is identified as receiving life or medical benefits:
   a. primary
   b. beneficiary
   c. participant
   d. recipient

2. TEFRA of 1982 established the _____, which pays a fixed amount intended to cover the cost of treating a typical patient for a particular DRG.
   a. OPPS
   b. NPI
   c. DRG
   d. PPS

3. The set of patient attributes that is used to define each MS-DRG consists of:
   a. principal diagnosis, secondary diagnosis, insurance policy rules, principal procedure, and patient age
   b. principal procedure, discharge status, patient age and sex, and principal diagnosis
   c. principal and secondary diagnosis, principal procedure, patient age and sex, and discharge status
   d. discharge status, principal and secondary diagnosis, principal procedure, sex

4. A four-digit classification system that identifies and explains services or procedures and the location in which they were rendered is called a(n):
   a. ancillary code
   b. revenue code
   c. billing code
   d. accommodation code

5. CMS delegates the daily operation of the Medicare program to:
   a. DHHS
   b. PRO
   c. RVU
   d. MACs

6. The Omnibus Budget Reconciliation Act of 1986 required a PPS-based payment system to replace the one based on existing outpatient hospital cost. This system is what classification system?
   a. MS-DRGs
   b. APCs
   c. CPT
   d. ICD-9-CM

7. This part of Medicare covers the inpatient hospital portion:
   a. Part A
   b. Part B
   c. Part C
   d. Part D

8. This issue of the *Federal Register* contains outpatient facility changes for CMS programs for the coming year:
   a. October/November
   b. November/December
   c. December/October
   d. November/August

9. Using the UB-04 claim form in Figure 2-10, choose the fields in which the patient's name, address, and date of birth would be placed.
   a. 10, 5, and 14
   b. 12, 13, and 18
   c. 1, 2, and 3
   d. 8, 9, and 10

10. Entity responsible for development of the plan that outlines monitoring of the Medicare program:
    a. MACs
    b. OIG
    c. DHSS
    d. HEW

REIMBURSEMENT QUIZ ANSWERS

1. b	6. b
2. d	7. a
3. d	8. b
4. b	9. d
5. d	10. b

Overview of CPT, ICD-9-CM, and HCPCS Coding

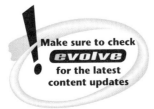

Make sure to check **evolve** for the latest content updates

■ INTRODUCTION TO MEDICAL CODING

Translates services/procedures/supplies/drugs into CPT/HCPCS/ICD-9-CM procedural codes

Translates diagnosis(es) into ICD-9-CM codes

Three Levels of Service Codes

1. Level I CPT

2. Level II HCPCS, National Codes

3. Level III Local Codes—phased out with implementation of HIPAA code sets

Diagnosis Codes, ICD-9-CM

ICD-9-CM, Volumes 1 and 2, *International Classification of Diseases,* 9th ed., Clinical Modification

Volume 1, Tabular List

Volume 2, Alphabetic List

Volume 3, Index and Tabular of Procedures

- Classification system

- The diagnosis explains why service was provided

- Specific in nature and may be up to five numeric or alphanumeric places

- Diabetes becomes 250.XX

■ CPT

Developed by the AMA in 1966

Five-digit codes to report services provided to patients

Updated each November for use January 1

Incorrect Coding

Results in providers being paid inappropriately (either overpayment or underpayment)

Inpatient Services

Reported on standardized insurance form

- CMS-1450/Universal Billing Form 04 (UB-04) (see Figure 2-11)

Outpatient Services

Reported on CMS-1500

CPT/HCPCS Level I Modifiers

Indicates anatomical site of procedure or service

Alters CPT or HCPCS code

Full list, CPT, Appendix A

- Two separate lists
    1. One for physicians to use
    2. One for hospital outpatient facilities to use

Modifier Functions

Altered (i.e., more or less)

Bilateral

Multiple

Only portions of service (i.e., professional service only)

More than one surgeon

ASC Modifiers

-25 Significant, Separately Identifiable E/M Service, by Same Physician on the Same Day of Procedure or Other Service

Documentation must support service

Example: Patient seen for sinus congestion; hospital-based physician performs H&P, prescribes decongestant, notes lesion on back, and removes it

Code: E/M-25 + Procedure

-27 Multiple Outpatient Hospital E/M Encounters on the Same Day

Separate and distinct E/M encounters

Performed in multiple outpatient hospital settings

Used only with E/M services

-50 Bilateral Procedure

Body is bilateral

Example: Procedure on hands

Caution: Some codes describe bilateral procedures

Typically not used on integumentary codes when reporting services

NOTE: Modifier -51 is not used when reporting facility services

-52 Reduced Services

Services reduced from those in code description

There is no other code that accurately reflects the service actually provided

Physician directed reduction

Documentation substantiates reduction

Procedure discontinued after IV sedation administered

Not for patient unable to pay

-58 Staged or Related Procedure by the Same Physician During the Postoperative Period

Subsequent procedure planned at time of initial surgery

- During postoperative period of previous surgery in series

    Example: Multiple skin grafts completed in several sessions

- Do not use when code describes a session

    Example: 67208 lesion destruction of retina, one or more sessions

- Therapeutic procedure performed during the global period of a diagnostic procedure

    Example: Surgical biopsy of breast followed by subsequent mastectomy

-59 Distinct Procedural Service

Used to report services not normally reported together

Different session or encounter

Different procedure

Different site

Separate incision, excision, lesion, injury

    Example: Physician removes several lesions from patient's leg, also notes a suspicious lesion on torso and biopsies the torso lesion

- Excision code for lesion removal + biopsy code for torso lesion with -59

- Indicates biopsy as distinct procedure, not part of lesion removal

-73 Discontinued Outpatient Hospital/Ambulatory Surgery Center (ASC) Procedure Prior to the Administration of Anesthesia

Procedure stopped due to patient's condition

After surgical preparation and sedation

Prior to administration of anesthesia

-74 Discontinued Outpatient Hospital/Ambulatory Surgery Center (ASC) Procedure after Administration of Anesthesia

Procedure stopped due to patient's condition

After administration of anesthesia

May be after procedure begins

    Example: Intubation started or incision was made

-76 Repeat Procedure or Service by Same Physician

NOTE: "Same Physician"

Used to indicate necessary service

> *Example:* X-rays before and after fracture repair

-77 Repeat Procedure by Another Physician

NOTE: "Another Physician"

Performed by one physician, repeated by another physician

Submitted with written report to establish medical necessity

-78 Unplanned Return to Operating/Procedure Room by the Same Physician Following Initial Procedure for a Related Procedure During Postoperative Period

For complication of first procedure

> *Example:* Patient has outpatient procedure in morning, returned to operating room in afternoon with severe hemorrhage

Indicates charge is not typographical error

- Medical record must specifically document need for service provided

-79 Unrelated Procedure or Service by Same Physician During Postoperative Period

> *Example:* Several days after discharge for procedure, patient returns for unrelated problem

- Diagnosis code would also be different

-91 Repeat Clinical Diagnostic Laboratory Test

Repeat same laboratory tests on same day for multiple test results

- e.g., serial troponin levels for acute MI confirmation

No tests rerun to confirm original test results

No malfunction of equipment or technician error

HCPCS Level II Modifiers

Examples of Anatomical Modifiers

-LT Left side

-RT Right side

-E1 Upper left, eyelid

-E2 Lower left, eyelid

-E3 Upper right, eyelid

-E4 Lower right, eyelid

-FA Left hand, thumb

-F1   Left hand, second digit

-F2   Left hand, third digit

-F3   Left hand, fourth digit

-F4   Left hand, fifth digit

-F5   Right hand, thumb

-F6   Right hand, second digit

-F7   Right hand, third digit

-F8   Right hand, fourth digit

-F9   Right hand, fifth digit

-TA   Left foot, great toe

-T1   Left foot, second digit

-T2   Left foot, third digit

-T3   Left foot, fourth digit

-T4   Left foot, fifth digit

-T5   Right foot, great toe

-T6   Right foot, second digit

-T7   Right foot, third digit

-T8   Right foot, fourth digit

-T9   Right foot, fifth digit

-LC   Left circumflex, coronary artery

-LD   Left anterior descending coronary artery

-RC   Right coronary artery

Anatomical modifiers are not used with skin procedures

> ***Example:*** Removal of skin tags, any area

Exception is with codes that indicate feet, hands, fingers, legs, arms, and eyelids

The Index

Used to locate service/procedure terms and codes

Speeds up code location

Serves as a dictionary

- First entries and last entries on top of page
- Code display in index
  - Single code: 38115
  - Multiple codes: 26645, 26650
  - Range of codes: 22305-22325

Location Methods

Service/procedure: Repair, excision

Anatomical site: Medial nerve, elbow

Condition or disease: Cleft lip, clot

Synonym: Toe and interphalangeal joint

Eponym: Jones Procedure, Heller Operation

Abbreviation: ECG, PEEP (Positive end-expiratory pressure)

"See" in index

Cross-reference terms: "Look here for code"

Index: Stem, Brain: *See* Brainstem

Appendices of CPT

Appendix A: Modifiers and Modifiers for ASC

Appendix B: Additions, Deletions, Revisions

Appendix C: Clinical Examples, E/M Codes

Appendix D: Add-On Codes

Appendix E: -51 Exempt Codes

Appendix F: -63 Exempt Codes

Appendix G: Conscious (Moderate) Sedation

Appendix H: Performance Measures, Category II Modifiers

Appendix I: Genetic Testing Modifiers

Appendix J: Electrodiagnostic Medicine Listing of Sensory, Motor, and Mixed Nerves

Appendix K: Products Pending FDA Approval

Appendix L: Vascular Families

Appendix M: Crosswalk to Deleted CPT Codes

Be certain to review information in CPT appendices before the examination

■ EVALUATION AND MANAGEMENT (E/M) SECTION (99201-99499)

Outpatient

One who has not been admitted to a health care facility

Example: Patient receives services at clinic or same-day surgery center

Inpatient

One who has been formally admitted to a health care facility

Example: Patient admitted to hospital or nursing home

Physician dictates

• Admission orders

- H&P (history and physical)

- Requests for consultations

Emergency Department (ED) Services (99281-99285)
No distinction between new and established patients

To qualify as ED (ER), facility must be open 24 hours a day

5 ED codes do not report all ED services

- The codes report only physician services during an encounter, not all interventions provided during encounter (Figure 3-1)

- Services provided in addition to the interventions are reported separately

  - For example, sutures, debridement, etc., are reported in addition to the ED CPT code

  - Each ED develops its own method of implementation of charge grid

Level 1—99281	Level 2—99282	Level 3—99283
1. Initial (triage) assessment 2. Suture removal 3. Wound recheck 4. Note for work or school 5. Simple discharge information	Interventions from previous level plus any of the following: 1. OTC med administration 2. Tetanus booster 3. Bedside diagnostic tests (stool hemoccult, glucometer) 4. Visual acuity 5. Orthostatic vital signs 6. Simple trauma not requiring x-ray 7. Simple discharge information	Interventions from previous level plus any of the following: 1. Heparin/saline lock 2. Crystalloid IV therapy 3. X-ray, one area 4. RX med administration 5. Fluorescein stain 6. Quick cath 7. Foley cath 8. Receipt of ambulance patient 9. Mental health emergencies (mild) not requiring parenteral medications or admission 10. Moderate complexity discharge instructions 11. Intermediate layered and complex laceration repair
Level 4—99284	**Level 5—99285**	**Critical Care 99291, 99292**
Interventions from previous level plus any of the following: 1. X-ray, multiple areas 2. Special imaging studies (CT, MRI, ultrasound) 3. Cardiac monitoring 4. Multiple reassessments of patient 5. Parenteral[1] medications (including insulin) 6. Nebulizer treatment (1 or 2) 7. NG placement 8. Pelvic exam 9. Mental health emergencies (moderate). May require parenteral medications but not admission 10. Administration of IV medications [1]*not through the alimentary canal but rather by injection through some other route, such as subcutaneous, intramuscular, intraorbital, intracapsular, intraspinal, intrasternal, or intravenous*	Interventions from previous level plus any of the following: 1. Monitor/stabilize patient during in hospital transport and/or testing (CT, MRI, ultrasound) 2. Vasoactive medication 3. Administration (dopamine, dobutamine, multiple) nebulizer treatments (3 or more) 4. Conscious sedation 5. Lumbar puncture 6. Thoracentesis 7. Sexual assault exam 8. Admission to hospital 9. Mental health emergency (severe) psychotic and/or agitated/combative 10. Requires admission 11. Fracture/dislocation reduction 12. Suicide precautions 13. Gastric lavage 14. Complex discharge instructions	Interventions from any previous level plus any of the following: 1. Multiple parenteral medications 2. Continuous monitoring 3. Major trauma care 4. Chest tube insertion 5. CPR 6. Defibrillation/cardioversion 7. Delivery of baby 8. Control of major hemorrhage 9. Administration of blood or blood products

Figure **3-1** Example of ED acuity sheet.

Example:

1. One ED may develop method in which when two elements in Level 3 are provided and one element in Level 4 is provided, Level 4 (99284) is reported

2. Second ED may develop method in which when two elements in Level 3 are provided and one element in Level 4 is provided, Level 3 (99283) is reported

For the purposes of the worktext, the level is assigned based on the highest level of service provided, as in Example 1

Critical Care (99289-99300) and ED Codes
ED services often require additional codes from Critical Care Services

Example: Multiple organ failure

Critical Care Services are provided to patients in life-threatening (critically ill or injured) situations

- 99281-99285 collapse into Level 1, 2, or 3 under APC system
  - Hospital determines what level the codes are in

    For example,

    99281 = Level 1

    99282 & 99283 = Level 2

    99284 & 99285 = Level 3

  OR

    99281 & 99282 = Level 1

    99283 & 99284 = Level 2

    99285 = Level 3

- Levels are reimbursed at different rates by CMS
  - For example, for ED levels reimbursed
    - Level 1 ED $74.70
    - Level 2 ED $130.77
    - Level 3 ED $226.30
- Both Critical Care codes (99291 & 99292) are included in Critical Care and reimbursed at $491.01 (not a time-based payment)

APC (Ambulatory Patient Classification) Levels of Service

Facilities report ED services for non-OPPS patients using CPT codes

- There are five ED CPT codes (99281-99285) (see Figure 3-1)

For Medicare only under OPPS, these five codes collapse into 3 levels

- Three levels are 610, 611, and 612

Number of levels is dependent upon facility protocol

Example:

- 610 Low Level Emergency Visits (would be equal to 99281 and 99282)
- 611 Mid Level Emergency Visits (would be equal to 99283 and 99284)
- 612 High Level Emergency Visits (would be equal to 99285)

Another facility may define the levels as follows

- 610 Low Level Emergency Visits (would be equal to 99281)
- 611 Mid Level Emergency Visits (would be equal to 99282 and 99283)
- 612 High Level Emergency Visits (would be equal to 99284 and 99285)

Each level includes a baseline level of service

- Baseline services are
  - Registration
  - Initial Nursing Assessment
  - Periodic Vital Signs
  - Discharge Instructions
  - Exam Room setup/cleanup
  - Limited intervention using

Minimal resources

- 10 Minutes or less staff contact

  Examples:
  - Administration of oral medications
  - Initiation of oxygen therapy
  - Obtaining lab specimens

Levels ascend based upon

- Increase in staff time
- Additional interventions

  Examples:
  - Extended initial nursing assessment or discharge
  - Starting an IV
  - Insertions of tubes (catheters, Foleys, or nasogastric)

Each hospital creates its own set of internal guidelines to determine in which level each Critical Care and ED CPT code is included

- CMS directs only that the system is reasonable and relates to resource intensity
- Does not direct which CPT codes go in each APC level

Critical care codes collapse into 1 APC

- 620 Critical Care

Uses of Anesthesia

Relieve pain

Manage unconscious patients, life functions, and resuscitation

Analgesia

Relief of pain

Some Methods of Anesthesia

Endotracheal: Through mouth

Local: Application to area (injection or topical)

Epidural: Between vertebral spaces

Regional: Field or nerve

MAC: Monitored anesthesia care

Patient-Controlled Analgesia (PCA)

Patient administers drug

Used to relieve chronic pain or temporarily for severe pain following surgery

Moderate (Conscious) Sedation

To be used when surgeon administers sedation himself/herself

- No anesthesia personnel are present

Decreased level of consciousness

Report with 99143-99145 (Medicine)

Presence of trained observer, such as a nurse, is required

Second physician administered sedation, report 99148-99150

SURGERY SECTION (10021-69990)

Largest CPT section

Each year CMS publishes a list of CPT surgery codes that are paid only as an inpatient procedure

- For example, 33300-33335, repair of wounds of the heart and great vessels, are inpatient procedures
  - Whereas 33282-33284, implantation or removal of cardiac event recorders, are paid as outpatient procedures
- Inpatient procedures reported with Volume 3 procedure codes
- Outpatient procedures reported with CPT surgery codes

Section Format

Divided by subspecialty (e.g., integumentary, cardiovascular)

Notes and Guidelines

Throughout section

Information varied and extensive

"Must" reading

Subsection notes apply to entire subsection

Subheading notes apply to entire subheading

Category notes apply to entire category

Parenthetical information (Figure 3-2)

Unlisted Procedure Codes

Used only when more specific code not found in Category I or Category III

Written report accompanies submission

Each unlisted code service paid on case-by-case basis

Separate Procedures

"(Separate procedure)" follows code description

Usually minor surgical procedure

Incidental to more major procedure

- Breast biopsy

- Biopsy before radical mastectomy would not be coded

- Appendectomy performed routinely when other abdominal surgery is performed

Separate procedures reported when

- Only procedure performed

- With another procedure

  - On different site

  - Unrelated to major procedure

GENERAL SUBSECTION (10021, 10022)

Fine needle aspirations with or without (w/wo) imaging guidance

Pathology 88172 and 88173 for evaluation of aspirate

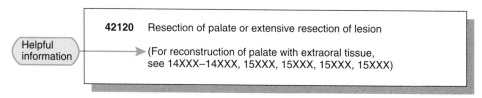

Figure **3-2** Parenthetical information in the CPT manual.

INTEGUMENTARY SYSTEM SUBSECTION (10040-19499)

Often used in all specialties of medicine

Used not just by surgeons or dermatologists but by a wide range of physicians

Subheadings of Integumentary Subsection

- Skin, Subcutaneous, and Accessory Structures
- Nails
- Repair (Closure)
- Introduction
- Destruction
- Breast

Skin, Subcutaneous, and Accessory Structures (10040-11646)

Incision and Drainage (10040-10180)

I&D of abscess, carbuncle, boil, cyst, infection, hematoma, pilonidal cyst

- Lancing (cutting of skin)
- Aspiration (removal by puncturing lesion with a needle and withdrawing fluid)

Gauze or tube may be inserted for continued drainage

Pilonidal cyst

- Also known as a pilonidal abscess
- May be incised and drained (10080, 10081) or excised (11770-11772)

Excision—Debridement (11000-11044)

Dead tissue cut away and washed away with sterile saline

11000-11001 Eczematous or infected skin

11004-11006 Debridement of infected area based on location and **depth** of necrotizing tissue (subcutaneous, muscle, fascia)

+11008 Removal of prosthetic material or mesh from abdominal wall

11010-11012 Foreign material with fracture or dislocation

11040-11044 Skin, subcutaneous muscle, bone

Paring or Cutting (11055-11057)

Removal by scraping or peeling (e.g., removal of corn or callus)

Codes indicate number: 1, 2-4, 4+

Biopsy (11100-11101)

Skin, subcutaneous tissue, or mucous membrane biopsy

Not all of lesion removed

- All of lesion removed = excision

Codes indicate number: 1 or each additional

Tissue that is removed during excision, shave, etc., and submitted to pathology is NOT reported separately as a biopsy

- Rather, it is included in the code for the excision

Skin Tag Removal (11200-11201)
Benign lesions

Removed with scissors, blade, chemicals, cryosurgery, electrosurgery, etc.

Codes indicate number: Up to 15 and each additional 10 lesions

Shaving of Lesions (11300-11313)
Removed by transverse incision or sliced horizontally

Based on

- Size (e.g., 1.1-2.0 cm)

- Location (e.g., arm, hand, nose)

Does not require suture closure

Benign/Malignant Lesions (11400-11646)
Codes divided: Benign or malignant

Physician assesses lesion as benign or malignant

Codes include local anesthesia and simple closure

Report each excised lesion separately

Lesion size

- Taken from physician's notes

- Includes greatest diameter plus margins (Figure 3-3)

  Example: A benign lesion measuring 0.5 cm at widest point is removed with 0.5 cm-margin at narrowest point (each side, 0.5 + 0.5 = 1.0 cm). Reported as 1.5-cm lesion excision (11402)

  - Do not take size from pathology report—storage solution shrinks tissue

  - Includes greatest diameter plus margins

  - Margins (healthy tissue) are also taken for comparison with unhealthy tissue

  Example: 1-cm lesion with 2-cm margin left and right of lesion

  1 + 2 + 2 = 5 cm

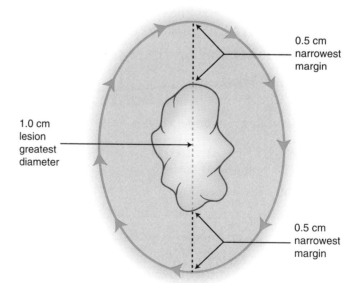

Figure **3-3** Calculating the size of a lesion.

- Re-excisions following initial excision of malignant lesion coded as excision of malignant lesion

All excised tissue pathologically examined

Codes 11400-11646 report excision of lesion

Codes 17000-17286 report destruction

Destroyed lesions have no pathology samples

> *Example:* Laser, cryosurgery, or chemical destruction (lysis)

Lesion closure

- Simple or subcutaneous closure included in removal

- Reported separately

  - Layered or intermediate, 12031-12057 (Repair—Intermediate)

  - Complex, 13100-13153 (Repair—Complex)

Nails (11719-11765)

Includes toes and fingers

Types of services

- Trimming, debridement, removal, biopsy, repair

Introduction (11900-11983)

Types of Services
- Lesion injections (therapeutic or diagnostic), tattooing, tissue expansion, contraceptive insertion/removal, hormone implantation services, and insertion/removal of nonbiodegradable drug-delivery implant

Repair (12001-13160)

Repair Factors in Wound Repair
As types of wounds vary, types of wound repair also vary

Length, complexity (simple, intermediate, complex), and site must be documented

- Length measured in centimeters

- Measured prior to closure

Types of Wound Repair
Simple: Superficial, epidermis, dermis, or subcutaneous tissue

- One-layer closure

- Dermabond closure

- Medicare patients report Dermabond closure with G0168

Intermediate: Layered closure of deeper layers of subcutaneous tissue and superficial fascia with skin closure

- Single-layer closure can be coded as intermediate if extensive debridement is required

Complex: Greater than layered; may include multiple layers of tissue and fascia or extensive debridement

> *Example:* Scar revision, complicated debridement, extensive undermining, stents, extensive retention sutures

Included in Wound Repair Codes
Simple ligation of vessels in an open wound

Simple exploration of nerves, blood vessels, and exposed tendons

Normal debridement

- Additional codes for debridement can be used when
  - Gross contamination requires prolonged cleaning
  - Appreciable amounts of devitalized/contaminated tissue are removed to expose healthy tissue
  - Debridement is provided without immediate primary closure

Grouping of Wound Repair
Add together lengths by

- Complexity of wound
  - Simple, intermediate, complex
- Location of wound
  - e.g., face, ears, eyelids, nose, lips

1 inch = 2.54 cm

> *Example:* **Same complexity, same codes description location:**
> Intermediate repairs of 2.9-cm laceration of leg and 1.1-cm laceration of buttocks. 2.9 + 1.1 = 4.0 cm (12032)

> *Example:* **Different complexity:** Intermediate repair of 2.9-cm laceration of leg and simple repair of 1.1-cm laceration of buttocks. 2.9-cm intermediate repair (12032) and 1.1-cm simple repair (12001)

> *Example:* **Same complexity, different code description locations:**
> Intermediate repair of 2.9-cm laceration of leg and intermediate repair of 1.1-cm laceration of nose. 2.9-cm intermediate repair of leg (12032) and 1.1-cm intermediate repair of nose (12051)

Do not Group Wound Repairs that are
Different complexities

> *Example:* Simple repair and complex repair

Different locations as stated in the code description

> *Example:* Simple repairs of scalp (12001) and nose (12011)

Adjacent Tissue Transfer, Flaps, and Grafts (14000-15776)

Information Needed to Code Graft
Type of graft—adjacent, free, flap, etc.

Donor site (from)

Recipient site (to)

Any repair to donor site

Size of graft

Adjacent Tissue Transfer/Rearrangement (14000-14300)
Includes excision and/or repair (e.g., Z-plasty, W-plasty, V-plasty, Y-plasty, rotation flap, advancement flap)

Codes based on size and location of graft

Measure site of defect from excision plus size of defect from flap design for total size

Skin Replacement Surgery and Skin Substitutes (15002-15431)
15002-15005 Site preparation based on size and site

15040 Harvest for tissue culture

15050-15431 Graft codes by type

Split-thickness: Epidermis and some dermis (Figure 3-4)

Full-thickness: Epidermis and all dermis

Grafts (15300-15431)
Bilaminate skin substitute

• Artificial skin, such as silicone covered nylon mesh

Allograft: Donor graft

Xenograft: Nonhuman donor

Code is based on recipient site, not donor site

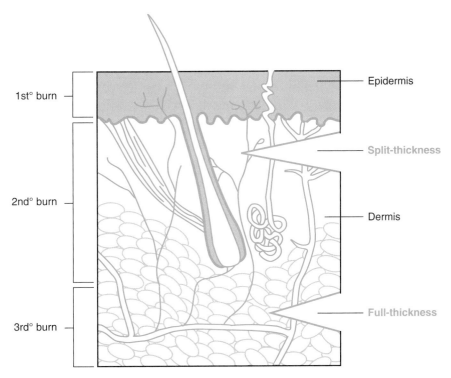

Figure **3-4** Split-thickness and full-thickness skin grafts.

Flap (15570-15776)
Some skin left attached to blood supply

• Keeps flap viable

Donor site may be far from recipient site

Flaps may be in stages

Codes divided by location and size

Formation of flap (15570-15576)

• Based on recipient location: Trunk, scalp, nose, etc.

Transfer of flap (15650): Previously placed flap released from donor site

• Also known as walking or walk up of flap

Muscle, Myocutaneous, or Fasciocutaneous Flaps (15732-15738)

• Based on recipient location: head and neck, trunk, upper or lower extremity

• Repairs made with

  • Muscle

  • Muscle and skin

  • Fascia and skin

• Flaps rotated from donor to recipient site

• Includes closure donor site

Other Procedures (15780-15879)
Many cosmetic procedures including:

• Dermabrasion

• Chemical peel

• Blepharoplasty

• Rhytidectomy

• Excessive skin excision

Pressure (Decubitus) Ulcers (15920-15999)
Excision and various closures

• Primary, skin flap, muscle, etc.

Many codes "with ostectomy"

• Bone removal

Locations

• Coccygeal (end of spine)

• Sacral (between hips)

• Ischial (lower hip)

• Trochanteric (outer hip)

Site preparation only: 15936, 15946, or 15956

• Defect repair of donor site reported separately

Burns Treatment (16000-16036)
Codes for small, medium, and large

Must calculate percentage of body burned using the Rule of Nines for adults (Figure 3-5)

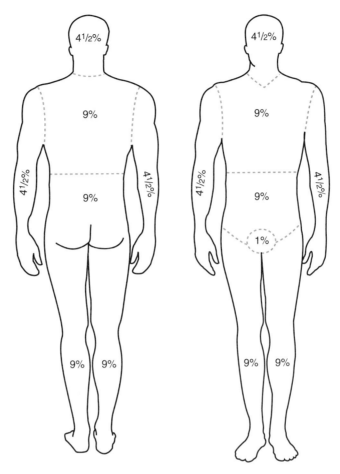

Figure **3-5** The Rule of Nines is used to calculate burn area on an adult.

- <5% = small
- 5% to 10% = medium
- >10% = large

Lund-Browder for children (Figure 3-6)

- Proportions of children differ from those of adults
- Heads are larger

Often require multiple debridements and redressing

Based on

- Initial treatment of 1st-degree burn (16000)
- Size

Report percent of burn and depth

Escharotomies are performed only on an inpatient basis (16035-16036)

Destruction (17000-17286)
Ablation (destruction) of tissue

- Laser, electrosurgery, cryosurgery, chemosurgery, etc.
- Benign/premalignant or malignant tissue
- Malignant tissue is based on location and size
- Benign/premalignant is based on the number of lesions removed

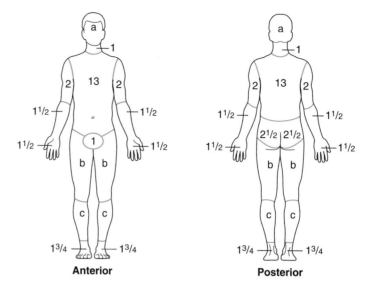

Relative percentage of body surface areas (% BSA) affected by growth

	0 yr	1 yr	5 yr	10 yr	15 yr
a – 1/2 of head	9 1/2	8 1/2	6 1/2	5 1/2	4 1/2
b – 1/2 of 1 thigh	2 3/4	3 1/4	4	4 1/4	4 1/2
c – 1/2 of lower leg	2 1/2	2 1/2	2 3/4	3	3 1/4

Figure **3-6** Lund-Browder chart for estimating the extent of burns on children.

Mohs' Microscope Surgery (17311-17315)
Surgeon acts as pathologist and surgeon

Removes one layer of lesion at a time

Continues until no malignant cells remain

Based on stages and number of specimens per stage indicated in medical record

Other Procedures (17340-17999)
Treatment of acne

- Cryotherapy

- Chemical exfoliation

- Electrolysis

- Unlisted procedures

Breast Procedures (19000-19499)
Divided based on procedure

- Incision

- Excision

- Introduction

- Mastectomy procedures

- Repair/Reconstruction

Use excision of lesion codes if entire lesion is removed during incisional biopsy

Use additional codes for placement of radiological markers

- Code each marker placement separately

Mastectomies based on extent of procedure

- Wide excision
  - Removal of neoplasm, capsule, and surrounding margins
- Radical
  - Wide excision and anatomical structure surrounding neoplasm

  Example: Muscle or fascia
  - Performed on an inpatient basis
- Conservative partial mastectomy in which lesion is removed with adequate margins, 19301
- Axillary dissection and partial mastectomy, 19302
- Radical and modified radical, 19305, 19306, and 19307, based on extent

Confirm whether pectoral muscles, axillary, or internal lymph nodes were removed

19307 most common and includes breast and axillary lymph node removal

Code removal of lymph nodes separately unless included in code description

Bilateral procedures, use -50

Biopsy/Removal of Lesion

Incisional biopsy: Incision made into lesion and small portion of lesion removed

Excisional biopsy: Entire lesion removed

Open incisional biopsy most complex (19101)

Percutaneous core needle biopsy with imaging guidance (19100)

- Same procedure without imaging guidance is 19102

Automated vacuum assisted or rotating biopsy device described in 19103 is the use of advanced breast biopsy instrumentation

- Image guidance performed by physician reported separately
- Complete, simple removal of a mass is reported with 19120

Lesion may be preoperatively marked by placing thin wire (radiologic marker) down to lesion

- Wire placement reported separately (19290)
- Additional wires reported with 19291
- Metallic localization clips may be placed during biopsy operative session so the site can be located later, if necessary
- Placement of clip reported with 19295, once for each clip placed
- Image guidance performed by physician reported separately

MUSCULOSKELETAL SYSTEM SUBSECTION (20000-29999)

Subsection divided: Anatomical site, then service (e.g., excision)

Used extensively by orthopedic surgeons

- Many codes commonly used by variety of physicians

Extensive notes

Most common

- Fracture and dislocation treatments
- "General" subheading
- Arthroscopic procedures
- Casting and strapping

Eponyms are "things" named after "people"

> **Example:** Barr procedure is a tendon transfer of the lower leg (27690-27692), and Mitchell Chevron procedure is a complex metatarsal osteotomy (bunion correction) (28296)

- Procedures are often referred to with eponyms
- Check the index of the CPT manual for directions to eponym codes

Fracture Treatment

Type of treatment depends on type and severity of fracture

Diagnosis codes must support the procedure codes and document the medical necessity

Open: Surgically opened to view or remotely opened to place nail across fracture site

- Open reduction with internal fixation is ORIF

Closed: Not surgically opened

Percutaneous: Insertion of devices through skin or a remote site

Treatment terms should not be confused with **types** of fractures:

- Open fracture: Fractured bone penetrates skin
- Closed fracture: Fractured bone does not penetrate skin

Traction

- Application of force to align bone
- Force applied by internal device (e.g., wire, pin) inserted into bone (skeletal fixation)
- Application of force by means of adhesion to skin (skin traction)

Manipulation
Use of force to return bone back to normal alignment

Codes often divided based on whether manipulation was or was not used

Dislocation
Bone displaced from normal joint position

Treatment: Return bone to normal joint location

Subheading "General"
Begins "Incision" (20000-20005)

Depth makes difference between choice of Integumentary or Musculoskeletal incision codes

Musculoskeletal code used when underlying bone or muscle is involved

Wound Exploration (20100-20103)

Traumatic penetrating wounds

Divided on wound location

Includes

- Surgical exploration

- Enlargement

- Debridement

- Removal of foreign body (bodies)

- Ligation

- Repair of tissue and muscle

Use additional code for repair of major structures or blood vessels

Not used for integumentary repairs

- Unless the repair requires extension, enlargement, or exploration

Excision (20150-20251)

Biopsies for bone and muscle

Divided by

- Type of biopsy (bone/muscle)

- Depth

- Some by method

Can be percutaneous needle or excisional

Does not include tumor excision, which is coded separately

Biopsy with excision: Code only excision

Introduction or Removal (20500-20694)

Codes for

- Injections

- Aspirations

- Insertions

- Applications

- Removals

- Adjustments

Therapeutic sinus tract injection procedures

- Not nasal sinus

- Abscess or cyst with passage (sinus tract) to skin

- Antibiotic injected with use of radiographic guidance

Removal of foreign bodies lodged in muscle or tendon sheath

Integumentary removal codes for removal from skin

Injection into

- Tendon sheath
- Tendon origin
- Ligament
- Ganglion cyst
- Trigger points

Placement of needles or catheters into muscle and/or soft tissue

- For interstitial radioelement application

Arthrocentesis injection "and/or" aspiration of a joint

- Both aspiration and injection reported with one code (20600-20610)
- Codes based on joint size: Small, intermediate, major
- Do not unbundle and report aspiration/injection with two codes

External Fixation (20690-20694)

Device that holds bone in place

- Application, adjustment, removal under anesthesia

Code fracture treatment and external fixation

- Unless treatment and fixation both included in fracture care code description
- Adjustment to (20693) and removal of (20694) EID are coded separately

Replantation (20802-20838)

Used to report reattachment of amputated limb

Code by body area

Performed only on an inpatient basis

Grafts (20900-20938)

Autogenous Grafts

Used to report harvesting through separate incision of

- Bone
- Cartilage
- Tendon
- Fascia lata
- Tissue

Fascia lata grafts: From lower thigh where fascia is thickest

Some codes include obtaining grafting material (then, not coded separately)

Modifier -51 exempt

Other Procedures (20950-20999)

Monitoring muscle fluid pressure (interstitial for compartment syndrome, etc.)

- Pressure increases when blood supply decreases due to increased accumulation of fluids

Bone grafts identified by site taken from (donor site)

Free osseocutaneous flaps: Bone grafts

• Taken along with skin and tissue overlying bone

Electrical stimulation

• Used to speed bone healing

• Placement of stimulators externally or internally

• Ultrasound also used externally

Arthrodesis

Fixation of joint (arthro = joint, desis = fusion)

• Fixation with pins, wires, rods, etc. to immobilize the joint

Often performed with other procedure such as fracture repair

• Arthrodesis of the spine is also called spinal fusion

Subsequent Subheadings

After General subheading, divided by anatomical location

• Anatomical subheadings divided by type of procedure

   Example: Subheading "Head" divided by procedure

• Incision

• Excision

• Manipulation

• Head Prosthesis

• Introduction or Removal

• Repair, Revision, and/or Reconstruction

• Other Procedures

• Fracture and/or Dislocation

Spinal Instrumentation and Fixation

Insertion of spinal instrumentation reported in addition to arthrodesis (fusion)

Many codes are add-on and are reported in addition to definitive procedure

Spine (Ventral Column), 22100-22855, divided by repair location

• Cervical (C1-C7)

   • C1 = Atlas

   • C2 = Axis

• Thoracic (T1-T12)

• Lumbar (L1-L5)

• Sacral (S1)

Coccyx (tailbone)

Vertebral segment: Single complete vertebral bone with articular processes and laminae

Vertebral interspace: Non-bony compartment between two vertebral bodies which contains the disk

Single level = two vertebrae and the disk that separates them

Percutaneous vertebroplasty

- Use of polymethylmethacrylate injected into the vertebral space

- Polymethylmethacrylate is a type of bone cement/glue like silicone but not silicone

- Adheres bone fragments together

- Fills vertebral body defects

Types of spinal instrumentation

Segmental: Devices at each end of repair area plus at least one other attachment

Nonsegmental: Devices at each end of defect only

Approach: Pay special attention to the approach used to perform the surgery

- Several different approaches to spine: Most common anterior (front) and posterior (back)

- Most spinal instrumentation codes divided based on approach

Spinal instrumentation procedures are performed only on an inpatient basis

Casting and Strapping (29000-29799)

Replacement procedure or initial placement to stabilize when provided without additional restorative treatment

> *Example:* Application of wrist splint or cast for wrist sprain

Initial fracture treatment includes placement and removal of first cast

- Subsequent cast applications coded separately

- Payers have strict individual reimbursement policies for subsequent casting

Application not coded when part of surgical procedure

> *Example:* Repair of radial fracture includes application of cast or splint

Ace bandage applications not billed separately

Removal bundled into surgical procedure

Supplies reported separately

Endoscopy/Arthroscopy (29800-29999)

Surgical arthroscopy always includes diagnostic arthroscopy

Codes divided by joint

- Subdivided by procedure

- Be aware of subterms and bundled procedures within code descriptions

NOTE: Parenthetical information following codes indicates codes to use if procedure was an open procedure

RESPIRATORY SYSTEM SUBSECTION (30000-32999)

Anatomical site arrangement:

- Nose

- Larynx

Further subdivided by procedure:

- Incision
- Excision

Endoscopy

Endoscopy in all subheadings except Nose

Each preceded by "Notes"

Endoscopy Rule One
Code full extent

> *Example:* Procedure begins at mouth and ends at bronchial tube

Bronchial tube = full extent

Endoscopy Rule Two
Code correct approach

> *Example:* For removal:

- Interior lung lesion via endoscopy inserted through mouth
- Exterior lung lesion via laparoscope inserted through skin

Incorrect approach = incorrect code = incorrect reimbursement

Endoscopy Rule Three
Diagnostic always included in surgical

> *Examples:*

- Diagnostic bronchial endoscopy begins
- Identifies foreign body
- Removed foreign body (surgical endoscopy)

Multiple Procedures

Frequent in respiratory coding

- **Watch for bundled services**

Sequence primary procedure first, no modifier

Sequence secondary procedures next

Bilateral procedures often performed, use -50

Remember: Modifier -51 is not used in facility coding

Format for reporting chosen by payer

> *Example:* Nasal lavage

- 31000-50

Nose (30000-30999)

Used extensively by otorhinolaryngologists (ear, nose, and throat [ENT] specialists)

Also wide variety of trained physicians in other specialties

Approach to nose

• External approach, use Integumentary System

• Internal approaches, use Respiratory System

Incision (30000, 30020)
Bundled into Incision codes are drain or gauze insertion and removal

Supplies reported separately

Excision (30100-30160)
Contains intranasal biopsy codes

Polyp excision coded by complexity

• Excision includes any method of destruction, even laser

• Use -50 (bilateral) for both sides

Turbinate excision and resection

• Three turbinates: Superior, middle, inferior

• Excision of inferior turbinate, 30130

• Excision of superior or middle turbinate, 30999

• Submucous resection of inferior turbinate, 30140

   Reduction of inferior turbinates, 30140-52

• Submucous resection of superior or middle turbinate, 30999

Introduction (30200-30220)
Common procedures

   Example: Injections to shrink nasal tissue or displacement therapy (saline flushes) to remove mucus

Displacement therapy performed through nose

Removal of Foreign Body (30300-30320)
Distinguished by the site of removal, whether at office or in hospital (requires general anesthesia)

Repair (30400-30630)
Many plastic procedures, e.g.,

• Rhinoplasty (reshaping nose internal and/or external)

• Septoplasty (rearrangement or plastic repair of nasal septum)

Destruction (30801-30802)
Use of cauterization or ablation (removing by cutting)

Used for removal of excess nasal mucosa or to reduce inferior turbinate inflammation

Based on intramural or superficial extent of destruction

• **Intramural:** Deeper mucosa

• **Superficial:** Outer layer of mucosa

350

Other Procedures (30901-30999)
Control of nasal hemorrhage

- Packing

- Ligation

- Cauterization

Anterior packing for less severe bleeding

Posterior packing for more severe bleeding

Accessory Sinuses, Incision, Excision, Endoscopy (31000-31294)

Codes for lavage (washing) of sinuses

- Cannula (hollow tube) placed into sinus

- Sterile saline solution flushed through

Codes are divided by surgical approach: Incision, Excision, or Endoscopy

Procedures may involve multiple codes when multiple locations are accessed

> *Example:* 31020, sinusotomy, maxillary, can be coded with 31050 sinusotomy, sphenoid, and 31070 sinusotomy, frontal

Repair of fractures occurring during procedure may be coded separately if not included in code description

Use -50 (bilateral) for both sides

Maxillary sinusotomy may use an external and intranasal approach to creating passage between sinus and nose

- Used to clear blocked or infected sinus

- Intranasal sinusotomy, 31020

- External sinusotomy, radical (such as Caldwell-Luc)

  Access through mouth

  Incision above eyetooth

  Sinus is cleaned

  New opening created or old opening enlarged

Larynx (31000-31599)

Excision (31300-31420)
Laryngotomy: Open surgical procedure to expose larynx

- For removal procedure (e.g., tumor)

May be confused with Trachea/Bronchi codes for tracheostomy used to establish air flow

Introduction (31500-31502)
Used to establish, maintain, and protect air flow

Endotracheal intubation, establishment of airway

Based on planned (ventilation support) or emergency procedure

Laryngoscopic (Endoscopy) Procedures (31505-31579)
Uses terms *indirect* and *direct*

- **Indirect:** Tongue depressor with mirror used to view larynx

- **Direct:** Endoscope passed into larynx, physician directly views vocal cords

Repair (31580-31590)
Several plastic procedures and fracture repairs

Laryngoplasty procedures based on purpose

Fracture codes based on whether manipulation used

Trachea and Bronchi (31600-31899)

Incision (31600-31614)
Tracheostomy divided by

- Planned (ventilation support)

- Emergency

Divided by type

- Transtracheal or cricothyroid (location of incision)

Endoscopy (31615-31656)
Bronchoscopy tube may be inserted into nose or mouth

Rigid endoscopy performed under general anesthesia

Flexible endoscopy usually performed under local or conscious (moderate) sedation

Introduction (31715-31730)
Catheterization

Instillation

Injection

Aspiration

Tracheal tube placement

Some include inhaled gas as contrast material

Excision/Repair (31750-31830)
Plastic repairs of tracheoplasty and bronchoplasty

Lungs and Pleura (32035-32999)

Incision (32035-32225)
Thoracotomy. Surgical opening of chest to expose to view; used for

- Biopsy

- Cyst

- Foreign body removal

- Cardiac massage, etc.

Excision/Removal (32310-32540)
Biopsy codes in both Excision and Incision categories

- Excisional biopsy with percutaneous needle
- Incisional biopsy with chest open

Also services of pleurectomy, pneumocentesis, and lung removal

- **Segmentectomy:** 1 segment
- **Lobectomy:** 1 lobe
- **Bilobectomy:** 2 lobes
- **Total Pneumonectomy:** 1 lung

Thoracentesis. Needle inserted into pleural space for aspiration (withdrawal) of fluid or air (32421, 32422)

Introduction (32550, 32551)
- Insertion of indwelling tunneled pleural catheter
- Tube thoracostomy

Destruction (32560)
- Chemical pleurodesis

CARDIOVASCULAR (CV) SYSTEM SUBSECTION (33010-37799)

Cardiology Coding Terminology

Both Medicine and Surgery sections contain invasive procedures

Invasive: Enters body by the following methods

- Incisional

    Example: Opening chest for removal (e.g., tumor on heart)

- Percutaneously
    - Placement of catheter into artery or vein by means of

    Example: PTCA (percutaneous transluminal coronary artery) procedure

    - Wire threaded through needle and catheter slid over wire
    - Cut down—small nick made and catheter inserted

    Example: Catheter inserted into femoral or brachial artery

Common catheters are

- Broviac
- Hickman
- HydroCath
- Arrow multi-lumen
- Groshong
- Dual-lumen
- Triple-lumen

Noninvasive: Procedures that do not break skin

    Example: Electrocardiogram

Electrophysiology (EPS): Study of electrical system of heart

    Example: Study of irregular heartbeat (arrhythmia)

Nuclear Cardiology: Diagnostic and treatment specialty; uses radioactive substances to diagnose cardiac conditions

Example: MRI

■ Cardiovascular in Surgery Section

Codes for Procedures

Heart/Pericardium (33010-33999)

- Pacemakers, valve disorders

Arteries/Veins (34001-37799)

Heart/Pericardium (33010-33999)

Both percutaneous and open surgical

- Cardiologists often use percutaneous intervention; cardiovascular or thoracic surgeons often use open surgical procedures

Extensive notes throughout

Frequent changes with medical advances

Examples of categories of Heart/Pericardium subheading

- Pericardium
- Cardiac Tumor
- Pacemaker or Pacing Cardioverter-Defibrillator

Examples of services

- Pericardiocentesis: Percutaneous withdrawal of fluid from pericardial space (pericarditis)
- Cardiac Tumor: Open surgical procedure for removal of tumor on heart

Pacemakers and Cardioverter-Defibrillators (33202-33249)

Devices that assist heart in electrical function

- Differentiate between temporary and permanent devices
- Differentiate between one-chamber and dual-chamber devices

Divided by where pacer placed, approach, and type of service

Patient record indicates revision or replacement

- Pacemaker pulse generator is also called a battery
- Pacemaker leads are also called electrodes
- Usual follow-up 90 days (global period)

Placed

Atrium (single chamber)

- Pulse generator and one electrode in atrium (single-chamber pacemaker)

Ventricle (single chamber)

- Pulse generator and one electrode in ventricle (single-chamber pacemaker)

Both (dual chamber)

- Pulse generator and one electrode in right ventricle and one electrode in right atrium

Biventricular, both ventricles and atrium (uses 3 leads)

- Pulse generator and one electrode in right ventricle, one electrode in right atrium, and one electrode in left ventricle via the coronary sinus

Approach

Epicardial: Open procedure to place on heart

Transvenous: Through vein to place in heart

Type of service

Initial placement or replacement of all or part of device

Number of leads placed is important in code selection

Electrophysiologic Operative Procedures (33250-33266)

Surgeon repairs defect causing abnormal rhythm

Chest opened to full view

- Cardiopulmonary (CP) bypass usually used

Endoscopy procedure

- Without cardiopulmonary bypass

Codes based on reason for procedure and if CP bypass used

- Performed only on an inpatient basis

Patient-Activated Event Recorder (33282, 33284)

Also known as cardiac event recorder, Holter monitor, or loop recorder

Internal surgical implantation required

Divided based on whether device is being implanted or removed

Cardiac Valves (33400-33496)

Divided by valve

- Aortic
- Mitral
- Tricuspid
- Pulmonary

Subdivided by whether replacement, repair, or excision is completed (all done with bypass machine)

Code descriptions are all similar, requiring careful reading

Performed only on an inpatient basis

Coronary Artery Bypass Graft (CABG)

CAB performed for bypassing severely obstructed coronary arteries (atherosclerosis or arteriosclerosis)

Performed only on an inpatient basis

Determine what was used in repair

- Vein (33510-33516)
- Artery (33533-33536)
- Both artery and vein (33517-33523 and 33533-33536)

Based on number of bypass grafts performed and if combined venous and arterial grafts are used

Venous Grafting Only for Coronary Artery Bypass (33510-33516)
Based on number of grafts being replaced

> *Example:* Three venous grafts = 33512

Combined Arterial-Venous Grafting (33517-33530)
Divided based on number of grafts and whether procedure initial or reoperation

Procuring saphenous vein included, unless performed endoscopically

These codes are never used alone

Arterial-Venous codes (33517-33523) report only **venous** graft portion of procedure

Always used with Arterial Grafting codes (33533-33536)

> *Example:* 3 vein grafts and 2 arterial grafts = 33519 and 33534

Open procurement of saphenous vein is included in procedure (not coded separately)

Code harvesting of saphenous vein graft separately when endoscopic video-assisted procurement is performed (33508)

Code harvesting separately for upper extremity or femoral vessels

Arterial Grafting for Coronary Artery Bypass (33533-33536)
Divided based on number of grafts

Obtaining artery for grafting included in codes, except

- Procuring upper-extremity artery (i.e., radial artery), coded separately

Several codes (33542-33548) for myocardial resection, repair of ventricular septal defect (VSD), and ventricular restoration

Endovascular Repair of Descending Thoracic Aorta (33880-33891)

Placement of an endovascular aortic prosthesis for repair of descending thoracic aorta

- Less invasive than traditional approach of chest or abdominal incision

Synthetic aortic prosthesis placed via catheter

- Report fluoroscopic guidance separately (75956-75959)

   Includes diagnostic imaging prior to placement and intraprocedurally

Stent-graft (endoprosthesis) is deployed to reinforce weakened area

Arteries and Veins Subheading (34001-37799)

Only for noncoronary vessels

- Divided based on whether artery or vein involved

   Example: Different codes for embolectomy, depending on whether artery or vein involved

Catheters placed into vessels for monitoring, removal, repair

Nonselective or selective catheter placement

- **Nonselective:** Direct placement without further manipulation

- **Selective:** Place and then manipulate into further order(s)

  - Selective placement includes nonselective placement

Catheter Placement Example

- **Nonselective:** 36000 Introduction of needle into vein

- **Selective:** 36012 Placement of catheter into second-order venous system

Vascular Families are Like a Tree
First-order (main) branch (tree trunk)

Second-order branch (tree limb)

Third-order branch (tree branch)

Brachiocephalic Vascular Family (Figure 3-7)

- Report farthest extent of catheter placement in a vascular family; labor intensity is increased with the extent of catheter placement

Embolectomy and Thrombectomy (34001-34490)
Embolus: Dislodged thrombus

Thrombus: Mass of material in vessel located in place of formation

- May be removed by dissection or balloon

Balloon: Threaded into vessel, inflated under mass, pulled out with mass

- Codes are divided by site of incision and artery/vein

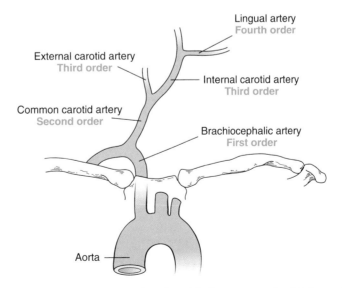

Figure **3-7** Brachiocephalic vascular family with first-, second-, third-, and fourth-order vessels.

Venous Reconstruction—CV Repairs (34501-34530)
Types of repairs
- Valve of the femoral vein

- Vena cava

- Saphenopopliteal vein anastomosis

Aneurysm

Aneurysm: Weakened arterial wall causing a bulge or ballooning

Repair by removal, bypass, or coil placement

Endovascular repair (34800-34900) from inside vessel

Direct (35001-35162) from outside vessel

Endovascular Repair of Abdominal Aortic Aneurysm (34800-34834)

Performed only on an inpatient basis

Repair Arteriovenous Fistula (35180-35190)

Abnormal passage from artery or vein

Divided based on fistula type

- Congenital

- Acquired/Traumatic

- By site

Repair methods

- Autogenous graft—fistula created artery to vein

- Non-auto fistula—biocompatible tube connecting artery to vein

Angioplasty and Atherectomy (35450-35495)

Divided by whether open or percutaneous and by vessel

- **Transluminal:** By way of vessel

- **Transluminal Angioplasty:** Catheter passed into vessel and stretched

  - Placement of eluding or non-eluding stents coded in addition to catheter placement

- **Transluminal Atherectomy:** Guide wire threaded into vessel and clots destroyed

Noncoronary Bypass Grafts (35500-35671)

Divided by

- Vein

- In Situ Vein (veins repaired in their original place)

- Other Than Vein

Code by type of graft and vessels being used to bypass

   Example: 35506, Bypass graft, with vein; carotid-subclavian

- Graft attached to carotid and to subclavian, bypassing defect of subclavian

Procurement of saphenous vein graft is included and not reported separately

Harvesting of upper-extremity vein or femoropopliteal vein is reported separately

Vascular Injection Procedures (36000-36522)

Divided into

- Intravenous

- Intra-Arterial—Intra-Aortic

- Venous

Used for many procedures, including

- Local anesthesia

- Introduction of needle

- Injection of contrast material

- Preoperative and postoperative care

  Example: Injection of opaque substance for venography (radiography of vein)

- Bypass grafts are performed only on an inpatient basis

- Harvesting of veins for bypass grafts can be performed on outpatient basis

Central Venous Access (CVA) Procedures

Peripheral = long term, used for medication/chemotherapy administration

Central = short term, used for monitoring

Categories

1. Insertion

2. Repair

3. Replacement, partial or complete

4. Removal

5. Other central venous access

6. Guidance for vascular access

Insertion (36555-36571)

Insertion of newly established venous access

- Tunneled under skin (e.g., Hickman, Broviac, Groshong)

- Nontunneled (e.g., Hohn catheter, triple lumen, PICC)

- Central (e.g., subclavian, intrajugular, femoral, inferior vena cava)

- Peripheral (anything else)

Codes divided by tunneled/non-tunneled, with port or without port, central/peripheral, and age

Repair (36575, 36576)

Repair of malfunction without replacement

Repair of central venous access device

No differentiation between age of patient or central/peripheral insertion

Replacement (Partial or Complete) (36578-36585)

Partial (36578) is replacement of catheter only

Complete (36580-36585) is replacement through same venous access site

Differentiated by tunneled/non-tunneled, central/peripheral, and with or without subcutaneous port or pump

Removal (36589, 36590)
To be used for tunneled catheter

Removal of non-tunneled catheter is not reported separately

Other Central Venous Access (36591-36598)
Collection of blood specimen

Declotting of catheter by thrombolytic agent

Mechanical removal of obstructive material from catheter

Guidance for Vascular Access
77001, fluoroscopic guidance for central venous access device placement, replacement, or removal

Reported in addition to primary procedure

76937, ultrasound guidance for vascular access

Reported in addition to primary procedure

Transcatheter Procedures (37184-37216)
Arterial mechanical thrombectomy (37184-37186)

- Removal of thrombus by means of mechanical device

  From artery or arterial bypass graft

Venous mechanical thrombectomy (37187, 37188)

- Removal of a thrombus by means of a mechanical device

  From vein

Arterial and venous mechanical thrombectomy may be performed as primary procedure or add-on

- Includes

  Introduction of device into thrombus

  Thrombus removal

  Injection of thrombolytic drug(s), if used

  Fluoroscopic and contrast guidance

  Follow-up angiography

- Report separately

  Diagnostic angiography

  Catheter placement(s)

  Diagnostic studies

  Pharmacologic thrombolytic infusion before or after (37201, 75896)

  Other interventions

Other Procedures (37195-37216)

- Used to report a variety of transcatheter procedures

  Example: Transcatheter biopsy, therapy, infusion, retrieval, and intravascular stents

HEMIC AND LYMPHATIC SYSTEM SUBSECTION (38100-38999)

Divisions

- Spleen
- General
- Lymph Nodes and Lymphatic Channels

Spleen Subheading (38100-38200)

Spleen easily ruptured, causing massive and potentially lethal hemorrhage

Excision:

- Splenectomy: Total or partial/open or laparoscopic

Often done as part of more major procedure

- Bundled into major procedure
- Repair
- Laparoscopy

General (38204-38242)

Bone Marrow
Codes divided based on

- Presentation
- Preparation
- Purification
- Aspiration
- Biopsy
- Harvesting
- Transplantation

Stem Cells
Immature blood cells originating in bone marrow

Used in treatment of leukemia

Types of stem cells
Allogenic: Same species

Autologous: Patient's own

Lymph Nodes and Lymphatic Channels Subheading (38300-38999)

Two types of lymphadenectomies

- **Limited:** Lymph nodes only for staging
- **Radical:** Lymph nodes and surrounding tissue

Often bundled into more major procedure (e.g., prostatectomy)

Do not unbundle and report lymphadenectomy separately

MEDIASTINUM SUBSECTION (39000-39499)

Incision codes for foreign body removal, biopsy, or drainage

Excision codes for removal of cyst or tumor

All procedures, except for 39400 (mediastinoscopy), are performed on an inpatient basis

DIAPHRAGM SUBSECTION (39501-39599)

Only category: Repair

Includes hernia or laceration repairs

DIGESTIVE SYSTEM SUBSECTION (40490-49999)

Divided by anatomical site from mouth to anus + organs that aid digestive process

Example: Liver and gallbladder

Many bundled procedures

Endoscopy

Diagnostic endoscopy is always bundled into a surgical endoscopy

Code to furthest extent of procedure

Endoscopy Terminology

Notes define specific terminology

Code descriptions are specific regarding

- Technique and depth of scope

  Esophagoscopy: Esophagus only

  Esophagogastroscopy: Esophagus and past diaphragm

  Esophagogastroduodenoscopy: Esophagus and beyond pyloric channel

- Proctosigmoidoscopy: Rectum and sigmoid colon (6-25 cm)
- Sigmoidoscopy: Entire rectum, sigmoid colon, and may include part of descending colon (26-60 cm)
- Colonoscopy: Entire colon, rectum to cecum, and may include terminal ileum (greater than 60 cm)

Laparoscopy and Endoscopy

Some subheadings have both laparoscopy (outside) and endoscopy (inside) procedures

Example: Subheading Esophagus

- Endoscopy views inside
- Laparoscopy inserted through umbilicus; views from outside
- Adjustment during 90-day post-op period included in surgery

Hemorrhoidectomy and Fistulectomy Codes (46221-46320)

Divided by

- Complexity
  - Simple: No plastic procedure involved
  - Complex: Includes plastic procedure and fissurectomy
- Anatomy
  - Subcutaneous: No muscle involvement
  - Submuscular: Sphincter muscle
  - Complex fistulectomy involves excision/incision of multiple fistulas

Hernia Codes (49491-49659)

Divided by

- Type of hernia

  Example: Inguinal, femoral, incisional, ventral

- Initial or subsequent repair
- Age of patient
- Clinical presentation:
  - **Strangulated:** Blood supply cut off
  - **Incarcerated:** Cannot be returned to cavity (not reducible)

Additional code is used for implantation of mesh or prosthesis

- Laparoscopy surgical procedures

URINARY SYSTEM SUBSECTION (50010-53899)

Anatomical division:

- Kidney
- Ureters
- Bladder
- Urethra

Further divided by procedure:

- Incision
- Excision
- Introduction
- Repair
- Laparoscopy
- Endoscopy

Kidney Subheading (50010-50593)

Endoscopy codes are used for procedures done through a previously established stoma or incision

Caution: Codes may be unilateral or bilateral

Introduction Category (50382-50398)
Codes divided by renal pelvis catheter procedures or other introduction procedures

Renal pelvis catheters further divided; internal dwelling or externally accessible

Catheters for drainage and injections for radiography

Aspirations

Insertion of guide wires

Tube changes

Usually reported with radiology component

Ureter Subheading (50600-50980)

Caution: Codes may be unilateral or bilateral

Divided by type of procedure

- Incision

- Excision

- Introduction

- Repair

- Laparoscopy

- Endoscopy

Bladder Subheading (51020-52700)

Includes codes for

- Incision

- Removal

- Excision

- Introduction

- Urodynamics

- Repair

- Laparoscopy

- Endoscopy

  - Cystoscopy

  - Urethroscopy

  - Cystourethroscopy

- Transurethral surgery

Many bundled codes

Example: Urethral dilation is included with insertion of cystoscope

Read all descriptions carefully

Urodynamics (51725-51798)
Procedures relate to motion and flow of urine

Used to diagnose urine flow obstructions

Bundled: All usual, necessary instruments, equipment, supplies, and technical assistance

Vesical Neck and Prostate (52400-52700)
Contains codes for transurethral resection of the prostate (TURP)

Example: 52601 reports a complete transurethral electrosurgical resection of the prostate and includes vasectomy, meatotomy, cystourethroscopy, urethral calibration and/or dilation, internal urethrotomy, and control of any postoperative bleeding

Other approaches are reported with 55801-55845

Example: 55801 reports removal of the prostate gland (prostatectomy) through an incision in the perineum and includes vasectomy, meatotomy, urethral calibration and/or dilation, internal urethrotomy, and control of any postoperative bleeding

MALE GENITAL SYSTEM SUBSECTION (54000-55899)

- Penis (most codes)
- Testis
- Epididymis
- Tunica Vaginalis
- Scrotum
- Vas Deferens
- Spermatic Cord
- Seminal Vesicles
- Prostate

Biopsy Codes

Located in anatomical subheading to which the codes refer

Example: Biopsy codes in subheadings

- Epididymis (Excision)

Example: 54800, needle biopsy of epididymis

- Testis (Excision)

Example: 54500, needle biopsy of testis

Penis (54000-54450)

Incision codes (54000-54015) differ from Integumentary System codes

- Penis incision codes used for deeper structures

Destruction (54050-54065)
Codes divided by

- Extent: Simple or extensive

- Method of destruction (e.g., chemical, cryosurgery)

Extensive destruction can be by any method

Excision (54100-54164)
Commonly used codes for biopsy and circumcision

Introduction (54200-54250)
Many procedures for corpora cavernosum (spongy body of penis)

- Injection procedures for Peyronie disease (toughening of corpora cavernosum)

- Treatments for erectile dysfunction

Repair (54300-54440)
Many plastic repairs

Some repairs are staged (more than one stage)

- Stage indicated in code description

FEMALE GENITAL SYSTEM SUBSECTION (56405-58999)

Anatomical division: From vulva to ovaries

- Many bundled services

Vulva, Perineum, and Introitus (56405-56821)

Skene's gland coded with Urinary System, Incision or Excision codes

- Group of small mucous glands, lower end of urethra

  - Paraurethral duct

Incision (56405-56442)
I&D of abscess: Vulva, perineal area, or Bartholin's gland

Marsupialization
Cyst incised

Drained

Edges sutured to sides to keep cyst open, creating a pouchlike repair

Destruction (56501, 56515)
Lesions destroyed by variety of methods

- Destruction = Eradication, not to be confused with excision; excision is removal

Divided by whether destruction is simple or extensive

- Complexity based on physician's judgment

- Stated in medical record

Destruction has no pathology report

Excision (56605-56740)
Biopsy includes

- Local anesthetic

- Biopsy

- Simple closure

- Code based on number of lesions biopsied

Vulvectomy: Surgical Removal of Portion of Vulva (56620-56640)
Based on extent and size of area removed

Extent:

- Simple: Skin and superficial subcutaneous tissues

- Radical: Skin and deep subcutaneous tissues

Size:

- Partial: <80% vulvar area

- Complete: >80% vulvar area

Extent and size indicated in operative report

Repair (56800-56810)
Many plastic repairs

Read notes following category

- If repair procedure involves wound of genitalia, use Integumentary System code

Endoscopy (56820-56821)
By means of a colposcopy with or without biopsy

Vagina (57000-57425)

Codes divided based on service (e.g., incision, excision)

Introduction (57150-57180)
Includes vaginal irrigation, insertion of devices, diaphragm, cervical caps

Report the inserted device separately

- 99070 or HCPCS National Level II code, such as A4261 (cervical cap)

Repair (57200-57335)
For nonobstetric repairs

- For obstetric repairs, use Maternity Care and Delivery codes

Manipulation (57400-57415)
Dilation: Speculum inserted into vagina and enlarged using dilator

Endoscopy (57420-57425)
Colposcopy codes based on purpose

- e.g., biopsy, diagnostic

- Includes code for laparoscopic approach for repair of paravaginal defect

Cervix Uteri (57452-57800)

Cervix uteri, narrow lower end of uterus

Services include excision, manipulation, repair

Excision (57500-57558)
Conization codes

- **Conization:** Removal of cone of tissue from cervix

LEEP (loop electrocautery excision procedure) technology can be used for conizations

Corpus Uteri (58100-58579)

Many complex procedures

- Often very similar wording in code descriptions

- Requires careful reading

Excision (58100-58294)
Dilation & curettage (D&C, 58120) of uterus

- After dilation, curette scrapes uterus

- Coded according to circumstances: obstetrical or nonobstetrical

Do not report postpartum hemorrhage service with 58120

- Use 59160—Maternity and Delivery code

Many hysterectomy codes

- Based on approach (vaginal, abdominal) and extent (uterus, fallopian tubes, etc.)

Often secondary procedures performed with hysterectomy

Do not code secondary, related minor procedures separately

Only 58110 (endometrial biopsy), 58120 (dilation and curettage), and 58145 (myomectomy, vaginal approach) are performed on an outpatient basis

Laparoscopy/Hysteroscopy (58541-58579)
Laparoscopic approach for:

- Removal of myomas

- Hysterectomies

Codes divided by tissue removed and weight

Introduction (58300-58356)
Common procedures

- e.g., insertion of an IUD

Report supply of device separately

Specialized services

- e.g., artificial insemination procedures

Used to report physician component of service

Component coding

- Necessary with catheter procedures for hysterosonography
- Notes following codes indicate radiology guidance component codes

Oviduct/Ovary (58600-58770)

Oviduct. Fallopian Tube

Incision category contains tubal ligations

- When it occurs during the same hospitalization but not at same session as delivery, ligation is coded separately

Laparoscopy (58660-58679)
Through abdominal wall

Codes in the laparoscopy and hysteroscopy section are divided by approach

- Then by purpose of procedure, e.g., lysis, lesion removal

Caution: If only diagnostic laparoscopy

- Do not use Female Genital System codes
- Use 49320, Digestive System

Many codes can be reported separately with appropriate modifiers

> **Example:** 58660 Laparoscopy, surgical, with lysis of adhesions, can be coded with any of the indented codes that follow 58660 (58661, 58662, 58670)

Ovary (58800-58960)

Two categories only: Incision and Excision

- **Incision:** Primarily for drainage of cysts and abscesses
  - Divided by surgical approach
- **Excision:** Biopsy, wedge resection, and oophorectomy

In Vitro Fertilization (58970-58976)

Specialized codes usually used by physicians trained in fertilization procedures

- Codes divided by type of procedure and method used

MATERNITY CARE & DELIVERY SUBSECTION (59000-59899)

Divided by service

- Antepartum services
  Amniocentesis
  Fetal non-stress test
  Fetal monitoring during labor
- Type of delivery
  Vaginal delivery
  C-section
  Delivery after a previous C-section
- Abortion

Gestation

Fetal gestation: Approximately 266 days (40 weeks)

EDD: Estimated Date of Delivery

- 280 days from last menstrual period (LMP)

Trimesters
First, LMP to Week 12

Second, Weeks 13-27

Third, Week 28 to EDD

Excision (59100-59160)
Postpartum curettage: Removes remaining pieces of placenta or clotted blood (59160)

Nonobstetric curettage: 58120 (Corpus Uteri, Excision)

Introduction (59200)
Insertion of cervical dilator: Used to prepare cervix for an abortive procedure or delivery (for abortive procedures, see 59855)

Cervical ripening agents may be introduced to prepare cervix

- Is a "separate procedure" and not reported when part of more major procedure

Repair (59300-59350)
Only for repairs during pregnancy

Repairs done as a result of delivery or during pregnancy

Episiotomy or vaginal repair by other than attending

Suture repair (cerclage) of cervix or uterus (hysterorrhaphy)

Abortion Services (59812-59857)

Spontaneous: Happens naturally (for a complete spontaneous abortion, report with a code from the E/M section)

Incomplete: Requires medical intervention

Missed: Fetus dies naturally during first 22 weeks' gestation

Septic: Abortion with infection

Medical intervention:

- Dilation and curettage or evacuation (suction removal)
- Intra-amniotic injections (saline or urea)
- Vaginal suppositories (prostaglandin)

ENDOCRINE SYSTEM SUBSECTION (60000-60699)

Nine glands in endocrine system; only four included in subsection

1. Thyroid
2. Parathyroid

3. Thymus

4. Adrenal

Pituitary and Pineal. *See* Nervous System subsection

Pancreas. Digestive System

Ovaries and Testes. Respective genital systems

Divided into two subheadings

- Thyroid Gland

- Parathyroid, Thymus, Adrenal Glands, and Carotid Body

Carotid Body
Refers to area adjacent to carotid artery

Can be site of tumors

Thyroid Gland, Excision Category (60100-60281)

Code descriptions often refer to

- Lobectomy (partial or subtotal): Something less than total

- Thyroidectomy (total): All

Thyroid, 1 gland with 2 lobes

NERVOUS SYSTEM SUBSECTION (61000-64999)

Divided anatomically:

- Skull, Meninges, and Brain

- Spine and Spinal Cord

- Extracranial Nerves, Peripheral Nerves, and Autonomic Nervous System

Skull, Meninges, and Brain Subheading (61000-62258)

Categories
Injection, Drainage, or Aspiration

Twist Drills, Burr Hole(s), or Trephination

Conditions that Require Openings into Brain to
- Relieve pressure

- Insert monitoring devices

- Place tubing

- Inject contrast material

Craniectomy or Craniotomy Category (61304-61576)
Removal of portion of skull, usually as operative site, performed emergently to prevent herniation of brain into the brainstem

Codes divided by site and condition for which procedure is performed

Performed only on an inpatient basis

Surgery of Skull Base Category (61580-61619)
Skull base: Area at base of cranium

- Lesion removal from this area very complex

Surgery of Skull Base Terminology
Approach procedure used to gain exposure of lesion

Definitive procedure is what is done to lesion

Repair/reconstruction procedure reported separately only if extensive repair

Surgery of Skull Base (61580-61619)
Approach procedure and definitive procedure coded separately

Example: Removal of an intradural lesion using middle cranial fossa approach

- 61590 approach procedure, middle cranial fossa and

- 61608 definitive procedure of intradural resection of lesion

Most of these procedures are performed only on an inpatient basis

Cerebrospinal Fluid (CSF) Shunt Category (62180-62258)
Used to drain fluid

Codes describe placement of

- Devices

- Repair

- Replacement

- Removal of shunting devices

Most performed only on an inpatient basis

Spine and Spinal Cord Subheading (62263-63746)
Codes divided by condition and approach

Often used are

- Unilateral or bilateral procedures (-50)

- Radiologic supervision and fluoroscopic guidance coded separately

Includes codes for

- Spinal anesthetic injections 62310-62319

- Intrathecal catheter placement/implantation 62350-62355

Introduction/Injection of Anesthetic Agent (Nerve Block), Diagnostic or Therapeutic Category (64400-64530)
Includes codes for

- Nerve blocks 64400-64450

- Facet joint injections 64470-64476

- Epidural injections 64479-64484

  - Used to provide pain relief

  - As compared to an epidural catheter placement used for anesthetic purposes

EYE AND OCULAR ADNEXA SUBSECTION (65091-68899)

Terminology extremely important

- Code descriptions often vary only slightly

Understanding of eye anatomy is necessary for proper coding in this subsection

Codes divided anatomically, e.g.,

- Eyeball
- Anterior segment
- Posterior segment
- Ocular adnexa
- Conjunctiva

Some codes specifically for previous surgery

Example: Insertion of ocular implant, secondary 65130

Much bundling:

Example: Subheading Posterior Segment, Prophylaxis category notes indicate:

- "The following descriptors (67141, 67145) are intended to include all sessions in defined treatment period."

Cataracts

Method used depends on type of cataract and surgeon preference

Nuclear cataract: Most common, center of lens (nucleus), due to aging process

Cortical cataract: Forms in lens of cortex and extends outward; frequent in diabetics

Subcapsular cataract: Forms at back of lens

Removal and lens replacement (66830-66986)

- Extracapsular cataract extraction (ECCE) is partial removal

Removes hard nucleus in one piece

Removes soft cortex in multiple pieces

- Intracapsular cataract extraction (ICCE) is total removal

Removes lens and capsule in one piece

- Phacoemulsification

Small incision into eye and introduction of probe

High-frequency waves fragment cataract; then suctioned out

Lens placed through same small incision

Eyelids (67700-67999)

Blepharotomy (67700)

- Incision into eyelid for drainage of abscess

373

Blepharoplasty

- Repair of eyelid
- Codes in Integumentary System (15820-15823)
- Codes in Eye and Ocular Adnexa (67916, 67917, 67923, 67924)

These codes strictly for ectropion and entropion

Selection of code depends on technique used to repair eyelid

- Blephoroplasty coded with specific techniques (67901-67908)

AUDITORY SYSTEM SUBSECTION (69000-69990)

Codes divided by

- External Ear (69000-69399)
- Middle Ear (69400-69799)
- Internal Ear (69801-69949)
- Temporal Bone, Middle Fossa Approach (69950-69979)

Understanding of ear anatomy is necessary for proper coding in this subsection

External, middle, and internal ear further divided by procedure

- Incision
- Excision
- Removal
- Repair

Myringotomy and tympanostomy

- Eustachian tube connects middle ear to back of throat for drainage
- Fluid collects in middle ear when tube does not function properly
- Prevents air from entering middle ear and pressure builds
- Surgical intervention

  Myringotomy (incision into tympanic membrane)

  Tympanostomy (placement of PE tube [pressure equalization])

Operating Microscope (+69990)

Employed with procedures using microsurgical techniques

Code in addition to primary procedure performed

Do not report separately when primary procedure description includes microsurgical techniques

Example: 15758, Free fascial flap with microvascular anastomosis

Note that following 15758 is the statement:

"(Do not report code 69990 in addition to code 15758)" indicating to the coder not to report the use of operating microscope separately

■ HCPCS CODING

Developed by Centers for Medicare and Medicaid Services (CMS)

• Formerly HCFA

HCPCS developed in 1983

CPT did not contain all codes necessary for Medicare services reporting.

One of Two Levels of Codes

1. Level I, CPT

2. Level II, HCPCS, also known as national codes

Phased out Level III, Local Codes

Developed by Medicare and other carriers for use at local level

Varied by locale

Discontinued October 2002 due to HIPAA code set regulations

• Some codes incorporated into HCPCS Level I and Level II

Level II, National Codes

Codes for wide variety of providers

• Physicians

• Hospital outpatient facilities

• Orthodontists

Codes for wide variety of services

• Specific drugs

• Durable medical equipment (DME)

• Ambulance services

Format

Begins with letter, followed by four digits

   Example: E0605, vaporizer, room type

Each letter represents group codes

   Example: "J" codes used to report drugs, J0585, Botox, per unit

Temporary Codes

Certain letters indicate temporary codes

   Example: K0552, Supplies for external drug infusion pump

• K codes are temporary codes

Code book published every January, but codes are added and deleted throughout the year and providers are notified through carrier bulletins

HCPCS National Level II Index

Directs coder to specific codes

Do not code directly from index

Reference main portion of text before assigning code

Alphabetical order

Ambulance Modifiers

Origin and destination used in combination

- First letter: Origin
- Second letter: Destination

  Example:

  - -R = Residence
  - -H = Hospital
  - -RH origin (first letter), residence, and destination (second letter), hospital

PET Modifiers

Positron Emission Tomography: Noninvasive Imaging Procedure
Assesses metabolic organ activity

Table of Drugs

Listed by generic name, not brand name

Often used when reporting immunizations or injections

■ AN OVERVIEW OF THE ICD-9-CM

On the CCS examination, you will be assigning ICD-9-CM codes to both inpatient and outpatient (ASC) services using Volumes 1-3.

INTRODUCTION

Morbidity (illness)

Mortality (death)

CM = Clinical Modification

Provides continuity of data

World Health Organization's ICD-9 used globally

1977: U.S. develops ICD-9 version

- Has more code subsets
- Data collapse back to ICD-9 for uniformity of data

Medicare

Medicare Catastrophic Act of 1988

- Required use of ICD-9-CM codes for outpatient claims

Act abolished but codes still used

Uses of ICD-9-CM

Facilitate payment of health services

Evaluate patients' use of health services

Fiscal entities track health care costs

Research

- Health care quality
- Future needs
- Newer cancer center built if patient use warrants
- Predict health care trends
- Plan for future health care needs

ICD-9-CM on Insurance Forms (Figure 3-8)

Diagnoses establish medical necessity

Services and diagnoses must correlate

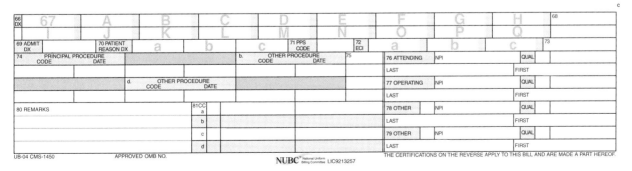

Figure **3-8** Blocks 66-81 of CMS-1450/UB-04. (Courtesy U.S. Department of Health and Human Services, Centers for Medicare and Medicaid Services.)

FORMAT OF ICD-9-CM

Volume 1, Diseases, Tabular List

Volume 2, Diseases, Alphabetic Index

Volume 3, Procedures, Tabular and Alphabetic Index

Volume 1, Diseases, Tabular List

Contains code numbers

001.0-999.9 Diagnosis codes describe condition

V & E codes = supplemental information

Volume 2, Diseases, Alphabetic Index

Appears first in book

Refers coder to code numbers in Volume 1

Never code directly from Index!

Volume 3, Procedures, Tabular List, and Alphabetic Index

Index and Tabular List used for procedures and therapies

Inpatient settings

Procedures and therapies

ICD-9-CM CONVENTIONS

Symbols, abbreviations, punctuation, and notations

NEC: Not elsewhere classifiable

- No more-specific code exists

NOS: Not otherwise specified

- Unspecified in documentation

[ ] Brackets

Enclose synonyms, alternative wording, or explanatory phrases

Helpful, additional information

Can affect code

Found in Tabular List (001.0-999.9)

( ) Parentheses

Contain nonessential modifiers

- Take them or leave them

Found in Tabular List and Index

Do not affect code

Colon & Brace

: Colon: Tabular List, completes statement with one or more modifiers

} Brace: Tabular List, modifying statements to right of brace

Lozenge, Section Mark, & Bold Type

☐ Lozenge: Can indicate codes unique to ICD-9-CM

§ Section: Can be footnote indicator

Bold type: Codes and code titles in Tabular List, Volume 1

Italicized Type

All excludes notes

Codes NOT used as principal diagnosis

Slanted Brackets [ ]

Enclose manifestations of underlying condition

Code underlying condition first

Includes, Excludes, Use Additional Code

Includes notes: In chapter, section, or category

Excludes notes: Conditions are coded elsewhere

Use additional code: Assignment of other code(s) is necessary

And/With

And: Means and/or

With: One condition with (in addition to) another condition

Code, if Applicable, any Causal Condition First

May be principal diagnosis if no causal condition applicable or known

> *Example:* 707.10, Ulcer of lower limb, except decubitus; states
> • Chronic venous hypertension with ulcer (459.31)

If ulcer caused by chronic venous hypertension

• **First:** 459.31 chronic venous hypertension

• **Second:** 707.10 ulcer of lower limb

VOLUME 2, ALPHABETIC INDEX

Nonessential modifiers: Have no effect on code selection

Enclosed in parentheses

Clarify diagnosis

> *Example:* Ileus (adynamic) (bowel) . . .

Terms

Main terms (bold typeface)

- Subterms

- Indented two spaces to right

- Not bold

Cross References

Directs you: *see, see also*

- *"see"* directs you to specific term

   Example: Panotitis—*see* Otitis media

"see also" directs you to another term for more information

   Example: Perivaginitis (*see also* Vesiculitis)

"see category" Volume 1, Tabular List, specific information about use of code

   Example: Mesencephalitis (*see also* Encephalitis) 323.9; late effect—*see* category 326

Notes

Define terms

Give further coding instructions

   Example: Index: "Melanoma"

   NOTE: "Except where otherwise indicated . . ."

Mandatory fifth digits also appear as notes (one reason never to code from Index)

Eponyms

Disease or syndromes named for person

   Example: Arnold-Chiari (*see also* Spina bifida)

Etiology and Manifestation of Disease

Etiology = cause of disease

Manifestation = symptom

Combination codes = etiology and manifestation in one code

Neoplasm

In Volume 2, Index, locate Neoplasm Table under the alphabetic entry "N"

SECTIONS

Section 1, Index to Diseases

Section 2, Table of Drugs and Chemicals

Section 3, Index to External Causes of Injuries and Poisonings (E Codes)

Section 1, Index to Diseases

Largest part of Volume 2—Index

First step in coding, locate main term in Index by sign, symptom, or disease— not body area

Subterms indented two spaces to right

May have more than one subterm

Section 2, Table of Drugs and Chemicals

Located after the Index of Diseases

Contains classification of drugs and substances to identify poisoning and adverse effects

- Adverse effect occurs when substance is taken correctly but has a negative reaction to substance

Condition E code for drug found under "therapeutic" column

- Poisoning occurs when substance is incorrectly taken

   Example: Amoxicillin prescribed for bronchitis causes rash (adverse effect); or rather than one tablet of prescribed amoxicillin, patient takes 4 tablets and nausea results (poisoning)

Drug name placed alphabetically on left under heading "Substance" (Figure 3-9)

First column: "Poisoning" code for substance involved if not related to an adverse effect

E codes identify how poisoning occurred

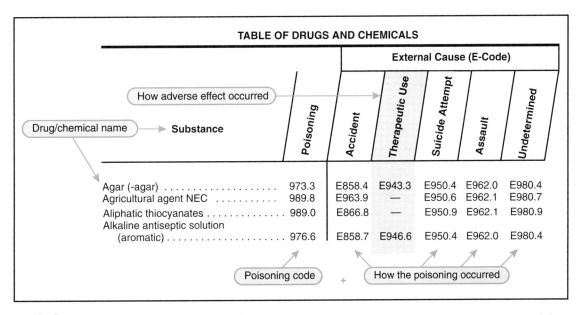

TABLE OF DRUGS AND CHEMICALS

Substance	Poisoning	Accident	Therapeutic Use	Suicide Attempt	Assault	Undetermined
Agar (-agar)	973.3	E858.4	E943.3	E950.4	E962.0	E980.4
Agricultural agent NEC	989.8	E963.9	—	E950.6	E962.1	E980.7
Aliphatic thiocyanates	989.0	E866.8	—	E950.9	E962.1	E980.9
Alkaline antiseptic solution (aromatic)	976.6	E858.7	E946.6	E950.4	E962.0	E980.4

Figure **3-9** Section 2, Table of Drugs and Chemicals. (From *International Classification of Diseases*, 9th Revision. U.S. Department of Health and Human Services, Public Health Service, Center for Medicare and Medicaid Services.)

Headings

Accident: Unintentional

Therapeutic: Correct dosage, correctly administered with adverse effects **(This is the only E code reported on the CCS examination)**

Suicide attempt: Self-inflicted

Assault: Intentionally inflicted by another person

Undetermined: Unknown cause

Section 3, E Codes

Alphabetic Index to External Causes of Injuries and Poisonings

Provides additional information about the nature of the injury/poisoning and locality

Never principal (inpatient) or primary (outpatient) diagnosis

Separate Index to External Causes

- Alphabetical, main terms in bold

- Subterms indented 2 spaces to right under main term

A Word of Caution about the Alphabetic Index

Some words in Index do not appear in Tabular—saves space

Exact word may not be in code description in Tabular

- Usually found in Alphabetic Index

- Must locate term in Index and then locate in Tabular

- Additional coding instructions found in Tabular

VOLUME 1, TABULAR LIST

Two Major Divisions

1. Classification of Diseases and Injuries (codes 001.0-999.9)

2. Supplementary Classification (V codes and E codes)

Classification of Diseases and Injuries

Main portion of ICD-9-CM

Codes from 001.0 to 999.9

Most chapters are body systems

   Example:
   - Digestive System
   - Respiratory System

Divisions of Classification of Diseases and Injuries

Chapters 1 through 17

Section: A group of related conditions

Category: Represents single disease/condition

Subcategory: More specific

Subclassification: Most specific

Remember
Assign to highest level of specificity, based on documentation
    If 4-digit code exists, do not report 3-digit code
    If 5-digit code exists, do not report 4-digit code

Volumes 1, 2, and 3 are required for the CCS certification examination

---

■ USING THE ICD-9-CM

Guidelines developed by Cooperating Parties

- American Hospital Association (AHA)
- American Health Information Management Association (AHIMA)
- Centers for Medicare and Medicaid Services (CMS)
- National Center for Health Statistics (NCHS)

GENERAL GUIDELINES

Appendix A of this text contains *Official Guidelines for Coding and Reporting*

You must know and follow Guidelines when assigning diagnoses codes

- All certification examinations adhere to the Guidelines
- As you review this ICD-9-CM material, locate the information in the Guidelines of your ICD-9-CM
- In this way, you will become familiar with the location of Guidelines content to be able to quickly reference the Guidelines during the examination

Guidelines for Following Labels

"(I)" indicates inpatient setting guidelines

"(O)" indicates outpatient setting guidelines

"(I/O)" guidelines apply to both inpatient and outpatient settings

You have to be able to code inpatient and outpatient facility services on the CCS certification examination

STEPS TO DIAGNOSIS CODING (I/O)

Identify MAIN term(s) in diagnosis

Locate MAIN term(s) in Index

Review subterms

Follow cross-reference instructions (e.g., *see, see also*)

Verify code(s) in Tabular

Remember (I/O)

Read Tabular notes

Code to highest specificity

NEVER CODE FROM INDEX!

Guideline Section I.B.3. Level of Detail in Coding (I/O)

Assign diagnosis to highest level of specificity

Do NOT use 3-digit code if there is 4th

Do NOT use 4-digit code if there is 5th

Section I.A.2. Other (NEC) and Unspecified (NOS) (I/O)

NEC = Not elsewhere classifiable

• More specific code does NOT exist

NOS = Not otherwise specified (Means "unspecified")

• Available information NOT specific enough

• Use ONLY if more specific code NOT available

Section I.B.10. and 10.3. Acute and Chronic Conditions (I/O)

Exists alone or together

May be separate or combination codes

If two codes, code acute first

   Example: Acute (577.0) and chronic (577.1) pancreatitis

When two separate codes exist, code

• Acute cystitis 595.0

• Chronic cystitis 595.2

Combination code: Both acute and chronic conditions

• Diarrhea (acute) (chronic) 787.91

• Acute and subacute bacterial endocarditis 421.0

• Otitis, acute and subacute 382.9

Section I.B.11. Combination Code (I/O)

Always use combination code if one exists

   Example: Encephalomyelitis (diagnosis) due to rubella (manifestation), 056.01

Section I.B.9. Multiple Diagnoses Coding (I/O) for Single Condition

Etiology (cause)

Manifestation (symptom)

- Slanted brackets *[ ]*

    Example: Retinopathy, diabetic 250.5 *[362.01]*

- Must check Tabular notes to assign correct fifth digit for diabetes

- Tabular: 362.0, Diabetic retinopathy, instructs to "Code first Diabetes 250.5"

Section II.H. Uncertain Conditions (I)

If diagnosis at time of discharge states

probable,

suspected,

likely,

questionable,

possible,

rule out,

Code condition as if condition existed, until proven otherwise

Example: "Cough and fever, probably pneumonia" (I/O)

- Inpatient: Code pneumonia, do NOT code cough and fever

- Outpatient: Code cough and fever, do NOT code pneumonia

Section I.B.13. Impending or Threatened Condition (I)

Code any condition described at time of discharge as impending or threatened

- Did occur: Code as confirmed

- Did NOT occur: Code as impending or threatened (MAIN terms)

SELECTION OF PRINCIPAL DIAGNOSIS (I)

Condition established after study (tests)

Responsible for patient admission

SELECTION OF PRIMARY DIAGNOSIS (O)

Condition for encounter

Documented

Responsible for services provided

Also list coexisting condition(s) or comorbidity(ies)

DIAGNOSIS AND SERVICES (I/O)

Diagnosis and procedure MUST correlate

Medical necessity established

No correlation = No reimbursement

Section II.A. Symptoms, Signs, and Ill-Defined Conditions (I)

Inpatient coders do NOT use when definitive diagnosis has been established

Can be the provisional diagnosis if a more specific diagnosis is not available

Section I.A.6. Codes in Brackets (I/O)

Never sequence as principal diagnosis

Always sequence in order listed

> ***Example:*** Index lists: Diabetes, gangrene 250.7 *[785.4]*

- 785.4 = gangrene

Tabular: 785.4 indicates "Code first any associated underlying condition: diabetes (250.7X). . . ."

- Code first diabetes, then gangrene
- 250.7X = diabetes (X = fifth digit)
- 785.4 = Gangrene

Section II.B. Two or More Interrelated Conditions (I/O)

When two or more interrelated conditions exist and either could be the principal diagnosis, either is sequenced first

> ***Example:*** Patient with mitral valve stenosis and coronary artery disease (two interrelated conditions)

- Either can be principal diagnosis and sequenced first
- Resource intensiveness affects choice

Section II.C. Two or More Equal Diagnoses (I/O)

Either can be sequenced first

> ***Example:*** Diagnosis of viral gastroenteritis and dehydration

Section II.D. Comparative or Contrasting Conditions (I)

"Either/or" diagnoses coded as confirmed

If determination CANNOT be made, either can be sequenced first

- Pneumonia or lung cancer
- Lung cancer or pneumonia

Section II.E. Symptom(s) Followed by Contrasting/ Comparative Diagnosis (I)

Symptom code sequenced first

Then, other diagnoses

Section I.C.18. Observation and Evaluation for Suspected Conditions Not Found (I/O)

V71.0-V71.9

Assigned as principal diagnosis for

- Admissions for evaluation

- Following an accident that would ordinarily result in health problem, BUT there is none

  Example: Car accident, driver hits head, no apparent injury, admit to R/O head trauma

Section II.F. Original Treatment Plan Not Carried Out (I)

Principal diagnosis becomes

- Condition that after study was reason for admission

Treatment does NOT have to be carried out for condition

  Example: Patient admitted for elective surgery, develops pneumonia; surgery canceled

- Code reason for surgery first

- Code "Surgical or other procedure NOT carried out because of contraindication" (V64.1)

- Also code pneumonia

V CODES

Located after 999.9 in Tabular

Two digits before decimal (e.g., V10.10)

Index for V codes, Alphabetic Index to Diseases

Main terms: Contraception, counseling, dialysis, status, examination

Uses of V Codes (I/O)

Not sick BUT receives health care (e.g., vaccination)

Services for known disease/injury (e.g., chemotherapy)

A circumstance/problem that influences patient's health BUT NOT current illness/injury

  Example: Organ transplant status

  Example: Birth status and outcome of delivery (newborn)

Special Note about "History of" (I/O)

Index to Disease, MAIN term "History"

Entries between "family" and "visual loss V19.0" = "family history of"

Entries before "family" and after "visual loss V19.0" = "personal history of"

Special Note About "History of"
Section I.18.e. of Guidelines contains the V Code Table

- Identifies how V codes can be listed (first, first/additional, additional only)

History V Code Categories in Tabular
V10   Personal history of malignant neoplasm

V12   Personal history of certain other diseases

V13   Personal history of other diseases

   Except: V13.4 Personal history of arthritis, and V13.6, Personal history of congenital malformations. These conditions are life-long so are not true history codes

V14   Personal history of allergy to medicinal agents

V15.8   Other personal history presenting hazards to health

   Except: V15.7 Personal history of contraception

V16   Family history of malignant neoplasm

V17   Family history of certain chronic disabling diseases

V18   Family history of certain other specific diseases

V19   Family history of other conditions

SECTION I.B.12. LATE EFFECTS (I/O)

Late effect residual of (remaining from) previous illness/injury

- e.g., Burn that leaves scar

Residual coded first (scar)

Cause (burn) coded second

Late effect codes are not in a separate chapter; rather, throughout Tabular

Reference the term "Late" in the Index

There is no time limit on developing a residual

There may be more than one residual

   Example: Patient has a stroke (434.91) and develops paralysis on dominant side (hemiparesis, 438.21) and loss of ability to communicate (aphasia, 438.11)

ICD-9-CM, CHAPTER 1, INFECTIOUS AND PARASITIC DISEASES (I/O)

Divided based on etiology (cause of disease)

Many combination codes

   Example: 112.0 candidiasis infection of mouth, which reports both the organism and condition with one code

Multiple Codes (I/O)

Sequencing must be considered.

- UTI due to *Escherichia coli*
- 599.0 (UTI) etiology
- 041.4 (*E. coli*) organism (in this order)

Human Immunodeficiency Virus (I/O)

Code HIV or HIV-related illness ONLY if stated as confirmed in diagnostic statement

- 042 HIV or HIV-related illness
- V08 Asymptomatic HIV status
- 795.71 Nonspecific HIV serology

Previously Diagnosed HIV-Related Illness (I/O)

Code prior diagnosis HIV-related disease 042 (HIV)

NEVER assign these patients to

- V08 (Asymptomatic) or
- 795.71 (Nonspecific serologic evidence of HIV)

Patient with HIV admitted for unrelated condition

HIV Sequencing (I)

If admitted for HIV-related illness (e.g., pneumonia)

- Code 042 (HIV)
- Followed by current illness (pneumonia)

If admitted for other than HIV-related illness

- Code reason for admittance
- Then 042 (HIV)

Sequencing (O)

- Sequence first reason most responsible for encounter
- Followed by secondary diagnosis that affects encounter or patient care

HIV and Pregnancy (I/O)

This is an exception to HIV sequencing

During pregnancy, childbirth, or puerperium, code:

- 647.6X (Other specified infections and parasitic diseases)
- Followed by 042 (HIV)

Asymptomatic HIV during pregnancy, childbirth, or puerperium

- 647.6X (Other specified infections and parasitic diseases)
- V08 (Asymptomatic HIV infection status)

- Reporting asymptomatic HIV varies by state
  - Check the state's reporting laws

Inconclusive Laboratory Test for HIV (I/O)

795.71 (Inconclusive serologic test for HIV)

- Reporting inconclusive laboratory HIV tests varies by state
  - Check the state's reporting laws

HIV Screening (I/O)

Code V73.89 (Screening for other specified viral disease)

- Patient in high-risk group for HIV
- V69.8 (Other problems related to lifestyle)

Patients returning for HIV screening results = V65.44 (HIV counseling)

Caution (I/O)

Incorrectly applying these HIV coding rules can cause patient hardship

Insurance claims for patients with HIV usually need patient's written agreement to disclosure

Section I.C.1.b. Septicemia, Systemic Inflammatory Response Syndrome (SIRS) Sepsis, Severe Sepsis, and Septic Shock

Sepsis: Assign systemic infection code as first listed when sepsis is present

- Assign a sepsis code as secondary when sepsis develops during encounter

Septicemia/Sepsis: Usually a 038 septicemia code and a 995.9x SIRS code (in this order)

- Code the organ system dysfunction by the SIRS (e.g., 518.81 respiratory failure followed by 995.92)

Septic Shock: Organ dysfunction associated with severe sepsis

- Code underlying systemic infection (e.g., 038.xx) followed by the SIRS code (995.92)

ICD-9-CM, CHAPTER 2, NEOPLASMS (I/O)

Two steps for coding neoplasms

- Incorrectly applying these neoplasm codes can also cause patient hardship
  1. Index: Locate histologic type of neoplasm (e.g., sarcoma, melanoma); review all instructions
  2. Locate code identified (usually in Neoplasm Table in Index) by body site

Neoplasm Table divided into columns:

- Malignant (primary, secondary, ca in situ)
- Benign

- Uncertain behavior
- Unspecified

Example: Pathology report confirmed diagnosis stated in operative report of primary malignant neoplasm of the bladder neck. ICD-9-CM Index, Neoplasm Table, bladder, neck, under Primary column, 188.5. Code then referenced in Tabular to ensure accurate assignment.

Coded as primary site unless specified as secondary site (metastasis)

Bone	Meninges	Brain
Peritoneum	Diaphragm	Pleura
Heart	Retroperitoneum	Liver
Lymph nodes	Spinal cord	Mediastinum

Unknown status of neoplasm is always reported with 199.1

Types of neoplasms are associated with morphology behavior codes (M codes)

Section I.C.2. Neoplasms (I/O)

Treatment directed at malignancy: Neoplasm is principal diagnosis

- Except for chemotherapy or radiotherapy:
  - Therapy (treatment), list first
  - Neoplasm, list second

Chemotherapy: V58.11

Radiotherapy: V58.0

First-Listed Diagnosis, Neoplasms (I/O)

Surgical removal of neoplasm and subsequent chemotherapy or radiotherapy

- Code malignancy as principal diagnosis

Surgery to determine extent of malignancy

- Code malignancy as principal diagnosis

History and Secondary Metastasis of Neoplasms (I/O)

V10, "Personal history of malignant neoplasm," if

- Neoplasm was previously destroyed
- No longer being treated

If patient receives treatment for secondary neoplasm (metastasis)

- Secondary neoplasm is principal diagnosis
- Even though primary is known

Admission for Neoplasms (I)

Admission for symptoms of primary or secondary neoplasm

- Malignancy principal diagnosis

Do NOT code symptoms or signs

Anemia and Complications with/of Neoplasm (I/O)

Patient treated for anemia or dehydration due to neoplasm or therapy

- Code
- Anemia or dehydration, followed by neoplasm
- Neoplasm
- E code for antineoplasm drug adverse effect

Patient admitted to repair complication of surgery for an intestinal malignancy

- Complication, principal diagnosis
- Complication is reason for encounter
- Malignancy, secondary diagnosis

V Codes and Neoplasms (I/O)

Patient receiving chemotherapy or radiotherapy post-op removal of neoplasm code:

- Therapy
- Active neoplasm

Do NOT report H/O (history of) neoplasm

ICD-9-CM, CHAPTER 3, ENDOCRINE, NUTRITIONAL, AND METABOLIC DISEASES AND IMMUNITY DISORDERS (I/O)

Disorders of Other Endocrine Glands (I/O)

Diabetes Mellitus 250 coded frequently

- Often requires two codes

  Example:
  - Diabetic iritis 250.5X for diabetes (etiology)
  - *[364.42]* for iritis (manifestation)

5th digit indicates type of diabetes

0 type II or unspecified type, not stated as uncontrolled

Fifth-digit 0 is for use for type II patients, even if the patient requires insulin

1 type I [juvenile type], not stated as uncontrolled

2 type II or unspecified type, uncontrolled

Fifth-digit 2 is for use for type II diabetic patients, even if the patient requires insulin

3 type I [juvenile type], uncontrolled

V58.67 used in addition to diabetes code to show long-term use of insulin

If type not indicated, report type II

Patient with type II diabetes may receive insulin for periods when diabetes is uncontrolled

Type I diabetic is one who is insulin-dependent

Other Metabolic and Immunity Disorders Section (I/O)

Disorders such as gout and dehydration

Disorders often have many names

- 242.0X Toxic diffuse goiter also known as
  - Basedow's disease
  - Graves' disease
  - Primary thyroid hyperplasia

ICD-9-CM, CHAPTER 4, DISEASES OF BLOOD AND BLOOD-FORMING ORGANS (I/O)

Short chapter with 10 sections

Includes anemia, blood disorders, coagulation defects

Often used code: Anemia

Many different types of anemia

- Hereditary hemolytic (282)
- Iron deficiency (280)
- Acquired hemolytic (283)
- Aplastic (284)
- Other and Unspecified (285)

Multiple coding often necessary

Identify underlying disease condition

ICD-9-CM, CHAPTER 5, MENTAL DISORDERS (I/O)

Includes codes for

- Personality disorders
- Stress disorders
- Neuroses
- Psychoses
- Sexual dysfunction, etc.

5th digit = status of episode

Example: 304.2 Drug dependence, cocaine, has following 5th digits

- 0 unspecified (episode)
- 1 continuous
- 2 episodic
- 3 in remission

ICD-9-CM, CHAPTER 6, DISEASES OF NERVOUS SYSTEM AND SENSE ORGANS (I/O)

Central Nervous System

Peripheral Nervous System

Disorders of Eye

Diseases of Ear

Pain—Category 338

Acute or chronic pain not elsewhere classified due to:

- Trama

- Neoplasm

- Post-operative

- Psychosocial dysfunction

Principal/Primary diagnosis

- When definitive diagnosis not established

- Pain management is reason for encounter/admission

ICD-9-CM, CHAPTER 7, DISEASES OF CIRCULATORY SYSTEM (I/O)

Three types of hypertension

1. Malignant accelerated, severe, poor prognosis

2. Benign continuous, mild, controllable

3. Unspecified, NOT indicated as either malignant or benign

Hypertension table located in Index of ICD-9-CM

- Under "H," Hypertension

- Codes divided based on type (malignant, benign, unspecified)

Section I.C.7.a.1. Hypertension, Essential, or NOS (I/O)

Assign hypertension (arterial, essential, primary, systemic, NOS) to 401

Fourth digit to indicate type

- 0 Malignant

- 1 Benign

- 9 Unspecified

Section I.C.7.a.2. Hypertension with Heart Disease (I/O)

402 Category

- Certain heart conditions when stated "due to hypertension" or implied ("hypertensive")

- Add 4th digit for type

- Use additional code to specify type of heart failure (428)

Section I.C.7.a.3. Hypertensive Chronic Kidney Disease with Chronic Kidney Failure (I/O)

Cause-and-effect relationship assumed in chronic kidney failure with hypertension

Category 403, Hypertensive chronic kidney disease, used when following present

- Chronic kidney disease (585.X)
- Kidney failure, unspecified (586)
- Kidney sclerosis, unspecified (587)

Fifth digit assignment required for stage of CKD

- 0 CKD stage I through IV
- 1 CKD stage V or end stage

Section I.C.7.a.4. Hypertensive Heart and Chronic Kidney Disease (I/O)

Assign 404 when both hypertensive chronic kidney disease and hypertensive heart disease stated

Assume cause-and-effect relationship

Assign 5th digit for mention of stage of chronic kidney disease and/or congestive heart failure

- Use additional code to specify type of heart failure (428)

Section I.C.7.a.5. Hypertensive Cerebrovascular Disease (I/O)

Code

- Cerebrovascular disease (430-438)
- Type of hypertension (401-405)

Section I.C.7.a.6. Hypertensive Retinopathy (I/O)

Code

- Hypertensive retinopathy (362.11)
- Type of hypertension (401-405)

Section I.C.7.a.7. Hypertension, Secondary (I/O)

Hypertension caused by an underlying condition

Code

- Underlying condition
- Type of hypertension (405)

Section I.C.7.a.8. Hypertension, Transient (I/O)

Transient hypertension: Temporary elevation of BP

Do NOT assign 401-405, Hypertensive Disease

- Hypertension diagnosis NOT established

- Use
  - 796.2, Elevated blood pressure
  - 642.3X, Transient hypertension of pregnancy

Section I.C.7.a.9. Hypertension, Controlled (I/O)

Hypertension controlled by therapy

- Assign code from 401-405

Section I.C.7.a.10. Hypertension, Uncontrolled (I/O)

Untreated hypertension

Uncontrolled hypertension

Documentation must state malignant hypertension to report 404

Assign code from 401-405

Section I.C.7.a.11. Elevated Blood Pressure (I/O)

Elevated blood pressure coded 796.2

- Elevated BP reading without hypertension is diagnosis
- Hypertension NOT stated, NOT coded to 401

ICD-9-CM, CHAPTER 8, DISEASES OF RESPIRATORY SYSTEM (I/O)

Watch for "Use additional code to identify infectious organism"

- Some codes indicate specific organism and do not need an additional code
- Respiratory Failure Sequencing

If the respiratory failure is due to an acute condition (such as MI [myocardial infarction]) or acute exacerbation of a chronic condition (such as COPD [chronic obstructive pulmonary disease]), sequence the acute condition first

Example: MI (acute condition) and respiratory failure

- Sequence MI first and respiratory failure second

If the respiratory failure (acute condition) is due to a chronic nonrespiratory condition (such as myasthenia gravis), sequence the respiratory failure first

Example: Acute respiratory failure (acute) and myasthenia gravis (chronic)

- Sequence acute respiratory failure first and myasthenia gravis second

Acute Respiratory Infection Section (I/O)

Frequently used codes, such as

- Common cold (460, acute nasopharyngitis)
- Sore throat (462, acute pharyngitis)
- Acute tonsillitis (463)
- Bronchitis (490-491)
- Acute upper respiratory infection (465, URI)

- Influenza (487, flu)

Read Guidelines for Chapter 8 for specifics on coding COPD and asthma

ICD-9-CM, CHAPTER 9, DISEASES OF DIGESTIVE SYSTEM (I/O)

Mouth to anus and accessory organs

Extensive subcategories

574 Cholelithiasis (10 subcategories)

- Each has 5th digit subclassification

Commonly used codes

- Ulcers (531-534)
  - Gastric (531)
  - Duodenal (532)
  - Peptic (533)
  - Gastrojejunal (534)
- Hernias (550-553)

ICD-9-CM, CHAPTER 10, DISEASES OF GENITOURINARY SYSTEM (I/O)

Commonly used codes

- Urinary tract infection (599.0)
- Inflammation of prostate (601)
- Disorders of menstruation (625-627)

Stages of chronic kidney disease

- Stage I: Blood flow through kidney increases, kidney enlarges (585.1)
- Stage II: (mild) Small amounts of blood protein (albumin) leak into urine (microalbuminuria) (585.2)
- Stage III: (moderate) Albumin and other protein losses increase. Patient may develop high blood pressure and kidney loses ability to filter waste (585.3)
- Stage IV: (severe) Large amounts of urine pass through kidney, blood pressure increases (585.4)
- Stage V: Ability to filter waste nearly stops (585.5)
- End-stage renal failure (585.6)

  When documentation indicates chronic renal disease (CKD) and ESRD, report ESRD

- Unspecified 585.9

Status post kidney transplant, assign V42.0

- Patient may still have CKD

ICD-9-CM, CHAPTER 11, COMPLICATIONS OF PREGNANCY, CHILDBIRTH, AND PUERPERIUM (I/O)

Extensive multiple coding with many 5th digit assignments and notes

Admission for pregnancy, complication

- Obstetric complication = primary diagnosis

Chapter 11 ICD-9-CM codes take precedence over codes from other chapters unless the documentation indicates the condition being treated is not affecting the management of the pregnancy

Codes 640-676.9 share same 5th digit subclassification

- Denotes current episode of care
- 0 Unspecified as to episode of care or not applicable
- 1 Delivered, with or without mention of antepartum condition
- 2 Delivered, with mention of postpartum complication
- 3 Antepartum condition or complication
- 4 Postpartum condition or complication

Section I.C.11.a.1. General Rules (I/O)

Not all encounters are pregnancy-related

Example: Pregnant woman, broken ankle; report

- Broken ankle
- V22.2 Pregnant state incidental

Must be documented in medical record that condition being treated not affecting pregnancy

Section I.C.11.a.2. Complications of Pregnancy, Childbirth, and Puerperium (I/O)

Chapter 11 codes (630-677)

- Used on mother's medical record
- Not on newborn medical record

Mother's record

- Outcome of delivery code (V27.0-V27.9) when delivered

Section I.C.11: Selection of Principal Diagnosis—Obstetric (I)

- No delivery: Principal diagnosis = principal complication
  - If more than one complication, sequence any first

Section I.C.11.b.1. and 2. Selection of Primary Diagnosis (O)

Routine prenatal visits, no complications:

- V22.0, Supervision, normal first pregnancy or
- V22.1, Supervision, other normal pregnancy

Prenatal outpatient visits for high-risk pregnancies

- V23, Supervision of high-risk pregnancy

Section I.C.11.a.3. and 4. Fifth Digit (I/O)

All categories EXCEPT 650 (Normal delivery)

Watch for

- Onset of delivery before 37 weeks' gestation (644.2X)
- Post-term pregnancy 40-42 weeks' gestation (645.1)
- Prolonged pregnancy beyond 42 weeks' gestation (645.2)

Requires 5th digit for

- Antepartum
- Postpartum
- If delivery has occurred

Appropriate 5th digit listed under each code

- 640.0 Threatened abortion
  - 0: Unspecified episode
  - 1: Delivered with or without complication
  - 3: Antepartum condition or complication

Section I.C.11. Normal Delivery, 650 (I)

Normal delivery includes

- Vaginal delivery
- Minimal or no assistance
- With or without episiotomy
- No fetal manipulation or instrumentation
- Full-term, single, liveborn infant

No complications, principal diagnosis = 650

With complications = NOT 650

V27.0 (Single liveborn)

- Only outcome for 650 (Normal delivery)

Delivery Procedure Codes (I)

If delivered prior to admission

- In ambulance
- At home
- In ED

Do NOT code delivery

Code any postpartum repairs

Postpartum Period (I/O)

After delivery and continues for 6 weeks

Abortions (I/O)

No identifiable fetus

500 grams or less

Less than 22 weeks' gestation

Codes 634-637 require 5th digits

- 0: Unspecified
- 1: Incomplete POC (product of conception), NOT expelled (may retain part or all of placenta or fetus)
- 2: Complete, all POC expelled prior to care

Abortions with Liveborn Fetus (I/O)

Attempted abortion results in liveborn fetus

- 644.21 (Early onset of delivery) appropriately

Use V27.X (Outcome of delivery)

Attempted abortion code also assigned

ICD-9-CM, CHAPTER 12, DISEASES OF SKIN AND SUBCUTANEOUS TISSUE (I/O)

Skin

Epidermis

Dermis

Subcutaneous tissue

Infectious skin/Subcutaneous tissue

Scar tissue

Accessory Organs

Sweat glands

Sebaceous glands

Nails

Hair and hair follicles

Other

> ***Example:*** Cellulitis due to *Staphylococcus*, report:
> - Cellulitis 682.X
> - Staph 041.X

ICD-9-CM, CHAPTER 13, DISEASES OF MUSCULOSKELETAL SYSTEM AND CONNECTIVE TISSUE (I/O)

Bone

Bursa

Cartilage

Fascia

Ligaments

Muscle

Synovia

Tendons

Chapter 13 Sections (I/O)

Arthropathies (joint disease) and related disorders

Dorsopathies (curvature of spine)

Rheumatism, Excluding Back

Osteopathies, Chondropathies, and Acquired Musculoskeletal Deformities

Extensive notes and 5th digits

ICD-9-CM, CHAPTERS 14 AND 15, CONGENITAL ANOMALIES AND CONDITIONS ORIGINATING IN PERINATAL PERIOD (I/O)

Congenital Anomalies (abnormalities at birth), 740-759

Conditions Originating in Perinatal Period

- Perinatal period through 28th day following birth
- Codes can be used after 28th day, if documented that condition originated during perinatal period

Chapter 17 codes are only for the newborn record; never on the maternal record

Assign V30-V39 as first listed according to type of birth

Use of Codes V29 (I/O)

V29 Observation and evaluation of newborn

Suspected of having an abnormal condition

Infant 28 days or less

Use of Codes V30-V39 (I)

V30-V39 Liveborn infant(s)

Example:

- V30 Single liveborn
- V31 Liveborn twins

Inpatient: Principal diagnosis

NOTE: V30 used ONLY once, hospital where baby delivered

Coding Additional Diagnosis (I)

Code conditions that require

- Treatment

- Further investigation
- Additional resource

Prolonged length of stay (LOS)

Implications for future care

Insignificant conditions, signs, symptoms

- Resolve with no treatment
- Need no code
- EVEN IF documented

Prematurity and Fetal Growth Retardation (I)

Codes from categories

- 764 (Slow fetal growth and fetal malnutrition) and
- 765 (Disorders relating to short gestation and unspecified low birthweight)

Not assigned solely on birthweight or gestational age

Use physician's assessment of maturity

Use additional code for weeks of gestation (765.20-765.29)

ICD-9-CM, CHAPTER 16, SYMPTOMS, SIGNS, AND ILL-DEFINED CONDITIONS

Do NOT code a sign or symptom if

- Definitive diagnosis made (symptoms are part of disease)

Used only if no specific diagnosis made

ICD-9-CM, CHAPTER 17, INJURY AND POISONING

Section Examples (I/O)

Fractures

Dislocations

Sprains and Strains

Intracranial Injury

- With or without loss of consciousness

Internal Injury

- Open or closed

Crushing Injury

Foreign Body

Burns

Late Effects

- Code manifestation or reason for treatment first

Poisoning

■ Index and Tabular

E code Index located in Section III

Directly before the Tabular

Not in the Index to Disease, Volume 2

E codes are located after the V codes in the Tabular

E Codes (I/O)

The only E codes assigned on the CCS examination are those for adverse effects of correct medication correctly given and correctly taken

Provide supplemental information

Never principal diagnosis

Identify

- Cause of an injury or poisoning
- Intent (unintentional or intentional)
- Place it occurred

General E Code Guidelines

Use with any code in Volume 1

Initial encounter

- Use E code

Subsequent encounter

- Use late effects E codes

Intent

Unknown, Undetermined (E980-E989)

Unspecified, Undetermined (E980-E989)

Questionable, Undetermined (E980-E989)

Table of Drugs and Chemicals (I/O)

Alphabetic listing with codes

Do NOT code directly from Table

Always reference Tabular

Late Effects of External Cause (I/O)

Should be used with late effect of a previous injury/poisoning

Should NOT be used with related current injury code

Sequence and Different Degree (I/O)

Do NOT code a sign/symptom if definitive diagnosis made

- Symptoms are part of disease

Use only if no specific diagnosis is made

Burns Classified (I/O)

According to extent of body surface involved

Burn site NOT specified

Additional data required

Category 948 (I/O)

4th digits = % body surface involved

5th digits = % body surface involved in 3rd-degree burns

Rule of Nines applies
  Burn Example: 3rd-degree burn of abdomen (10%) and 2nd-degree burn of thigh (5%) by hot water

- 942.33 Burn, abdomen, 3rd degree

- 945.26 Burn, thigh, 2nd degree

- 948.11 15% total burn area and 10% 3rd degree

- E924.0 Burn by hot liquid

Debridement of Wound, Infection, or Burn (I)

Excisional debridement (86.22)

- Cut away

- Performed by physician or other health care provider

Nonexcisional procedure (86.28)

- Shaved or scraped

- Performed by physician or

- Nonphysician

Coding for Multiple Injuries (I/O)

Separate code for each injury

Most serious injury first

Vessel and Nerve Damage (I/O)

Code primary injury first

- Use additional code if nerve damage minor

Primary injury = Nerve damage

- Code nerve damage first

Multiple Fractures (I/O)

Same coding principles as multiple injuries

Code multiple fractures by site

Sequenced by severity

Fractures (I/O)

Not indicated as closed or open = closed

Same bone fractured AND dislocated:

- Code fracture ONLY (highest level of injury)

Section IV, Diagnostic Coding and Reporting Guidelines for Outpatient Services (O)

Hospital-based outpatient services = OPPS

Part of Official Coding and Reporting Guidelines, Section IV

Guidelines A (O)
Use term *first-listed diagnosis* in lieu of *principal diagnosis*

Guideline B (O)
Use codes 001.0 through V86.1 to code diagnosis, symptoms, conditions, problems, complaints, or other reason(s) for visit

Guideline C (O)
Documentation should describe patient's condition using terminology that includes specific diagnoses as well as symptoms, problems, or reasons for encounter

Guideline D (O)
Selection of codes 001.0 through 999.9 (Chapters 1-17) will frequently be used to describe reason for encounter

Guideline E (O)
Codes that describe symptoms and signs, as opposed to diagnoses, are acceptable for reporting purposes when an established diagnosis has NOT been confirmed by physician

Guideline F (O)
V codes deal with encounters for circumstances other than disease or injury

> *Example:* Well-baby checkup

Guideline G (O)
Codes have three, four, or five digits

Fourth- and/or fifth-digit codes provide greater specificity

Three-digit code is used ONLY if there is NO fourth or fifth digit

Where fourth and/or fifth digits are provided, they must be assigned

Diagnoses NOT coded to full digits available are invalid

Guideline H (O)
List first code for diagnosis, condition, problem, or other reason for encounter/visit shown in medical record to be chiefly responsible for services provided

List additional codes that describe any significant co-existing conditions or conditions also being treated

Guideline I (O)
Do NOT code diagnoses documented as probable, suspected, questionable, ruled out, or working diagnoses

Rather, code condition(s) to highest degree of certainty for that encounter/visit, such as symptoms, signs, abnormal test results, or other reason for visit

Guideline J (O)
Chronic diseases treated on an ongoing basis may be coded and reported as many times as patient receives treatment and care for condition(s)

Guideline K (O)
Code all documented conditions that coexist at time of visit and that require or affect patient care, treatment, or management

Do NOT code conditions previously treated or no longer existing

"History of" codes (V10-V19) may be used as secondary codes if

- Affects current care or treatment

Guidelines L and M (O)
For patients receiving diagnostic or therapeutic services ONLY

Sequence first

- Diagnosis
- Condition
- Problem
- Other reason shown in medical record to be chiefly responsible for encounter

Codes for other diagnoses (e.g., chronic conditions)

- May be sequenced as secondary diagnoses

    Exception:
    - Patients receiving chemotherapy, radiation therapy, or rehabilitation
    - V code first diagnosis, problem for which service being performed second

Medical necessity principles apply

- Multiple tests require supporting diagnosis for each test

Guideline N (O)
For patients receiving preoperative evaluations ONLY

- Code from category V72.8 (Other specified examinations)
- Assign secondary code for reason for surgery
- Code also any findings related to preoperative evaluation

Guideline O (O)
Code diagnosis that required surgery

Pre- and post-op diagnosis different

- Code the post-op diagnosis

Guideline P (O)
Code routine prenatal visits with no complications

- V22.0 (Supervision of normal first pregnancy)

- V22.1 (Supervision of other normal pregnancy)

Do NOT use these codes with pregnancy complication codes

VOLUME 3, PROCEDURES

90% of codes refer to surgical procedures

10% refer to diagnostic and therapeutic procedures

- Volume 3 codes are used by hospitals to report facility services provided to inpatients
- Procedures done in physician's office or outpatient ASC are coded using CPT codes
- Surgeon uses CPT to report services to inpatients

VOLUME 3, TABLE OF CONTENTS

Operations on body systems

Miscellaneous Diagnostic and Therapeutic Procedures

Most nonsurgical codes

VOLUME 3, TABULAR LIST

Conventions in Volume 3 are the same as those in Volumes 1 and 2

"Code also . . ." appears in Volume 3 and Volume 2

Additional information about coding various components or special adjunctive services of procedure

VOLUME 3, ALPHABETIC INDEX

Index often contains terms that do not appear in Volume 3, Tabular List

Example: In Index, Volume 3, the entry Gastrostomy, subterm Janeway, directs you to 43.19

- Janeway not mentioned in Tabular List in the description of 43.19

Index terms in bold

- Subterms not in bold

Alphabetical arrangement

Ignores single spaces and hyphens

Example: Opening and open reduction

- "Opening" appears before "open reduction" because space between two words is ignored

Often necessary and permissible to code individual components of a procedure

Example: During a procedure, a portion of intestine was removed and reconstruction of urinary bladder was done

- Both reconstruction (57.87) and resection (45.51) coded

Cross-reference features included in Volume 3 are

- *see*
- *see also*
- *see category*

Many operations named for surgeon who developed procedure (eponyms)

- These procedures located under person's name or name of operation

   Example: Watson-Jones is located under main term "Watson-Jones" and also as a subterm under "Operation"

Never code directly from Index.

VOLUME 3, TABULAR LIST

Format same as Volume 1, Tabular List of Diseases, except Volume 3 codes have two digits before decimal

Category, subcategory, and subclassification

BUNDLING

Included in all surgical procedures

- Opening and closing of surgical site
- Approach, except where approach differs from code description

   Example: Microscopic approach used instead of described approach

- Do not unbundle and code these separately
- If closure takes place during separate surgical procedure, closure can be coded separately

Coding Challenge

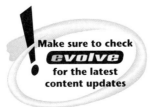

Make sure to check **evolve** for the latest content updates

EXAMINATIONS

You have three opportunities to practice taking an examination:

- Pre-Examination (before study)
- Post-Examination (after study)
- Final Examination (at the end of your complete program of study)

You should have a current edition of the following texts:

- ICD-9-CM, Volumes 1, 2, and 3 (*International Classification of Diseases,* 9th Edition, Clinical Modification)
- HCPCS (Healthcare Common Procedure Coding System)
- CPT *(Current Procedural Terminology)*

No other reference material, other than a medical dictionary, is allowed for any of the examinations.

- For the Pre-, Post-, and Final Examinations, you will need a computer that can use a CD-ROM and the three coding references listed above (ICD-9-CM, HCPCS, CPT).
- Each organization's certification examination has different scoring requirements, but as you take these examinations, you should strive for 80% to 90% on the Post-Examination and 75% as a minimum on the Final Examination.

NOTE: To enable the learner to calculate an examination score, minimums have been identified as "passing" within this text; however, this may or may not be the percentage identified by AHIMA as a "passing" grade. It is your responsibility to review all certification information published by AHIMA as they are the definitive source for information regarding the CCS certification examination.

GUIDELINES

Although there may be spaces for 6 procedure/service codes and 14 possible diagnosis codes, each case may or may not require this many codes to be correct or complete. However, no case will ever require more than that number of codes.

Do not assign E codes, M codes, or modifiers.

The Final Examination has more difficult questions and cases than the Pre-/Post-Examination to ensure that you have had adequate practice with the more complex coding cases.

PRE-EXAMINATION AND POST-EXAMINATION

The Pre-Examination contains 73 questions and is located on the CD-ROM. The purpose of the Pre-Examination is only to assess your beginning level of knowledge and skill—your starting place. Based on your scores, you can tailor your study to target your weakest areas and increase your scores. Take this examination before you begin your studies.

The multiple choice questions are located on the CD and answered on the computer screen. The cases are printed in this textbook in Unit IV. Read the case and assign all necessary service and diagnosis codes. These codes are then entered into the blocks on the computer. The software on the CD will calculate your score and retain this information for later use.

Immediately on completion of your study, you should complete the Post-Examination. Again the multiple choice questions from Part I are read and answered using the computer. The cases for Part II are printed in this textbook and answered on the computer. After you are finished, the CD will automatically compare your Pre-Examination scores with your Post-Examination scores, and will store the results for when you take the Final Examination. By comparing the results of the Pre-Examination and the Post-Examination, the software illustrates the improvements you have achieved.

Rationales for each question are available for review after you complete the Post-Examination. Study the questions for which you did not choose the right response. Did you misread the question, did you not know the material well enough to answer correctly, or did you run out of time? Knowing why you missed a question is an important step to improving your skill level.

Ideally, you should complete each examination in one sitting (4 hours, or 240 minutes); if time does not allow, spread the examination times over several periods. There are no time extensions in an actual examination setting, and learning how to judge the amount of time you spend on each question is an important part of this learning experience to prepare you for the real certification examination.

FINAL EXAMINATION

If you scored well on all areas of the Post-Examination (80%-90%), you are ready to move on to the Final Examination, which is on CD. The real certification examination is computer-based. Once you have completed the Final Examination, the software will compare all your scores to illustrate your improvement.

If you did not attain a minimum score on each section, you should develop a plan to restudy those particular areas where the examination indicates you are having difficulties. There are rationales for each question in the Final Examination, and you should review that information as well as material in the text. You can take any of the practice examinations again after your additional study.

GRADING OF THE EXAMINATION

Note: According to AHIMA guidelines, Part II of both the Pre-/Post- and Final Examinations does not include the assignment of modifiers.

The grading for the CCS is not published. AHIMA does a statistical analysis of the examination and determines if the examination is passing. For the purposes of this text, however, a grading method has been established.

The scoring for the CCS Final Examination includes deduction of points for unnecessary codes reported for conditions that the patient may have, but for which the physician rendered no treatment or management. For example, on an operative report, it was documented that the surgeon performed a mastectomy for a patient with diabetes. The surgeon mentioned that the patient had diabetes but provided no treatment or management for the condition. It would be unnecessary to report the diagnosis of diabetes, and if the student did report the diabetes, he/she would have 2 points deducted from the score for reporting an unnecessary diagnosis code. Conversely, if the surgeon requested a test in order to manage or render treatment for the diabetes (i.e., glucose level), it would be correct to report the diabetes, and if they didn't report the diagnosis code for the diabetes, they would have to deduct 2 points from the score for not reporting a necessary code.

The grading for the Pre-/Post-Examination includes 209 possible points as follows:

- Part I contains 60 questions
  - Each correct answer is worth 1 point
  - Possible points on Part I are 60
  - Strive for a minimum score of 74%, or 44 correct answers, to consider Part I successful
- Part II contains 13 coding cases
  - 136 points for codes or units (68 codes or units × 2 = 136)
  - 13 additional points for each correct first-listed diagnosis
  - Possible points to award on Part II are 149
  - Strive for a minimum score of 74%, or 110 points, to consider Part II successful

The grading for the Final Examination based on 229 points is as follows:

- Part I contains 60 questions
  - Each correct answer is worth 1 point
  - Possible points on Part I are 60
  - Strive for a minimum score of 74%, or 44 correct answers, to consider Part I successful
- Part II contains 13 coding cases
  - 156 points for codes or units (78 codes or units × 2 = 156)
  - 13 additional points for each correct first-listed diagnosis
  - Possible points on Part II are 169
  - Strive for a minimum score of 74%, or 125 points, to consider Part II successful

Calculating the score for Part II is based on:

Awarded	**Deducted**
2 points for each correct code or unit (Part II)	2 points for each incorrect or missing code or unit (Part II)
1 point for each primary/principal diagnosis correctly sequenced first (Part II)	2 points for each extra code or unit (Part II)

Let's look at how this is calculated by reviewing the examination results of a student who received the following scores on her final examination:

Awarded

Part I, 43 questions correct:	43 × 1 = +43
43 correct/60 possible	Part I, **72%**

Part II, 50 correct codes and units:	$50 \times 2 = +100$
Part II, 50 correct codes and units:	
13 correct first-listed diagnosis:	$\underline{13 \times 1 = +13}$
Awarded points for Part II:	$+113$
3 incorrect or missing codes and units:	$3 \times 2 = -6$
6 unnecessary codes and units:	$\underline{6 \times 2 = -12}$
Deducted points for Part II	-18

TOTAL: $113 - 18 = 95$ points from a possible 169 (95/169), or **56%**, for Part II

This student carefully reviewed the incorrect, missing, and unnecessary codes to determine her areas of weakness and then developed a plan to study those areas that had presented her with difficulties. One of these weaknesses was that she was overcoding the cases in Part II.

ACUITY SHEET

The following Emergency Department acuity sheet will be used throughout Part II when reporting ED services. Remove this acuity sheet from the text for easier reference.

Level 1—99281	Level 2—99282	Level 3—99283
1. Initial (triage) assessment 2. Suture removal 3. Wound recheck 4. Note for work or school 5. Simple discharge information	Interventions from previous level plus any of the following: 1. OTC med administration 2. Tetanus booster 3. Bedside diagnostic tests (stool hemoccult, glucometer) 4. Visual acuity 5. Orthostatic vital signs 6. Simple trauma not requiring x-ray 7. Simple discharge information	Interventions from previous level plus any of the following: 1. Heparin/saline lock 2. Crystalloid IV therapy 3. X-ray, one area 4. RX med administration 5. Fluorescein stain 6. Quick cath 7. Foley cath 8. Receipt of ambulance patient 9. Mental health emergencies (mild) not requiring parenteral medications or admission 10. Moderate complexity discharge instructions 11. Intermediate layered and complex laceration repair
Level 4—99284	**Level 5—99285**	**Critical Care 99291, 99292**
Interventions from previous level plus any of the following: 1. X-ray, multiple areas 2. Special imaging studies (CT, MRI, ultrasound) 3. Cardiac monitoring 4. Multiple reassessments of patient 5. Parenteral[1] medications (including insulin) 6. Nebulizer treatment (1 or 2) 7. NG placement 8. Pelvic exam 9. Mental health emergencies (moderate). May require parenteral medications but not admission 10. Administration of IV medications [1]*not through the alimentary canal but rather by injection through some other route, such as subcutaneous, intramuscular, intraorbital, intracapsular, intraspinal, intrasternal, or intravenous*	Interventions from previous level plus any of the following: 1. Monitor/stabilize patient during in hospital transport and/or testing (CT, MRI, ultrasound) 2. Vasoactive medication 3. Administration (dopamine, dobutamine, multiple) nebulizer treatments (3 or more) 4. Conscious sedation 5. Lumbar puncture 6. Thoracentesis 7. Sexual assault exam 8. Admission to hospital 9. Mental health emergency (severe) psychotic and/or agitated/combative 10. Requires admission 11. Fracture/dislocation reduction 12. Suicide precautions 13. Gastric lavage 14. Complex discharge instructions	Interventions from any previous level plus any of the following: 1. Multiple parenteral medications 2. Continuous monitoring 3. Major trauma care 4. Chest tube insertion 5. CPR 6. Defibrillation/cardioversion 7. Delivery of baby 8. Control of major hemorrhage 9. Administration of blood or blood products

■ PRE-/POST-EXAMINATION

PART II

With the use of a medical dictionary, CPT, and HCPCS and ICD-9-CM coding manuals, assign codes to the following:

1. **CASE 1**

   LOCATION: Inpatient hospital

   PREOPERATIVE DIAGNOSIS: Normal pressure hydrocephalus, Obstructed ventriculoperitoneal shunt

   PROCEDURE PERFORMED: Revision of shunt. Replacement of ventricular valve and peritoneal end. Entire shunt replacement.

   PROCEDURE: Under general anesthesia, the patient's head, neck, and abdomen were prepped and draped in the usual manner. An incision was made over the previous site where the shunt had been inserted in the posterior right occipital area. This shunt was found to be nonfunctioning and was removed. The problem was that we could not get the ventricular catheter out without probably producing bleeding, so it was left inside. The peritoneal end of the shunt was then pulled out through the same incision. Having done this, I placed a new ventricular catheter into the ventricle. I then attached this to a medium-pressure bulb valve and secured this with 3-0 silk to the subcutaneous tissue. We then went to the abdomen and made an incision below the previous site, and we were able to trocar the peritoneal end of the shunt by making a stab wound in the neck, then connecting it up to the shunt. This was then connected to the shunt. By pumping on the shunt, we got fluid coming out the other end. I then inserted this end of the shunt into the abdomen by dividing the rectus fascia, splitting the muscle, and dividing the peritoneum and placing the shunt into the abdomen. One 2-0 chromic suture was used around the peritoneum. The wound was then closed with 2-0 Vicryl, 2-0 plain in the subcutaneous tissue, and surgical staples on the skin. The stab wound on the neck was closed with surgical staples. The head wound was closed with 2-0 Vicryl on the galea and surgical staples on the skin. A dressing was applied. The patient was discharged to the recovery room.

2. **CASE 2**

   LOCATION: ASC

   PREOPERATIVE DIAGNOSIS: Nasal obstruction with sleep apnea, septal deviation due to trauma, bilateral inferior turbinate hypertrophy, left middle turbinate hypertrophy, left concha bullosa

   POSTOPERATIVE DIAGNOSIS: Same

   PROCEDURE: Septoplasty, bilateral inferior turbinate reduction, and endoscopic excision of left concha bullosa

   PROCEDURE DESCRIPTION: Following informed consent from the patient, she was taken to the operating room and placed supine on the operating room table. The appropriate monitoring devices were placed on the patient, and general anesthesia was induced. She was orally intubated without difficulty. She was draped in the usual sterile fashion. The nose was packed bilaterally with Afrin-soaked gauze. The 0-degree endoscope was passed into the left nasal cavity after gauze removal. She was seen to have a left inferior septal spur somewhat anterior and a large left middle turbinate that was grossly widened. The concha bullosa was injected with approximately 0.5 cc of 1% Xylocaine with epinephrine. A sickle knife was used to incise through the base of the concha bullosa. Straight scissors were then used to further cut through the bony attachment of the concha bullosa to the middle turbinate. It was then removed in one thin section with the straight Wilde forceps. There was very little bleeding. I did repack the left ostiomeatal complex with Afrin-soaked gauze; after 2 minutes, this was removed, and there was no bleeding.

   The right and left nasal septa were each then injected with approximately 2 cc of Lidocaine with epinephrine. The nasal septum was seen to be deviated superiorly on the right and left septal spur with some left posterior deviation as well. An incision was made at the anterior end of the right nasal septum. A mucoperichondrial and mucoperiosteal flap were then elevated. A 7 × 12 mm section of septal cartilage in the midportion of the cartilaginous septum was then removed. A mucoperichondrial and mucoperiosteal flap were then removed. A mucoperichondrial and mucoperiosteal flap were then elevated on the left nasal septum. Some of the bony vomer contributing to left posterior septal deviation was removed. No tear in the septum was created during this procedure. I did use an osteotome to remove the left septal spur with good result. Some of the superior, anterior, and right septal deviation was removed. However, I did not remove all of it since quite a bit of the right septal deviation was superior and did not contribute to any deviation of the inferior nasal septum on the right side. A small incision was made on the right nasal septum to allow for hematoma prevention. The inferior edges of both inferior turbinates were then cauterized with the needle point cautery. The butter knife was used to outfracture the inferior turbinates bilaterally. The nasopharynx was suctioned of blood. The anterior end of the nasal septal mucosa was reapproximated with 4-0 chromic catgut in an interrupted fashion. Doyle splints were then applied to the right and left nasal cavities bilaterally. They were sutured anteriorly with a 3-0 Ethilon suture tied on the left side. The patient was then allowed to recover from general anesthesia. She was transferred to the recovery room in good condition. She tolerated the procedure well. Estimated blood loss was less than 20 cc.

3. **CASE 3**

HISTORY AND PHYSICAL

LOCATION: Inpatient hospital

DATE OF ADMISSION: July 24, 20XX

CHIEF COMPLAINT: Shortness of breath and back pain

HISTORY OF PRESENT ILLNESS: This is a 90-year-old female with known history of coronary artery disease who was recently admitted, on April 24, with a non-Q-wave myocardial infarction that was elected to be treated conservatively. Since that time, the patient has felt relatively okay, up until last night when the patient indicated that she felt like she had increasing shortness of breath with pain in her chest, which seemed to radiate into her back. The patient denied any associated diaphoresis or nausea, which she had had with her prior event. This pain came and went. It kind of resolved overnight. The patient's symptoms returned drastically this morning, and subsequently, the patient was essentially unable to move at home. She had her Meals-on-Wheels delivered, and the delivery person called for the ambulance for her. Subsequently, the patient presented to the emergency department.

In the emergency department, the patient received oxygen and nitroglycerin, which improved the patient's symptomatology.

Currently, patient denies any chest pain or chest pressure, or any nausea. The patient indicates that she is currently not short of breath. The patient denies any increased swelling in her legs.

ALLERGIES: Sulfa

PAST MEDICAL HISTORY:

1. Diabetes mellitus.

2. Glaucoma.

3. Coronary artery disease.

4. Hypertension.

MEDICATIONS:

1. Norvasc 5 mg daily.

2. Aspirin 81 mg daily.

3. Atenolol 50 mg daily.

4. Bumex 0.5 mg daily.

5. Plavix 75 mg daily.

6. Enalapril 40 mg daily.

7. Glyburide 2.5 mg daily.

8. Imdur 60 mg daily.

9. Xalatan eyedrops.

10. Protonix 40 mg daily.

11. Timolol eyedrops.

FAMILY HISTORY: Noncontributory

REVIEW OF SYSTEMS: General, GI, cardiovascular, respiratory, ENT, eyes, neurologic, musculoskeletal, psych, endocrine performed. With the exception of those noted in the HPI and chronic paresthesias in patient's feet, otherwise unremarkable.

EXAMINATION: Vitals today: Temperature 36.4°, pulse 65, respiratory rate 19, blood pressure 141/41, O₂ sats 91% in room air. Cardiovascular: S1 and S2. No S3 or S4. Heart sounds distant. Lungs: Bilateral breath sounds with crackles present. HEENT: Head is atraumatic. Extraocular movements are intact. Nonjaundiced sclera. Moist oral mucosal membranes. Neck is supple. Trachea is midline. The patient does have JVD. Abdomen is soft and nontender. Positive bowel sounds. No rebound tenderness or guarding. No masses palpated. Extremities: Trace edema. Musculoskeletal: Patient moves all four extremities symmetrically and to command. Neurologic: Minimally decreased sensation to light touch in the lower extremities. Psych: Patient alert and oriented. Integument: No obvious petechia or purpura.

PA portable chest x-ray, which I visualized in the emergency department, shows pulmonary edema and no opacities.

LABORATORY DATA: Platelet count 162,000, white count 12.31, hemoglobin 9.4, BUN 41, sodium 139, potassium 4.9, chloride 102, bicarb 24.7, glucose 256, creatinine 1.4, calcium 8.3, CPK 27, troponin 0.07.

IMPRESSION:

1. Acute pulmonary edema.
2. Unstable angina.
3. Diabetes mellitus.

PLAN: At this point, we will admit the patient. The patient indicates that she wishes to be a code level II. Will place the patient on nitroglycerin at 5 mcg initial rate, titrating until chest is pain free or systolic pressure is greater than 100. Provide the patient with Lovenox 1 mg/kg subcutaneously q12h. Will adjust dose for renal function as necessary. Keep the patient on aspirin. Keep the patient on beta blocker. Blood sugar checks q.i.d. Supplemental insulin scale. Continue the patient on glyburide. Serial cardiac enzymes. Obtain a UA and a UC.

RADIOLOGY REPORT

EXAMINATION OF: Chest

CLINICAL SYMPTOMS: Shortness of breath

CHEST: 1:15 PM: Findings: Comparison is made with the portable chest x-ray of last month. Cardiac enlargement is unchanged, given the difference in technique. Pulmonary vascularity is mildly elevated and has increased mildly since the previous study. No focal infiltrates. Slight fibrosis or atelectasis in the bases. Blunting of the right costophrenic angle is unchanged because of fluid or pleural thickening. No mediastinal widening.

PROGRESS REPORT

SUBJECTIVE: The patient indicates that she did have some chest discomfort last night, with some dyspnea. The patient received morphine, which improved her discomfort. The patient currently indicates that she is not short of breath. Her pain has resolved. The patient, however, feels fatigued at this point.

REVIEW OF SYSTEMS: General, gastrointestinal, cardiovascular, respiratory, and endocrine were performed, and, with the exception of those noted in the HPI, review was negative.

OBJECTIVE: Heart: Regular. No murmurs. Lungs: Bilateral breath sounds. No wheezes or rhonchi. Abdomen: Soft and nontender with positive bowel sounds. Extremities: No edema. Vitals: Pulse 56, blood pressure 97/43, respiratory rate 14. O_2 sats: 96% on 4 L. Psych: Alert and oriented.

IMPRESSION:

1. Non-Q-wave MI.

2. Pulmonary edema secondary to #1.

3. Diabetes mellitus.

4. Hypotension with history of hypertension.

5. Gastroesophageal reflux disease.

6. Overall poor prognosis.

PLAN: At this point, we did discuss with the patient the continued goal of conservative management, as recommended by Cardiology on admission. The patient is in agreement with this. Again, the patient has mild hypotension. We will decrease the patient's antihypertensive agents. We will continue the patient on Imdur at 60 mg twice a day. We will obtain a basic metabolic panel today. We will continue the patient on aspirin, beta blocker, and ACE inhibitor, although beta blocker needs to be given at a lower dose. We will continue the patient on Lovenox. We will obtain daily CBC and daily basic metabolic panel.

PROGRESS NOTE

SUBJECTIVE: The patient denies any chest pain, chest pressure, fever, chills, or nausea. The patient indicates that she is feeling better today. The patient did have a hyperglycemic reaction this morning. However, the patient indicates that this resolved.

REVIEW OF SYSTEMS: General, cardiovascular, respiratory, and endocrinology were performed. With the exception noted in the HPI, all are negative.

PHYSICAL EXAMINATION: VITALS: Today: Temp is 36.1. Blood pressure is 105/42. Pulse is 71. Respiratory rate is 18. O_2 sats are 97% on room air. Cardiovascular: S1 and S2. No S3, no S4. No murmurs, clicks, gallops, or rubs. Lungs: Bilateral breath sounds. No wheezes, rhonchi, or crackles. In general, a pleasant female lying comfortably in bed. The abdomen was soft and nontender. Positive bowel sounds. Psych: The patient is alert and oriented.

LABORATORY STUDIES: Blood sugars of 44, 120, 96, 88, and 102

Reviewed nurse's and physical therapy notes. The patient refused physical therapy yesterday.

IMPRESSION:

1. Non-Q-wave MI.

2. Diabetes mellitus with moderate hypoglycemic reaction, currently improved.

3. Hypertension, improving.

4. Acute pulmonary edema, resolving.

PLAN: At this point, continue the patient on current diabetes mellitus medications. Continue the patient on current conservative therapy for non-Q-wave MI and occupational and physical therapy. Have social service plan for discharge planning. It is possible that the patient may require nursing home placement given her poor functional status.

DISCHARGE SUMMARY

PRIMARY DIAGNOSES:

1. Acute myocardial infarction.
2. Pulmonary edema due to congestive heart failure.
3. Coronary artery disease.
4. Diabetes mellitus.
5. Anemia.
6. Hypertension.
7. Gastroesophageal reflux disease.
8. Chronic renal failure.

HOSPITAL COURSE: The patient was admitted with acute pulmonary edema. Serial cardiac enzymes showed the patient to have a non-Q-wave myocardial infarction with a troponin of 0.85. The patient subsequently diuresed. The patient's Imdur was increased. The patient did exhibit some hypotension. The patient's antihypertensive dosage was reduced. The patient was also found to be anemic. The patient did consent to blood transfusion. The patient received 2 units packed red blood cells. The patient's symptoms did improve.

The patient was also noted to have chronic renal failure. The patient's renal failure was monitored; it essentially remained unchanged during hospital stay with some fluctuation. Creatinine 1.4 on admission and creatinine 1.6 with discharge.

EXAMINATION ON THE DAY OF DISCHARGE: Alert and oriented female. Heart is regular. No murmurs. Lungs: Fine breath sounds. No wheezes or rhonchi. No crackles. Abdomen soft, nontender. Positive bowel sounds. Psychiatry: Patient alert and oriented.

The patient did have hemoglobin of 9 upon discharge.

DISCHARGE MEDICATIONS:

1. Aspirin 81 mg a day.
2. Atenolol 25 mg daily.
3. Plavix 75 mg daily.
4. Lasix 20 mg twice a day.
5. Glyburide 2.5 mg daily.
6. Imdur 60 mg twice a day.
7. Xalatan eyedrops.
8. Protonix 40 mg daily.
9. Enalapril 20 mg daily.
10. Timolol eyedrops.

DISCHARGE INSTRUCTIONS: The patient is discharged home. Follow up with Dr. Green in 1 to 2 weeks with CBC. If the patient has any difficulties, she should return to the emergency department or contact Dr. Green's office.

4. **CASE 4**

LOCATION: Inpatient hospital

PREOPERATIVE DIAGNOSIS: Ventilator dependency due to stenosis of the larynx, aspiration pneumonia

PROCEDURE PERFORMED: Tracheostomy, permanent

DESCRIPTION OF PROCEDURE: After consent was obtained, the patient was taken to the operating room and placed on the operating room table in the supine position. After an adequate level of general endotracheal anesthesia was obtained, the patient was positioned for tracheostomy. The patient's neck was prepped with Betadine and then draped in a sterile manner. A curvilinear incision was marked approximately a fingerbreadth above the sternal notch in an area just below the cricoid cartilage. This area was then infiltrated with 1% Xylocaine with 1:100,000 units of epinephrine. After several minutes, sharp dissection was carried down through the skin and subcutaneous tissue. The subcutaneous fat was removed down to the strap muscles. Strap muscles were divided in the midline and retracted laterally. The cricoid cartilage was then identified. The thyroid gland was divided in the midline with the Bovie, and then the two lobes were retracted laterally, exposing the anterior wall of the trachea. The space between the second and third tracheal rings was then identified. This was infiltrated with local solution. A cut was then made through the anterior wall. The endotracheal tube was then advanced superiorly. An inferior cut into the third tracheal ring was then done to make a flap. This was secured to the skin with 4-0 Vicryl suture. A No. 6 Shiley cuffed tracheostomy tube was then placed and secured to the skin with ties, as well as the tracheostomy strap. The patient tolerated the procedure well and was taken to the critical care unit in stable condition. Report the procedure(s) and diagnosis.

5. **CASE 5**

OPERATIVE REPORT

LOCATION: Ambulatory surgical center

PREOPERATIVE DIAGNOSIS: Gastrointestinal bleeding

POSTOPERATIVE DIAGNOSIS: Multiple serpiginous ulcers in the gastric antrum and body, not bleeding

FINDINGS: The video therapeutic double-channel endoscope was passed without difficulty into the oropharynx. The gastroesophageal junction was seen at 42 cm. Inspection of the esophagus revealed no erythema, ulceration, exudates, stricture, or other mucosal abnormalities. The stomach proper was entered. The endoscope was advanced to the second duodenum. Inspection of the second duodenum, first duodenum, duodenal bulb, and pylorus revealed no abnormalities. Retroflexion revealed no lesion along the cardia or lesser curvature. Inspection of the antrum, body, and fundus of the stomach revealed no abnormality, except that there were multiple serpiginous ulcerations in the gastric antrum and body. They were not bleeding. They had no recent stigmata of bleeding. Photographs and biopsies were obtained. The patient tolerated the procedure well.

6. **CASE 6**

OPERATIVE REPORT

LOCATION: Outpatient surgery center

DIAGNOSIS: Benign prostatic hypertrophy with bladder neck obstruction

PROCEDURE PERFORMED: Cystoscopy and transurethral resection of the prostate

The patient is a 78-year-old male with obstructive symptoms and subsequent urinary retention. The patient underwent the usual spinal anesthetic, was put in the dorsolithotomy position, and was prepped and draped in the usual fashion. Cystoscopic visualization showed a marked high-riding bladder. Median lobe enlargement was such that it was difficult even to get the cystoscope over. Inside the bladder, marked trabeculation was noted. No stones were present.

The urethra was well lubricated and dilated. The resectoscopic sheath was passed with the aid of obturator with some difficulty because of the median lobe. TURP of the median lobe was performed, getting several big loops of tissue, which helped to improve visualization. Anterior resection of the roof was carried out from the bladder neck. Bladder-wall resection was taken from 10 to 8 o'clock. This eliminated the rest of the median lobe tissue as well. The patient tolerated the procedure well. Code the procedure(s) performed and the diagnosis.

7. **CASE 7**

LOCATION: Outpatient surgery center

PREOPERATIVE DIAGNOSIS: Right inguinal hernia

POSTOPERATIVE DIAGNOSIS: Right direct and right indirect inguinal hernia

PROCEDURE: This 50-year-old patient was brought to the operating room and placed in a supine position on the operating table. After satisfactory general anesthesia had been induced, the patient's abdomen and groin were prepped and draped in a sterile manner. A short transverse incision was made over the right inguinal area. Subcutaneous tissue was divided sharply. Ties and cautery were used for hemostasis. The external oblique aponeurosis was identified and opened from above downward. The ilioinguinal nerve was identified and protected. The patient had a direct inguinal hernia about 1 cm superior and medial to the internal ring. It was properitoneal fat pushed through a very small opening of about 0.5 cm in size. We reduced this and closed the hole with interrupted Ethibond, which gave a solid closure without tension. We then dissected up the round ligament and ligated it distally. Proximally, we then separated the round ligament from a small sac. We ligated the round ligament from a small internal sac. We then closed the internal ring with Ethibond suture in a Bassini repair. This gave us a solid repair and fixed the hernias. We then irrigated the wound with neomycin. Final sponge and needle counts were taken; they were correct. We then closed the external oblique aponeurosis with Vicryl. Subcutaneous tissue was closed with chromic and skin with nylon. Blood loss during the procedure was minimal. The patient tolerated the procedure well and left for the recovery room in stable condition.

8. **CASE 8**

   LOCATION: Inpatient hospital

   PREOPERATIVE DIAGNOSIS: Bleeding from splenic laceration with hemodynamic instability

   POSTOPERATIVE DIAGNOSIS: Bleeding from splenic laceration which extended into the parenchyma

   PROCEDURE PERFORMED: Exploratory laparotomy and splenectomy

   SPECIMEN: Spleen

   OPERATIVE FINDINGS: There was a small grade 1 laceration of the left lobe of the liver that was not bleeding. There was a grade 4 laceration of the spleen with extension into the parenchyma, with active bleeding. There was 1200 cc of blood in the abdomen. There was no other solid or hollow viscous injury. After good general endotracheal anesthesia, the patient was prepped and draped in the usual sterile fashion. A midline incision was made from the xiphoid process down to the umbilicus. The abdomen was entered, and the hemoperitoneum was released. This was evacuated, and the abdomen was packed off in four quadrants. We then inspected for bleeding. The liver was inspected, and there was a small amount of bleeding laceration of the edge of the left lobe. The bowel was run from the ligament of Treitz to the cecum, and no injury was noted. The ascending transverse and descending colon were inspected, as was the stomach, and no injuries were noted. There was no retroperitoneal hematoma noted. The spleen itself, however, was bleeding. There was a grade 4 laceration with extension into the parenchyma. It was quite enlarged. The spleen was taken down after blunt control was obtained at the hilum of the spleen. The splenic ligaments were divided with clamps and ties. After the spleen was fully mobilized and rotated toward the midline, the hilum was taken. Stick ties were used to secure the vessels at the hilum of the spleen, and it was divided. The organ was passed off as a specimen. Pelvic organs, including uterus and ovaries, were also inspected, and there was no injury here. The patient was then closed with running PDS and skin clips. She tolerated the procedure well.

9. **CASE 9**

   LOCATION: ASC

   PREOPERATIVE DIAGNOSIS: Granuloma, right inner cheek

   POSTOPERATIVE DIAGNOSIS: Granuloma, right inner cheek

   PROCEDURE PERFORMED: Excision of lesion from right buccal mucosa, likely benign

   PROCEDURE IN DETAIL: After informed consent from the patient's parents was obtained, the patient was taken to the operating room and placed supine on the operating table. The appropriate monitoring devices were placed on the patient, and general anesthetic was induced. It was maintained by inhalation mask technique. The mouth was opened once the child was asleep. There was a 7 × 7-mm pedunculated lesion on the right anterior buccal mucosa. The lesion was excised by cutting through its base. It came out in one piece. There was no bleeding. Great care was taken to be certain that there was no injury to the lips.

   The patient tolerated the procedure well. She was transferred to the recovery room in good condition.

10. **CASE 10**

    LOCATION: Inpatient hospital

    PREOPERATIVE DIAGNOSIS: Myasthenia gravis exacerbation

    POSTOPERATIVE DIAGNOSIS: Same

    PROCEDURE PERFORMED: Plasma exchange

    This is a 5'9", 270-pound man who has increasing muscle weakness thought to be related to myasthenia gravis, and plasma exchange was elected. His hematocrit was 45.5. His platelets were 190,000. His total blood volume was 5769, and the calculated plasma volume was a little above 3 liters, about 3125 or so. I targeted him for 1 plasma volume exchange of 3 liters using 5% albumin with 1 amp of calcium gluconate/liter, and did a 1-to-1 exchange. He started it at 14:30 and completed the exchange by 16:00. He had no medical complications throughout. His pressures were stable. Cardiac rate was stable. During the exchange, he was aggressively hydrated with an IV because at the time, I felt that he was still somewhat volume-contracted from his diarrhea. His pre-lab reflected this, and post-lab will be done. His final plasma value was 3575 on the machine. This was calculated from a 4297 total, minus the ACD-A of 722. The replacement volume was calculated at 3281 because there are not exactly 500 in each bottle of albumin; I was fairly close, and I was satisfied with this result. The patient will be reevaluated over the next 2 days with special attention paid to his renal status prior to continuing the next plasma exchange planned in 3 days, unless there are other problems that we have to deal with.

11. **CASE 11**

    LOCATION: Outpatient surgery center

    PROCEDURE NOTE: Jake is in for a vasectomy, having previously undergone counseling earlier today. Patient was placed in a supine position, and the scrotal area was shaved. Under sterile technique, the scrotal area was prepped with Betadine, and the sterile drapes were applied. The right vas was localized and under sterile technique was infiltrated with 1% Xylocaine. The vas was externalized, and a 1.5-cm portion of the tube was removed. Proximal and distal stumps were doubly ligated with 4-0 silk. There was a small blood vessel in the skin that was oozing and was clamped. Attention was directed to the left side, where a similar procedure was performed. With hemostasis intact, the proximal and distal stumps on the left were retracted into the scrotum, and attention was directed to the right side, where there was slight oozing from the skin edge; with pressure, this did resolve, and the proximal and distal stumps were retracted into the scrotum.

    ASSESSMENT: Vasectomy

    PLAN: The patient had been given the postvasectomy instruction sheet, and bacitracin and a gauze dressing were applied. He is to apply antibiotics a couple of times a day with gauze, and he was given an instruction sheet to have sperm counts done in 2 months' time, and to take contraceptive precautions in the meantime.

12. **CASE 12**

EMERGENCY DEPARTMENT REPORT

SUBJECTIVE: The patient is an 80-year-old male in acute respiratory distress. He is from the New York City area and was just about to take a train to go there today. He had sudden onset of shortness of breath and presents now because of it. He denies any chest pain or tightness. He has had no recent cough. He is bringing up frothy sputum as he arrives here.

PAST MEDICAL HISTORY:

Surgical:

1. Bypass surgery.

2. Angioplasty and stent.

3. Pacemaker.

Illnesses: The patient has a previous history of congestive heart failure and has been intubated in the past, most recently 4 months ago, with this same problem.

Family history, social history, and review of systems were not obtainable for this patient.

OBJECTIVE: This alert 80-year-old male appears to be in acute respiratory distress. Oxygen saturation is 72%. Blood pressure is 210/107. Respirations are 36. Pulse is 120. Telemetry shows a paced wide complexed rhythm. HEENT: Frothy pink sputum coming out of his mouth. Neck is supple without lymphadenopathy. His jugular veins are full. Respirations are labored. Lungs: Rales throughout. Heart: Rapid rate and rhythm. Abdomen: Soft and nontender with normal bowel sounds. Extremities: No peripheral edema is noted. No clubbing.

ASSESSMENT: Pulmonary edema

PLAN: He was immediately given Lasix 80 mg IV, given Nitro spray, and started on a Nitro drip. We gave him a few minutes to try to turn around. He was on 100% oxygen. He did not turn around and, in fact, he looked worse. We then talked about intubation with him and his wife and proceeded with it. He was bagged. He was given Versed IV, and he then was given succinylcholine 100 mg IV. He was then intubated without difficulty with an 8.0 ET tube to 24 cm. Breath sounds were heard bilaterally. CO_2 monitoring device confirmed placement. The patient was placed on the ventilator and transported to ICU in reasonably stable condition.

THORACIC MEDICINE/CRITICAL CARE CONSULTATION: I have been asked by Dr. Elhart to see the patient for ICU care. The patient was admitted with pulmonary edema, respiratory failure; he has chronic renal disease and is on Dr. Elhart's service—I would assume for the chronic renal disease, as well as respiratory failure, but that was secondary. The patient looks like he had a myocardial infarction with elevated troponins, CK-MBs, CPKs, and CKs. His pulmonary edema has started to clear. He was adjusted on the ventilator this morning. The CPAP went from 6 o'clock to 8 o'clock, and then he got too short of breath and went back on the ventilator. Since then, he has diuresed more, and I have him on CPAP at present. He is doing quite well, with a respiratory rate of 19 with good oxygenation. I think we have a fair chance of getting him extubated today.

The patient was visiting with relatives here in Manytown. He was trying to move some luggage, started to get diaphoretic, and did not feel well, and it started to become difficult to breathe. The wife felt he was gurgling, and he was sent to the emergency department, where he was found to be in pulmonary edema, and was intubated and placed on a ventilator.

The patient is intubated and on a ventilator, so I do not have a good family history, social history, past medical history, past surgical history, or review of systems. I got some things from the chart and some things from his wife. The patient's wife is fairly sure that he had stenting of the LAD done last year. We will send for those records. He had a coronary artery bypass graft done before that. It sounds fairly extensive. It seems to have been in 1989. He had at least three grafts, and the cardiologist has this outlined pretty well and what was done at that point. He also had a pacemaker. He has a history of renal artery disease status post renal artery stenosis, with history of hypertension, dyslipidemia, bradycardia, and chronic renal disease. He apparently has had some trouble with dye toxicity from an angiogram done a year ago and did not quite get over it. I guess there was partial clearing. It is difficult to tell without the records what went on.

PHYSICAL EXAMINATION: At the time I saw the patient, the physical examination reveals a patient who is alert, on a ventilator, and able to answer questions (yes and no, anyway). He certainly cannot verbalize it. HEENT: Benign. No blood is found in the posterior pharynx or the nose. Neck is supple. No JVD. Lungs actually show rales bilaterally but in the bases, not in the rest of the areas. Heart shows that S1 and S2 are regular without an S3 or S4. There is a systolic murmur at the fourth interspace midclavicular line that is somewhat difficult to hear. It is somewhat vague and soft, but I think it is present. Abdomen is soft and benign without hepatosplenomegaly. Normal bowel sounds are present. No bruits are heard in either flank; no masses are palpable; nontender. Extremities show no edema, rashes, clubbing, cyanosis, or tremor. Lymphatic system: No nodes in the neck, clavicular, or axillary area.

IMPRESSION:

1. Acute myocardial infarction with acute pulmonary edema and acute respiratory failure.

2. Chronic renal failure. You can see that on today's material, his BUN and creatinine levels are climbing. I am not sure what the plan is at this point. I am waiting for Cardiology to come by, but I think I can get him extubated later this afternoon. I will check his sputum. He does have a fair amount to suction, and it is somewhat thick, so I will make sure he does not have an infection. He is already on Unasyn for any sort of aspiration that might have occurred, although it is not well documented. We will check a 24-hour urine for creatinine clearance, get the records from the Manytown hospital to see what actually was done there, and then check on his lab in the morning. I will wait for Dr. Elhart to come by before we make any other plans, but hopefully, the patient will be extubated here shortly.

RADIOLOGY REPORT, CHEST

EXAMINATION OF: Chest

CLINICAL SYMPTOMS: Follow-up pulmonary edema

PORTABLE AP CHEST, 5:00 AM: FINDINGS: Comparison is made with yesterday morning's portable AP chest. Sternotomy with mediastinal clips. The endotracheal tube and NG tube have been removed. No appreciable change in heart size or pulmonary vascularity, given the difference in technique. Lungs are clear.

RADIOLOGY REPORT, CHEST

EXAMINATION OF: Chest

CLINICAL SYMPTOMS: Acute MI, pulmonary edema, acute respiratory failure, and renal disease

PORTABLE CHEST X-RAY: FINDINGS: Endotracheal tube and NG tube are not significantly changed. The cardiac silhouette is upper normal to mildly prominent but stable. Mild interstitial prominence remains in the infrahilar areas, but no other significant interval change is noted.

THORACIC MEDICINE/CRITICAL CARE PROGRESS REPORT

This is a follow-up for this patient with acute respiratory failure. He was extubated yesterday. He apparently had a cardiac catheterization in the past, and his kidneys were bad enough that they thought he might need dialysis, but then he recovered; but he certainly recovered incompletely because BUN today is 72, creatinine 2.6, and creatinine clearance is pending. Interestingly enough, potassium is low at 2.8, so we will replace that with oral potassium. We will check his basic metabolic panel in the morning and transfer him to the floor on telemetry. He does not want anything done here. He wants to go home by train, which is probably not the best idea because there is no guarantee that what happened to him this time will not happen again.

PHYSICAL EXAMINATION: Chest: Clear. Chest x-ray looks pretty good, too. Heart: Regular rhythm. Abdomen: Benign. Extremities: No edema. No clubbing.

LABORATORY DATA: All in good shape. Sputum showed greater than 25 white cells, less 10 squamous. No bugs were seen, so it may be just inflammation rather than true infection.

MEDICATIONS: He is on Unasyn at this point. We stopped the Unasyn today and put him on Augmentin. There is some question about whether he aspirated on it, but I certainly do not see anything on x-ray right now.

He is going to be talking to Dr. Elhart later today to decide what to do about whether to discharge or have the study done here. The patient is really positive that he wants to go back home in case things go wrong with his kidneys. At least he is at home and can undergo the dialysis closer to home. He is most comfortable with the situation there, as well as with his surroundings there, so we will leave that up to Dr. Elhart and the patient. But I still think it is a somewhat risky idea, so I imparted to the patient that particular idea. Otherwise, he can be discharged at Cardiology's leisure.

DISCHARGE SUMMARY: The patient was admitted with pulmonary edema, respiratory failure, and chronic renal disease. The patient looked like he has had myocardial infarction with elevated troponins. The patient was extubated after the pulmonary edema (less than 96 hours). Discussions with the patient and his family indicated that he did not want anything further done. He wanted further cardiac care done at home. We arranged for him to be discharged, and he was discharged Tuesday. It was advised that he have a cardiac catheterization to determine the extent of his myocardial infarction and whether anything could be fixed, but this is on top of somebody with chronic renal disease who most likely would suffer from the toxic effects of the dye and would probably have some difficulty with renal failure post cardiac catheterization if everything went wrong. Please see my drug note that outlined the drugs the patient was on when he was sent home.

429

DISCHARGE DIAGNOSES:

1. Acute respiratory failure.

2. Acute non-Q-wave myocardial infarction.

3. Congestive heart failure.

4. Chronic renal failure.

13. **CASE 13**

HISTORY AND PHYSICAL

REASON FOR ADMISSION: Renal failure, generalized edema, and coronary artery disease

The patient is a 66-year-old male I was asked to see in consultation in the office today by his primary care physician for a rising creatinine level. The patient has been having progressive shortness of breath. A stress test was done, which was positive. This was followed by a cardiac catheterization, where the patient was found to have multivessel coronary artery disease, including mid to right coronary artery, proximal LAD, and proximal circumflex with an ejection fraction of 66% without coarse regional motion abnormalities, with normal systolic function without any mitral regurgitation. The patient was supposed to have bypass surgery today; however, because his creatinine has gone up from 1.8 mg/dL to 2.3 mg/dL, his bypass surgery has been postponed. His BUN is 48, sodium 136, potassium 4.6, chloride 97, bicarb 29, creatinine 2.3, and calcium 8.6. His white count was 6000, with hemoglobin of 11.5, MCV of 101.7, and platelets 192,000. He has a normal Protime and INR.

The patient states that he had a 24-hour urine collection in the past, but he does not recall the results of that. We tried to get hold of the 24-hour urine taken by his primary care physician but were unsuccessful today.

The patient has been on Actos and recently was started on Crestor, which was a switch from Lipitor 40 mg daily.

For the past few months, he has been having progressive shortness of breath. For the past week or so, he has been getting more leg swelling where he cannot even tie his shoes because of his increased abdominal girth. He has been having exertional dyspnea. He cannot even walk half a block. He denies any PND. He has no chest pain. He has never had any chest pain. He has no palpitations, but he complains of massive leg edema.

PAST MEDICAL HISTORY IS SIGNIFICANT FOR THE FOLLOWING:

1. Long-standing hypertension.

2. Type II diabetes mellitus, on Lantus and Humalog insulin.

3. Diabetic retinopathy.

4. Right eye blindness.

5. Congestive heart failure, but normal ejection fraction as mentioned.

6. Obesity.

7. Hyperlipidemia.

8. Questionable diabetic nephropathy (again, I do not have any urinalysis or 24-hour urine collection).

9. Hypothyroidism.

SOCIAL HISTORY: He is single. He has a girlfriend, who was with him today. He quit smoking in 1986. He uses alcohol occasionally. He is retired. He used to work as a store manager at Maverick Discount. He is a native of New York.

FAMILY HISTORY: Father died of unclear reasons. Mother died of a myocardial infarction at age 65. One sister with breast cancer. One sister with lung cancer. No kidney disease, dialysis, or kidney transplantation.

ALLERGIES: Questionable Vasotec

CURRENT MEDICATIONS INCLUDE THE FOLLOWING:

1. Actos 15 mg daily.

2. Amitriptyline 50 mg daily.

3. Humalog 15 units t.i.d.

4. Lantus 56 units nightly.

5. Lisinopril 30 mg daily.

6. Multivitamin 1 daily.

7. Neurontin 300 mg 2 tabs b.i.d.

8. Prednisone eyedrops.

9. Synthroid 0.075 mg daily.

10. Torsemide 20 mg 2 tabs b.i.d.

11. Crestor 10 mg daily.

12. Isosorbide mononitrate 30 mg daily.

REVIEW OF SYSTEMS: Constitutional: Generalized weakness with fatigue. Eyes: He wears glasses. He has right-sided blindness. ENT: Negative. Cardiovascular: As mentioned. Respiratory: Negative. Gastrointestinal: Negative, except for constipation. Genitourinary: Negative. Musculoskeletal: Chronic intermittent back pain. Skin: Negative. Neuro: Numbness and tingling in the fingers and toes. Psychiatry: Negative. Endocrine: He has diabetes and hypothyroidism. Hematology: Anemia from yesterday's labs.

EXAMINATION: The patient was short of breath but not in any distress. His temperature was 101.8°. Respirations: 28 on room air. Pulse: 84/minute and regular. Weight: 296 pounds. Blood pressure on the right side, 108/45 sitting and 108/50 standing. On the left, 108/56 standing. He has right-sided blindness. He has increased jugular venous pressure with positive hepatojugular reflux. Lungs had good air entry bilaterally, but he had a few crackles in the bases. He has abdominal wall and lower extremity edema. He has 1 sacral edema. He had distinct heart sounds but no pericardial friction rub or murmurs. He did not have any carotid bruits.

His legs had palpable pulses, with edema in the lower extremities up to the thighs. No ulcerations. The patient was awake, alert, oriented ×3, without any focal neurological deficits. He had normal gait. He does have decreased sensations in his feet.

IMPRESSION:

1. Chronic renal failure with an estimated creatinine clearance of 13 mL/min.

2. Acute renal failure possibly related to his cardiac catheterization. This patient could have thromboembolic disease.

3. Chronic renal failure could be related to the diabetic nephropathy but also could be related to hypertension or renal vascular disease; again, without knowing whether he has proteinuria or not, it is difficult to say. In any case, the patient does have generalized edema, and that edema needs to be taken care of. He is on a long-acting diuretic, and he probably would benefit from a shorter-acting diuretic.

4. Anemia of acute and chronic renal failure.

5. Slight macrocytosis.

6. Type II diabetes.

7. Severe coronary artery disease that would require bypass surgery.

PLAN:

1. The patient was admitted to telemetry.

2. He is code Level I.

3. We will make sure he has adequate intake/output.

4. Fluid restriction 2 liters a day and also a salt restriction of 2 grams of sodium.

5. We will give him 2 mg of Bumex IV and start him at 0.125 mg an hour.

6. We will monitor his urine output hourly.

7. His surgery will be on hold until he is tuned up.

8. We will check potassium and magnesium every 6 hours and correct accordingly.

9. We will repeat his basic panel and CBC in the morning.

10. If his hemoglobin drops below 11, we will start him on Epo.

11. We will check iron studies and give him iron if need be.

12. Discontinue Crestor since his creatinine clearance is coming down.

13. Discontinue Actos since he has edema and it could be contributing to his massive edema and CHF symptoms.

14. Continue with his current insulin dose.

I had a long discussion with the patient about his renal function. I advised him that he might end up on dialysis either before or after his bypass surgery; however, he has severe coronary artery disease with a good ejection fraction, and he would benefit from bypass surgery. The patient understands that, and he agrees to dialysis if need be.

The option of what type of renal replacement therapy he would get will be discussed later.

The patient agrees to be admitted and diuresed. I discussed the case with Dr. Green on the phone, and he was in full agreement.

The total time I spent with this patient today was 65 minutes.

NEPHROLOGY/CRITICAL CARE PROGRESS NOTE

The patient is making good progress today as he made 1300 mL. Last night he had 32 and 850 output. His weight is 132.5 kg today, down from 133.4 kg yesterday. He has no complaints of chest pain or shortness of breath. He is awake, alert, oriented ×3 without any focal neurological deficits. His blood pressure is 124/57, temperature 36.9°, heart rate in the low 70s per minute, respirations 18 per minute, and sats 94% on room air.

His lungs are clear. He has regular rate and rhythm. He still has sacral abdominal wall and low extremity edema, probably 2+.

His BUN today is 53, down from 57, sodium 139, potassium 4.4, chloride 101, bicarb 27, glucose 149, creatinine 2.2, down from 2.6.

His urinalysis on admission showed no protein. His microscopic examination showed no blood.

Magnesium today is elevated at 2.3.

IMPRESSION:

1. Chronic renal failure with estimated creatinine clearance of 30 mL/min.

2. Acute renal failure secondary to probably his cardiac cath and possibly atheroembolic disease, possible contrast nephropathy.

3. The patient does not have proteinuria, so it is unlikely that he has diabetic nephropathy. He could have renal artery stenosis or hypertensive nephrosclerosis. I think it is important to figure out what he has because if he does have renal stenosis, this probably would need to be fixed prior to his bypass surgery.

4. Generalized edema and congestive heart failure, probably precipitated by Actos.

5. Anemia of acute and chronic renal failure.

6. Type II diabetes.

7. Severe coronary artery disease, which had required bypass surgery.

PLAN:

1. The patient will stay in the hospital for the time being.

2. Continue Bumex drip at 0.125 mg an hour.

3. Check spot urine protein and creatinine ratio.

4. Repeat labs in the morning to include BMP, CBC.

5. Renal ultrasound Monday morning because of the acute and chronic renal failure.

6. Will probably discharge him on Monday morning on oral Bumex.

7. The patient is already off Actos.

8. Will continue to monitor his potassium and magnesium every 6 hours and replace accordingly.

Discussed all of the above with the patient, including possible intervention on his renal arteries. He seems to understand and agree with the plan.

I discussed this case with the attending, and he was in agreement.

PROGRESS NOTE: The patient had no major events during the night. He is losing weight. He is diuresing very nicely. He had 341 in and 1000 out so far today. Yesterday, he had 1461 in and 3750 out. He has no complaints of chest pain or shortness of breath. He appears euvolemic. He still has a little bit of edema in the lower extremities. His vitals are stable. His BUN is down to 41, sodium 140, potassium 4.2, chloride 101, bicarbonate 28.7, creatinine down to 1.7, and calcium 8.4.

His white count is 3.6 K, hemoglobin 11.1, platelets 214,000.

IMPRESSION:

1. Acute on top of chronic renal failure.

2. Generalized edema and congestive heart failure, probably precipitated by Actos, all improving.

3. The patient could have renovascular disease. If he does, it needs to be fixed prior to his bypass surgery.

4. Anemia due to acute and chronic renal failure.

PLAN:

1. The patient did not have a ride today, so he will stay here tonight and will be discharged home tomorrow.

2. We will do an ultrasound before he is discharged.

3. Repeat labs in the morning, including basic panel, magnesium, and CBC.

4. We will schedule a renal MRA as an outpatient.

5. Continue with Bumex for the time being. He will be discharged home on p.o. Bumex. His lisinopril has been on hold and will continue to be on hold until renal MRA is done.

I discussed the above with the patient. He seems to understand and agrees with the plan.

DISCHARGE SUMMARY

DIAGNOSES:

1. Acute renal failure.

2. Congestive heart failure and generalized edema.

3. Chronic renal failure.

4. Severe coronary artery disease.

The patient is a 66-year-old male who is known to have coronary artery disease and was admitted because of generalized edema. The patient's creatinine has gone up to 2.3. He was found to have significant edema in bilateral lower extremities, thighs, and sacral area, and a few basilar crackles. His Actos and Crestor were both discontinued. He was given Bumex and then started on Bumex for a couple of days. The patient did well. He had no major problems during his hospitalization. He had no chest pain. His edema significantly improved. He had no proteinuria, so he does not seem to have diabetic nephropathy.

5. Hypertension.

   The patient was discharged in good general condition; code level I. The patient's creatinine improved, going down to 1.7 on date of discharge.

DISCHARGE PLAN:

1. Patient will follow up with Dr. Green. He will follow up with me as well when the basic panel and CBC results are known.

2. He will continue on Bumex 2 mg daily, fluid restriction, and salt restriction. He is off Actos and Crestor.

DISCHARGE MEDICATIONS:

1. Amitriptyline 50 mg daily.

2. Humalog 15 units t.i.d. with meals.

3. Lantus 56 units nightly.

4. Lisinopril has been discontinued for the time being.

5. Multivitamin 1 daily.

6. Neurontin 300 mg, 2 tablets b.i.d.

7. Prednisone eyedrops.

8. Synthroid 0.075 mg daily.

9. Torsemide discontinued.

10. Crestor discontinued.

11. Isosorbide mononitrate 30 mg daily.

12. Bumex 2 mg daily.

The patient agrees with all of the above.

FINAL EXAMINATION
PART II

With the use of a medical dictionary, CPT, and HCPCS and ICD-9-CM coding manuals, assign codes to the following:

1. **CASE 1**

   OPERATIVE REPORT

   PREOPERATIVE DIAGNOSIS: Right ureteral stricture

   POSTOPERATIVE DIAGNOSIS: Right ureteral stricture

   PROCEDURE PERFORMED: Cystoscopy, right ureteral stent change

   LOCATION: Outpatient surgery center

   PROCEDURE NOTE: The patient was placed in the lithotomy position after receiving IV sedation. He was prepped and draped in the lithotomy position. The 21-French cystoscope was passed into the bladder, and urine was collected for culture. Inspection of the bladder demonstrated findings consistent with radiation cystitis, which had been previously diagnosed. There was no frank neoplasia. The right ureteral stent was grasped and removed through the urethral meatus; under fluoroscopic control, a guide wire was advanced up the stent, and the stent was exchanged for a 7-French 26-cm stent under fluoroscopic control in the usual fashion. The patient tolerated the procedure well. Code for the outpatient facility services.

2. **CASE 2**

   OPERATIVE REPORT

   PREOPERATIVE DIAGNOSIS: Fever

   PROCEDURE PERFORMED: Lumbar puncture

   LOCATION: Emergency department

   DESCRIPTION OF PROCEDURE: The patient was placed in the lateral decubitus position with the left side up. The legs and hips were flexed into the fetal position. The lumbosacral area was sterilely prepped. It was then numbed with 1% Xylocaine. I then placed a 22-gauge spinal needle on the first pass into the intrathecal space between the L4 and L5 spinous processes. The fluid was minimally xanthochromic. I sent the fluid for cell count for differential, protein, glucose, Gram stain, and culture. The patient tolerated the procedure well without apparent complication. The needle was removed at the end of the procedure. The area was cleansed, and a Band-Aid was placed.

3. **CASE 3**

OPERATIVE REPORT

PREOPERATIVE DIAGNOSIS: Atelectasis of the left lower lobe

PROCEDURE PERFORMED: Fiberoptic bronchoscopy with brushings and cell washings

LOCATION: ASC

PROCEDURE: The patient was already sedated, on a ventilator, and intubated, so his bronchoscopy was done through the ET tube. It was passed easily down to the carina. About 2 to 2.5 cm above the carina, we could see the trachea, which appeared good, as was the carina. In the right lung, all segments were patent and entered, and no masses were seen. The left lung, however, had petechial ecchymotic areas scattered throughout the airways. The tissue was friable and swollen, but no mucous plugs were noted, and all the airways were open, just somewhat swollen. No abnormal secretions were noted at all. Brushings were taken, as well as washings, including some with Mucomyst to see whether we could get some distal mucous plug, but nothing really significant was returned. The specimens were sent to appropriate cytological and bacteriological studies. The patient tolerated the procedure fairly well.

Code the outpatient facility services.

4. **CASE 4**

OPERATIVE REPORT

PREOPERATIVE DIAGNOSIS: Abscess

PROCEDURE PERFORMED: Incision and drainage of left thigh abscess

LOCATION: Outpatient surgery center

OPERATIVE NOTE: With the patient under general anesthesia, he was placed in the lithotomy position. The area around the anus was carefully inspected, and we saw no evidence of communication with the perirectal space. This appears to have risen in the crease at the top of the leg, extending from the posterior buttocks region up toward the side of the base of the penis. In any event, the area was prepped and draped in a sterile manner. Then, we incised the area in fluctuation. We obtained a lot of very foul-smelling, almost stool-like material (it was not stool, but it was brown and very foul-smelling material). This was not the typical pus one sees with a *Staphylococcus aureus*–type infection. The incision was widened to allow us to probe the cavity fully. Again, I could see no evidence of communication to the rectum, but there was extension down the thigh and extension up into the groin crease. The fascia was darkened from the purulent material. I opened some of the fascia to make sure the underlying muscle was viable. This appeared viable. No gas was present. There was nothing to suggest a necrotizing fasciitis. The patient did have a very extensive inflammation within this abscess cavity. The abscess cavity was irrigated with peroxide and saline and was packed with gauze vaginal packing. The patient tolerated the procedure well and was discharged from the operating room in stable condition.

5. **CASE 5**

   EMERGENCY DEPARTMENT

   SUBJECTIVE: This is a 77-year-old male who presents with a finger laceration. He also has hypertension. He has no known allergies.

   He presents with a history of sustaining an avulsion laceration to his right third finger yesterday at about 1200 hours, when an air conditioner fell out of a window.

   OBJECTIVE: He is afebrile with stable vital signs. He states he is up-to-date for tetanus immunization. He last received that 6 years ago. He has a small, avulsed area on the fat pad surface of the distal right third finger. It measures about 3 mm in greatest diameter by about 4 to 5 mm. There is no bleeding currently. This was cleansed with saline and dressed with Bacitracin nonadherent dressing and tube gauze.

   ASSESSMENT: Avulsion laceration right third finger, as described above

   PLAN: Wound care instructions provided. Wound check and dressing change on Monday with his personal physician.

6. **CASE 6**

   LOCATION: Outpatient hospital

   EXAMINATION OF: Nephrostogram

   CONTRAST: Hand injection of contrast through the nephrostomy tube

   CLINICAL SYMPTOMS: Check placement of the nephrostomy tube

   NEPHROSTOGRAM HISTORY: This is a 76-year-old male with a history of prostate cancer, left ureteral obstruction, hydronephrosis, needing routine exchange of the nephrostomy tube.

   FINDINGS PRE–LEFT NEPHROSTOGRAM: Nephrostogram obtained demonstrates a preexisting 16-French nephrostomy tube within an upper pole calyx. Mild hydronephrosis is seen. No filling defects are identified. Ureteral coils are present.

   FINDINGS POST–LEFT NEPHROSTOGRAM: Final nephrostogram obtained demonstrates mild hydronephrosis. The new nephrostomy tube is present in the main renal pelvis with the tip of the pigtail into the ureteral pelvic junction. No contrast extravasation of filling defects is seen. Report both the nephrostogram and the radiologic supervision and interpretation of the test, in addition to the diagnosis.

7. **CASE 7**

   LOCATION: Outpatient hospital

   EXAMINATION OF: Right lower extremity ultrasound

   CLINICAL SYMPTOMS: Chronic ulcer, right lower extremity (calf)

   FINDINGS: Ultrasound examination of the deep venous system of the right lower extremity is negative for DVT. The right popliteal, greater saphenous, and femoral veins are patent and negative for thrombus. Unable to evaluate the open wound area.

8. **CASE 8**

HOSPITAL ADMISSION: This is an 82-year-old lady who presents with chief complaint of shortness of breath. Reason for admission: COPD, pneumonia, atrial fibrillation with rapid ventricular rate.

HISTORY OF PRESENT ILLNESS: This 82-year-old lady with known COPD is steroid-dependent and oxygen-dependent.

The patient has had a recent admission and discharge last Friday, when she had a stroke. The patient has known severe oxygen-requiring COPD. The patient has also been on chronic steroids, on high doses, about 15 mg per day. The patient was in good health until last night when, during the night, she readily developed more and more shortness of breath. The patient was transferred to the emergency department. The patient denies any fever or chills, but does admit to cough, although she says it is a chronic cough, for about a few months now; she says it really has not changed too much lately. She has minimal sputum. She did not have any chest pain, any nasal congestion, or any sore throat. This time, the patient remained alert and oriented. There was no change in mental status. The patient was given nebulizers in the ambulance and in the emergency room, and the saturations somewhat improved.

REVIEW OF SYSTEMS: Pulmonary: Shortness of breath, as above. This has developed overnight. Cardiovascular: No chest pain, no feeling of irregular heartbeat or rapid heartbeat. No fever, no chills. GI: No abdominal pain. The patient reports no cough with eating or difficulty swallowing. The patient's daughters also observed her eating prior and did not note any significant problems with swallowing. Neurologic: The patient had lately been admitted for possible stroke. The symptoms were lethargy, which resolved, and some word-finding difficulties. Psychiatric: No problem reported from the patient or from the patient's family. Hematology/Oncology: The patient does have diffuse bruises but no significant bleeding. Endocrine: No polyuria, no polydipsia. There is no mention of diabetes or glucose intolerance, even with steroid use. Extremities: The patient does have chronic lower extremity swelling, which is actually better today, as per patient's daughters.

PAST MEDICAL HISTORY:

1. The patient has severe oxygen-requiring COPD.

2. On recent CT, the patient was noted to have about a 2-cm soft tissue density in the left lung base. Prominent diffuse emphysematous changes were also seen.

3. Atrial fibrillation.

4. The patient was judged not to be a good candidate for anti-coagulation.

5. Vitamin B_{12} deficiency.

6. Crohn's disease.

7. Senile osteoporosis.

8. Venous insufficiency.

9. Left frontal region meningioma.

10. Right recent cerebellar stroke.

PAST SURGICAL HISTORY:

1. Bowel resection for Crohn's disease.

2. Cholecystectomy.

3. Bilateral cataracts.

FAMILY HISTORY: Mother had Hodgkin's disease. A sister and brother had lung cancer.

SOCIAL HISTORY: The patient quit smoking about 30 years ago but was a very heavy smoker. Occasional alcohol use.

ALLERGIES: No known allergies.

MEDICATIONS:

1. Amitriptyline 25 to 50 mg p.o. q h.s.

2. Augmentin 500 mg 3 times a day.

3. Aspirin 325 mg once a day.

4. Pulmicort 1 puff twice a day.

5. Calcium carbonate with vitamin D; 1 tablet twice a day.

6. Digoxin 0.25 mg once a day.

7. Diltiazem 120 mg once a day.

8. Folic acid 1 mg once a day.

9. Citrucel t.i.d. p.r.n.

10. DuoNeb nebulizers q 4 hours p.r.n.

11. Oxygen 1 to 4 liters.

12. Vitamin B_{12} 1000 mg/month.

13. Xalatan eye drops both eyes q h.s., 0.005%.

14. Prednisone 25 mg, then taper to 20 mg p.o. daily.

15. Serevent inhaler 1 puff twice a day.

16. Senokot 1 tablet twice a day.

17. Sulfasalazine 500 mg twice a day.

PHYSICAL EXAMINATION: Blood pressure 152/67. Heart rate 105, initial heart rate was in the 140s, the patient then was given Cardizem 15 mg IV; then, heart rates were in the 90s/low 100s. Temperature 36.0. Saturating 89% on 2 liters nasal cannula oxygen. The patient appears in no acute distress, appears actually very comfortable in the bed, joking with me. Psychiatric: Good mood, cooperative. Neurologic: Appears alert and oriented to place and person, can recall prior events; can move all extremities with no significant focal motor or sensory deficit. HEENT: Extraocular movements intact. Oropharynx, dry. Neck: Supple, no JVD, no lymph nodes palpable, no thyromegaly, no carotid bruit. Heart: Irregular S1 and S2. Maybe 1/VI systolic murmur, although blood pressure with the temperature and the irregularity, it is hard to say. Lungs: Bilateral lower area rhonchi. Back: No CVA tenderness. Abdomen: Soft, nontender, nondistended, positive bowel sounds. Lower extremities: bilateral 1+ edema. Skin: Bilateral extremities with superficial bruises. There is one small, about 3 mm in diameter, open wound with about 50% slough formation on the right lower extremity, lateral surface.

LABORATORY STUDIES: White blood cell count 12.1, this was 17.4 on the first; hemoglobin 11.0, platelets 270. Prior hemoglobins were 11.5 and 10.6. Differential includes 78% neutrophils. BUN 11, creatinine 0.6, sodium 144, potassium 3.2, chloride 95, bicarb above 41.8, glucose 81, creatinine 0.6. B natriuretic peptide 175. CK MB 0.6, CPK 13. Digoxin 1.1. INR 1.0. Magnesium 14. ABG: pH 7.44, pCO_2 69, pO_2 83 on nasal cannula oxygen at 5 liters. This equals a saturation of 97%. Troponin I less than 0.04. EKG evaluated by me shows atrial fibrillation with heart rate in 130s with incomplete right bundle branch block. Chest x-ray as evaluated by me shows right lower area atelectasis or infiltrate. This appears new or significantly worsened from the first of January. There is mild blunting of the sulci. The old medical records were reviewed. The case was discussed with the emergency room physician.

ASSESSMENT AND PLAN:

1. This lady who has known oxygen-dependent COPD presents with desaturating subjective shortness of breath and new x-ray changes. The patient will be admitted with the admitting diagnosis of pneumonia, COPD exacerbation. I will start the patient on higher dose of steroids. Will try to taper that fast since the patient has a history that she is poorly tolerating the steroids. She is usually awake and hyperactive from that. I will give the patient nebulizers, will continue the Serevent and Pulmicort. The patient will be on oxygen.

2. For the pneumonia, I will start patient on Claforan and azithromycin. Will follow for clinical improvement.

3. The patient had atrial fibrillation with rapid ventricular rate. This might be secondary to the pulmonary events and/or nebulizers. The patient was given 50 mg IV Cardizem, which brought down the heart rate to the 90s/low 100s. I will give the patient her Cardizem orally and will observe on telemetry for heart rate. The patient is noted not to be an anticoagulation candidate.

4. Hypokalemia will be replaced.

5. Possible left-sided pulmonary nodule. Follow-up CT will be done in a few months.

6. Crohn's disease, appears stable; in fact, patient is somewhat constipated now. Will give Citrucel and Senokot.

7. Osteoporosis, also on chronic steroid. Will give calcium and vitamin D. She might need further treatment as an outpatient for that, including, for example, Fosamax.

8. B_{12} deficiency. Hemoglobin appears stable since discharge.

9. History of stroke. Patient did not have real problem with word-finding difficulties, also motor functions appear good. There is no report of possible aspiration, although the location of the infiltrate would fit that, but will ask for aspiration precaution.

10. Code status was discussed with the patient; she wished to be code II. This is the same code status used when she was admitted last time as well.

RADIOLOGY REPORT

EXAMINATION OF: Chest

CLINICAL SYMPTOMS: Respiratory distress

CHEST: Findings: This examination is compared with a prior examination dated June 1. Heart size is prominent but unchanged when compared with the prior examination. Pulmonary vascular markings appear at the upper limits of normal. Abnormal focal pulmonary opacity is present within the right lower lung zone, as well as the left mid and left lower lung zones. Findings are most compatible with areas of infiltrate. Possibility of superimposed edematous change or atelectasis cannot be excluded. No pleural effusions are seen. There is atherosclerotic change of the thoracic aorta. Follow-up to document clearing is recommended.

PROGRESS NOTE

SUBJECTIVE: The patient indicates that her breathing is improved a little today. Daughter is at bedside. The patient indicates that she has a cough; however, it is not productive. The patient denies any chest pain or chest pressure. No fever or chills.

REVIEW OF SYSTEMS: General: Cardiovascular and respiratory were performed. With the exception noted in the HPI, are negative.

VITALS TODAY: Temp is 35.8 with T-max of 37.5 degrees. Pulse is 82. Respiratory rate is 16. Blood pressure is 142/78. O_2 sat is 98%. Cardiovascular: S1 and S2. No S3, no S4.

LUNGS: Bilateral breath sounds, occasional wheeze. Abdomen is soft and nontender. Positive bowel sounds.

PSYCH: The patient is alert.

IMPRESSION:

1. Pneumonia.

2. COPD exacerbation.

PLAN: At this point, continue the patient on current treatments. We will switch the patient to oral steroids, will start tapering dose. I will switch the patient to oral antibiotics. We will pursue discharge planning.

DISCHARGE SUMMARY

REASON FOR HOSPITALIZATION: The patient is an 82-year-old woman who presents to the emergency department with a complaint of shortness of breath. The patient has known chronic obstructive pulmonary disease. Also, on admission, she was found to have atrial fibrillation with a rapid ventricular rate, as well as right lower lobe pneumonia. The patient has not really had any fevers or chills, but she has been having quite a bit of coughing with minimal sputum production. In the ambulance on the way to the emergency department, the patient was given some nebulizers, and her oxygenation somewhat improved. She is on home O_2 and also has been found on a recent CT to have 2-cm soft tissue density in the left lung base.

Other medical conditions include:

1. Vitamin B_{12} deficiency.

2. Crohn's disease.

3. Osteoporosis.

4. Venous insufficiency.

5. Left frontal region meningioma.

6. Right recent cerebellar stroke.

7. History of cholecystectomy.

8. History of bilateral cataracts.

9. History of bowel resection for Crohn's disease.

On admission, the patient was started on Claforan and azithromycin for treatment of her pneumonia. She was also given a bolus of 50 mg IV of Cardizem to bring the heart rate back down. The patient was also found to be slightly hypokalemic, with potassium of 3.2 on admission. This was replaced. Over the course of her hospital stay, the patient has done well with improvement in her subjective sense of being short of breath. The patient has continued to have problems with dysphagia. She is status post a recent cerebrovascular accident. The patient was able to be switched to oral antibiotics on June 8. She has remained afebrile on this therapy and has continued to have good oxygen saturations on nasal cannula O_2. The patient will be discharged today in stable condition to the nursing home. Follow-up will be with her primary care physician in 1 week.

DISCHARGE MEDICATIONS:

1. Amitriptyline 25 mg p.o. q h.s.

2. Aspirin 325 mg once a day.

3. Zithromax 500 mg p.o. daily times 3 additional days.

4. Pulmicort 200 mcg inhaler b.i.d.

5. Calcium carbonate 500 mg p.o. b.i.d.

6. Vantin 200 mg p.o. b.i.d. for 14 additional days.

7. Digoxin 0.25 mg once a day.

8. Diltiazem CD 120 mg p.o. daily.

9. Folic acid 1 mg p.o. daily.

10. Ipratropium bromide inhaler 2.5 mL inhaled treatment.

11. Xalatan eye drops 1 drop in both eyes at bedtime.

12. Prednisone taper beginning at 40 mg p.o. daily for 4 days, then taper down to 30 mg daily for 2 days. Beginning third day, patient will be on 20 mg daily for 5 days.

13. Solu-Medrol Discus 1 puff b.i.d.

14. Senokot 1 tablet p.o. b.i.d.

15. Sulfasalazine enteric 1500-mg tablet p.o. b.i.d.

16. Ambien 5 mg p.o. q.h.s. p.r.n.

17. Citracal 19-gm packet p.o. b.i.d. p.r.n. for constipation.

DISCHARGE DIAGNOSES:

1. Oxygen-dependent chronic obstructive pulmonary disease with chronic obstructive pulmonary disease exacerbation.

2. Community-acquired pneumonia, right lower lobe.

3. Atrial fibrillation with rapid ventricular response, has responded to Cardizem, now rate controlled.

4. Hypokalemia, corrected.

5. Possible left-sided pulmonary nodule, follow-up CT will be needed in a couple of months.

6. Crohn's disease, stable.

7. Senile osteoporosis.

8. B_{12} deficiency.

9. History of cerebrovascular accident with residual dysphagia.

10. Venous insufficiency.

The patient will be discharged in stable condition to the nursing home.

Code for the diagnoses.

9. **CASE 9**

OBSERVATION

LOCATION: Hospital observation unit

REASON FOR ADMISSION: Exacerbation of COPD

HISTORY OF PRESENT ILLNESS: The patient is a 74-year-old male who comes in tonight complaining of progressive shortness of breath over the past 4 days. He had upper respiratory tract symptoms a week ago with nasal discharge and coldlike symptoms. It progressed to shortness of breath over the past 4 days. I was called by a family member of his earlier tonight, and I advised him to come to the Emergency Department, which he did. In the ED, he was wheezy and had oxygen saturation of 92%. He received a nebulizer treatment. A chest x-ray was done, which I reviewed myself; it showed no evidence of infiltrates. He had a large heart. The patient was admitted to the 6th floor. I proceeded by doing ABGs on him. His pH was 7.46, pCO_2 94, and bicarb 33.5 on 2 liters per nasal cannula. The patient had some cough with clear phlegm. No fever or chills now. He had some chills a week ago. The patient recently had an angiogram for his abdominal aortic aneurysm. He also had a stress test that apparently was positive. The patient is known to have chronic renal failure with a baseline creatinine of 2 to 2.2 with creatinine clearance of 32 mL per minute with a serum creatinine of 2.0 back in December. He does have severe congestive heart failure with ejection fraction less than 20%.

PAST MEDICAL HISTORY:

1. Chronic renal failure as mentioned.

2. Coronary artery disease, post two myocardial infarctions.

3. Post AICD placement.

4. Atrial fibrillation with rapid ventricular response, controlled.

5. Congestive heart failure with ejection fraction of less than 20%.

6. Abdominal aortic aneurysm, which is infrarenal measuring 6.2 cm.

7. Bilateral common iliac aneurysm, approximately 3.5 to 3.6 cm.

8. Left internal iliac artery aneurysm, questionably coiled lately.

9. COPD/asthma.

10. History of gouty arthritis with a recent gouty attack in his right first metatarsal phalangeal joint.

11. History of diverticulitis.

12. Hyperlipidemia.

13. Status post cholecystectomy, inguinal hernia repair, appendectomy.

14. Chronic renal failure, post PD catheter placement for peritoneal dialysis.

ALLERGIES: No known drug allergies.

MEDICATIONS:

1. Nebulizer at home.

2. Bumex 2 mg in the morning and 1 mg in the evening.

3. Coumadin 2 mg on Monday, 1 mg on other days.

4. Digoxin 0.125 mg p.o. b.i.d.

5. Potassium chloride 20 mEq p.o. b.i.d.

6. Zocor 10 mg p.o. qhs.

7. Coreg 25 mg p.o. b.i.d.

8. Allopurinol 100 mg p.o. daily.

9. Ranitidine 150 mg p.o. qhs.

FAMILY HISTORY: Mother died of pancreatitis. Father died at age 71. Otherwise, family history is noncontributory.

SOCIAL HISTORY: Lives here in town with his wife. She was not available today. He quit smoking 16 years ago.

REVIEW OF SYSTEMS: Constitutional: No fever, chills, or night sweats. ENT: Resolved upper respiratory tract symptoms. Respiratory: As mentioned. Cardiovascular: Exertional dyspnea. No chest pain. GI: Questionable dark stool but no diarrhea, nausea, or vomiting. He had some abdominal discomfort with coughing. Musculoskeletal: History of gouty arthritis that seems to be controlled. Skin: Trace edema. Neuro: Negative. Psychiatric: Negative.

PHYSICAL EXAMINATION: The patient was in mild respiratory distress. He was awake, oriented times three without any focal neurological deficits. His heart rate is in the 70s range, blood pressure has been 120s/80s, sats 92% when he came in, 98% on 2 liters per nasal cannula. Slightly increased jugular venous pressure. No cervical lymphadenopathy. Lungs: Good air entry bilaterally but expiratory wheezes bilaterally. No crackles. No sacral edema. Abdomen: Soft and nontender. He has PD catheter in the left lower quadrant. Small hematoma in the right inguinal area from his recent aortogram. Lower extremities: Very trace edema.

LABORATORY STUDIES: CBC tonight shows a white count of 8.6 thousand, hemoglobin 12.3, platelets 140,000, BUN 29, sodium 139, potassium 3.6, chloride 98, bicarb 31, creatinine 2.2, calcium 8.5. BNP 536 picogram/mL. INR 1.5 with a pro-time of 14.3. Digoxin 0.6. Troponin-I less than 0.04. His last uric acid level was 7.4.

IMPRESSION:

1. Exacerbation of COPD/asthma with wheezes.

2. Abdominal aortic aneurysm.

3. Noncompliance with medications and nebulizer treatments.

PLAN:

1. Albuterol MDI 2 puffs t.i.d.

2. Atrovent MDI 2 puffs t.i.d.

3. Azmacort MDI 2 puffs b.i.d.

4. Solu-Medrol 80 mg IV q 8 hours.

5. Continue the current p.o. medications.

6. Zithromax 500 mg IV daily.

7. The patient is code level I.

Discussed all of the above with the patient. He seems to understand and agrees with the plan. Will discuss further issues to his abdominal aortic aneurysm and further plans with his positive stress test when the rest of the family is available in the next couple of days.

OBSERVATION DISCHARGE SUMMARY

LOCATION: Hospital observation unit

DISCHARGE DIAGNOSIS: Exacerbation of COPD

The patient came in with wheezing. Oxygen saturations were 92%. He had no pulmonary edema. He had no infiltrates. Was given steroids, nebulizer therapy. He did well. His pO$_2$ was 94 on 2 liters. We walked him the next day. He was doing much better without any major complaints. He was discharged in reasonable general condition.

CODE LEVEL: I

DISCHARGE MEDICATIONS:

1. Albuterol inhaler two puffs three times a day p.r.n.

2. Allopurinol 100 mg p.o. daily.

3. Bumex 1 mg in the evening and 2 mg in the morning.

4. Coreg 25 mg p.o. b.i.d.

5. Digoxin 0.125 mg p.o. daily.

6. Zantac 150 mg p.o. daily.

7. Atrovent three times a day.

8. Potassium chloride 20 mEq p.o. b.i.d.

9. Zocor 10 mg p.o. daily.

10. Triamcinolone inhaler (Azmacort) two puffs three times a day.

11. Coumadin 2 mg every Monday and 1 mg on other 6 days of the week.

12. Prednisone 10 mg—he will take six pills for 3 days, then five pills for 3 days. He will go down by 10 mg every 3 days until off.

13. Zithromax 500 p.o. daily for 8 more days.

DISCHARGE PLAN: The patient will be scheduled in my clinic in 3 weeks with a basic panel, CBC, and Protime/INR.

Discussed all of the above with the patient. He seems to understand. I gave him the plan. Issues related to his aneurysm and cardiac status will be discussed in the clinic.

10. **CASE 10**

INITIAL HOSPITAL SERVICE: The patient, Stephen Moore, was brought to the hospital emergency department by air ambulance from Loganville. Stephen was involved in a motor vehicle rollover. Dr. Paul Sutton treated the patient in the emergency department and then contacted Dr. Sanchez, the general surgeon on call, who admitted the patient to the hospital.

LOCATION: Inpatient hospital

HISTORY: Mr. Moore is a 25-year-old young man who was involved in a motor vehicle rollover just outside of town. According to the paramedics who brought him down via air ambulance, the patient had arrested three times during the flight. The patient also was reported to be hypothermic with a temperature of 27°. The patient is transported with bilateral chest tubes in place. He also has no neck collar in place but is on a backboard with the neck stabilized with straps. There is no family available. The paramedics have no other history at the present time, other than that there is a possibility that after the rollover, he was immersed in cold water for approximately 5 to 10 minutes, but this history is speculative at the present time.

ROS, PAST, FAMILY, SOCIAL HISTORY: Unable to obtain because patient is unconscious.

PHYSICAL EXAM: The patient is hypotensive. His temperature is 27° with a blood pressure of 60 systolic. He has a tense distended abdomen. His pupils are fixed and dilated. He has no other obvious injuries.

ASSESSMENT:

1. Hypotension due to cold water.

2. Distended tight abdomen.

3. Hypothermia.

4. Dilated fixed pupils.

5. Possible major intra-abdominal injuries.

PLAN: He is going to be taken immediately to the operating room while we resuscitate him there in a more stable environment. X-ray had been asked previously to place a portable machine in the OR.

The patient is critically ill and is at high risk for mortality. The fixed dilated pupils are of concern, but control of his intra-abdominal bleeding and correction of the hypothermia are priorities.

OPERATIVE REPORT, LAPAROTOMY

LOCATION: Inpatient hospital

PREOPERATIVE DIAGNOSIS: Massive thoracic and abdominal injuries

POSTOPERATIVE DIAGNOSIS: Same

PROCEDURE PERFORMED: Damage control laparotomy with suture of a bleeding liver laceration

This young man presented with a temperature of 27° after he was involved in a rollover accident. During the transport down, he apparently arrested three times. The patient has a 60 systolic blood pressure at this stage. He had not had a collar placed during transport but was controlled on the backboard with his head stabilized. Immediately on arrival in the operating room, a cervical collar was placed. The patient had already been intubated. He had bilateral chest tubes in place.

Once he was on the operating room table, an attempt was made to get chest x-ray, but radiology could not get a plate under the patient. With good function of the chest tubes and the patient's continued severe hypotension, it was elected to proceed with the laparotomy and proceed with further evaluation as the case progressed. As the abdomen was being prepped, anesthesia was giving him fluids and blood and trying to warm him up. All fluids were run in warmers, including the blood that was being infused. Immediately upon having the abdomen prepped and draped, a long midline incision was made; the patient was found to have approximately a liter and one-half of blood present within the abdomen. He was cold. He had an actively bleeding liver tear that was on the dorsum, just lateral to the ligament teres. Several 0 chromic sutures were placed through this in figure-of-eight fashion, and this stopped the bleeding. This was done after we had immediately packed both the left and right upper quadrants, as well as the pelvis. After we were assured that his bleeding was controlled with the packing, anesthesia was continuously warming him and we used warm irrigation in the abdomen. The chest tubes were draining adequately. According to anesthesia, the patient still had fixed dilated pupils. By the end of the procedure, the patient's temperature was up to about 30°.

As the anesthesia was infusing the blood and fluids, and the patient's blood pressure was now coming up, we started looking at each of the quadrants. The patient was found to have a nonexpanding hematoma involving the pelvis, consistent with a pelvic fracture. This was repacked to make sure there was no active bleeding in this area, but there was no active bleeding. The packs were slowly removed from the left upper quadrant. The spleen was then visualized, and it had what appeared to be a grade one or two laceration; there was no active bleeding, this was repacked. The right side was then evaluated. Most of the blood was around the liver. The patient had a laceration at the dome of the liver, just to the right of the ligamentum teres; this was oversewn as noted above. At this point, because of the patient's hypothermia and instability, the abdomen was repacked. A Vac-Pac was quickly placed. The patient's pupils at this stage were still fixed and dilated. There was a question whether the fixed pupils were due to a primary head injury with an intracranial bleed, or whether this was just a hypoxic issue related to the original injury and the 3 arrests during transport. The patient was taken immediately from the operating room to the CAT scanner, with neurosurgeon available. CAT scan will be done immediately. If the patient does not have anything intracranial that needs to be fixed immediately, he will be taken to the intensive care unit, where we will continue resuscitation with warm fluids and blood as necessary. The patient is in critical condition. At the end of the procedure, the patient's blood pressure was up in the 80s systolic.

DISCHARGE SUMMARY

LOCATION: Inpatient hospital

DIAGNOSES:

1. Intracranial injury with fixed dilated pupils due to rollover car accident.

2. Liver laceration.

3. Hypotension.

4. Hypothermia.

5. Laceration spleen.

6. Cardiac arrest.

SUMMARY: The patient was admitted through the emergency department after being involved in a one-car rollover accident. Patient was an unrestrained driver. We took him immediately to surgery, and there we found abdominal bleeding and liver laceration. His abdominal injuries were repaired, and patient was then taken for a CT of his head to try to find cause of his unconscious state and dilation and fixation of his pupils. When I got to the CT room, the patient was not breathing. There was no chance for resuscitation, he just flat-lined immediately. There was nothing we could do for him, and the patient was pronounced dead at 2100 hours. His family was notified, and pastoral services were called in.

11. **CASE 11**

ADMISSION HISTORY AND PHYSICAL

CHIEF COMPLAINT: A 5-day-old male infant with elevated bilirubin and dehydration

HISTORY OF PRESENT ILLNESS: The patient was born at the hospital 5 days ago by C-section for an occiput posterior presentation. Mom had hypertension during labor and did receive magnesium sulfate. The baby did well following delivery and went home with mom 3 days later. Mom said her milk came in on Saturday, the day they were discharged from the hospital, and she expected baby to really be eating well, but he has not been. She said he typically nurses 20 minutes total and needs quite a bit of stimulation to keep on task. He has been sleepy at home. Today was their scheduled follow-up visit, and bilirubin in the office was 20.4. His birthweight was 9 pounds 3 ounces, and today, he weighed 7 pounds 12 ounces. That is a decrease of 15%.

PAST MEDICAL HISTORY: Significant only for receiving hepatitis B vaccine in the hospital. He is not on any medications and has no known drug allergies.

SOCIAL HISTORY: Mom, Dad, and baby are all living at home in suburbs currently, as Mom works as a lawyer and Dad is a truck driver. He will be going back on the road sometime next week. There is no tobacco use at home besides Dad's chewing tobacco and no pets at home.

FAMILY HISTORY: Mom and Dad are both alive and well. There are no siblings. Maternal grandfather has hypertension. Paternal grandfather has some sort of hypertrophic cardiac disease.

REVIEW OF SYSTEMS: Mom says the patient has had two wet diapers today. He has not had a bowel movement since Saturday about noon.

PHYSICAL EXAMINATION: General: The patient is sleeping with Mom, appears to be in no distress. Temperature has not been taken yet, but heart rate and respiratory rate are both within the normal range. I do not have a blood pressure yet either. HEENT examination: Fontanelle is soft, slightly sunken. Pupils are equal and reactive to light. Red reflexes intact in both eyes. External auditory ear canals and tympanic membranes are normal in appearance bilaterally. Mouth is dry but otherwise unremarkable. Neck is supple. Heart is regular in rate and rhythm with no murmur. Lungs are clear to auscultation bilaterally. Abdomen is soft and nontender. He is nondistended. He has active bowel sounds, and no masses are palpated. Umbilicus appears to be healing well. Extremities: He has 2+ femoral pulses bilaterally. Moves extremities spontaneously times four, although he does require a little stimulation to move very much. Genital examination: He is a circumcised male. Testes are descended bilaterally. Skin has no rashes, although he is very jaundiced in appearance.

LABS: Bilirubin was 20.4; this was done in the clinic.

ASSESSMENT:

1. Hyperbilirubinemia.

2. Dehydration.

PLAN: He will be started on IV fluids, D5 half-normal saline at 20 mL an hour and will be under triple phototherapy. Coombs and basic metabolic panel will both be drawn. Mom can breastfeed ad lib, and a repeat bilirubin will be done at 7 PM this evening.

PROGRESS NOTE: The patient is a 6-day-old infant. This is hospital day two. He was admitted for dehydration and hyperbilirubinemia.

SUBJECTIVE: Mom said that patient's color has definitely improved overnight. He is looking nice and pink this morning. She stated that feedings are still not going well. He will latch on and suck a couple of good sucks but then wants nothing to do with breastfeeding after that, will fuss and push away. She has been pumping and is able to pump 2 ounces every 2 to 3 hours. The baby has still been having several wet diapers and finally had a bowel movement yesterday—the first since Saturday.

OBJECTIVE: Weight today was 3.86 kg. That is up 12 ounces from yesterday. That makes him down 7.7% from birth. He was down 15% on admit. Feedings yesterday: It looks like he breastfed 5×, anywhere from 5 minutes to 15 minutes a side. Nursing also had to supplement 92 cc over the night. He received IV fluids, D5, normal saline at 20 cc/hour overnight, also a total of 155 cc of IV fluids since admit. Urine output since admit has been 1.25 cc/kg/hour. Heart rate has ranged in the 120s and 130s; respirations 30s and 40s. Blood pressure 91/55. He is maintaining his temperature well in the crib.

On **PHYSICAL EXAMINATION,** head is atraumatic, normocephalic. Fontanelle is flat this morning. Sclerae are still mildly icteric, but skin is otherwise nice and pink. Mouth and throat are moist and pink. Heart is regular in rate and rhythm. Lungs are clear to auscultation bilaterally. Abdomen is soft and nontender, nondistended. No masses are palpated. He has active bowel sounds. Umbilicus is healing well. Femoral pulses are strong bilaterally, circumcised male. Testes are descended bilaterally. He is much more active this morning, moving all four extremities spontaneously, and is wide awake with no tactile stimulation. Bilirubin this morning was 11.3. Basic metabolic panel this morning: Sodium is still elevated at 155, chloride 123.

ASSESSMENT:

1. Dehydration.

2. Hyperbilirubinemia.

3. Hypernatremia secondary to #1.

PLAN: We will go ahead and discontinue his phototherapy today. Lactation consultants have been consulted for assistance with breastfeeding. IV fluids will be decreased to maintenance at 14 cc/hour and changed to D5 half-normal saline, instead of D5 3/4 normal saline.

DISCHARGE SUMMARY

REASONS FOR HOSPITALIZATION: Dehydration, hyperbilirubinemia, and hypernatremia

SUMMARY OF HOSPITAL COURSE: The patient was admitted from the clinic at 5 days of age because of difficulty feeding at home, which had led to dehydration and hyperbilirubinemia. His ABO incompatibility test was negative. He was started on triple phototherapy and IV fluids at $1\frac{1}{2}$ times maintenance rate. Within 24 hours, his bilirubin had dropped from 20.4 down to 11.3. His sodium had dropped from 158 down to 155 on $\frac{1}{2}$ normal saline. Lactation consultants had been working with the patient and Mom on breastfeeding. He needed to be fed pumped breast milk most of the time because of impatience at the breast, but Mom wanted to keep trying. The patient's bilirubin had dropped to 9.9 after he had been off phototherapy for 24 hours. Sodium was down to 149, and the patient was having frequent wet diapers and stools. The patient was discharged home with instructions to Mom on keeping track of wet diapers and on attempting to breastfeed every 3 hours. They will follow up with Dr. Green in clinic next week.

INSTRUCTIONS TO THE PATIENT OR FAMILY: Activity ad lib. Medications: None. Diet: Attempt breastfeeding every 3 hours. If baby does not feed, Mom will feed pumped breast milk. Follow-up appointment will be next Wednesday, with Dr. Green in the clinic.

CONDITION ON DISCHARGE AS COMPARED TO CONDITION ON ADMISSION: The patient is continuing to improve following an episode of dehydration with hyperbilirubinemia and hypernatremia.

DISCHARGE DIAGNOSES:

1. Dehydration.

2. Hyperbilirubinemia secondary to #1.

3. Hypernatremia secondary to #1.

4. Difficulty breastfeeding.

12. **CASE 12**

ADMISSION HISTORY

CHIEF COMPLAINT: Chest pain

The patient was transferred from Othertown Hospital because of chest pain.

HISTORY OF PRESENT ILLNESS: The patient is a 65-year-old male with past medical history of diabetes mellitus, hypertension, chronic renal insufficiency, and esophageal cancer, status post resection with gastric pull-up. He also has a history of coronary artery disease and had CABG and aortic valve replacement about 7 years ago. He has been in reasonably stable health condition until at about 10 PM last night. He was lying in a recliner when he started having retrosternal chest discomfort. His chest discomfort was described as dull in character with an intensity of 5/10. It initially lasted for about 20 minutes before subsiding but has been waxing and waning since then. This morning at the time of presentation to Othertown Clinic, the intensity of the chest pain was 6/10. The chest pain is non-radiating and is not associated with diaphoresis, nausea, vomiting, shortness of breath, PND, or orthopnea. It was promptly relieved by administration of sublingual nitroglycerin at Othertown Hospital. At this time of evaluation, the patient has been chest pain free. He reports no other complaints. He has never had this type of chest pain over the past 7 years, and he does not think it is related to esophageal cancer. His exercise tolerance is less than one block and has been like that for some time. He does not think that it has changed recently with this event. He denies abdominal pain, hematemesis, or melena in stools. No change in urinary habits. His appetite has been good, although he intermittently has nausea. No headache, blurring of vision, or diplopia. He was seen last week at Nearby Clinic, where he had gone for medical follow-up. During that time, he had a CT scan of the chest, which was not different from the CT scan done at the hospital about 2 months ago. He follows with the medical oncology physician.

PAST MEDICAL HISTORY:

1. Coronary artery disease.
2. CABG.
3. Esophageal cancer.
4. Recent PE.
5. Diabetes mellitus type 2.
6. Hypertension.
7. Chronic renal insufficiency.
8. Chronic hyponatremia.
9. Anemia of chronic disease.
10. Thrombocytopenia.
11. Anticoagulation for mechanical heart valve.
12. Mechanical aortic valve.

PAST SURGICAL HISTORY:

1. Aortic valve replacement.

2. Hernia repair.

3. CABG 7 years ago.

4. Recent enteric tube for feeding.

MEDICATIONS:

1. Lopressor 25 mg daily.

2. Digoxin 0.125 mg daily.

3. Folic acid 1 mg daily.

4. Levothyroxine 0.1 mg daily.

5. Pantoprazole 40 mg daily.

6. Potassium chloride 3 mg b.i.d.

7. Sertraline 50 mg daily.

8. Ativan 0.5 mg q 8 hours p.r.n.

9. Ambien 5 mg at bedtime.

10. Lomotil 1 tablet four times daily as needed.

11. Iron 325 mg daily.

12. Multivitamin with mineral 1 tablet daily.

13. Kaopectate.

ALLERGIES: Penicillin and niacin

SOCIAL HISTORY: He lives with his wife in rural Anytown. He is a retired pharmacist. He smoked about 25 years, two to three packs a day, but quit in 1980. Alcohol is consumed on a social basis.

FAMILY HISTORY: His mother had asthma and an enlarged heart. His dad died at the age of 51 with heart disease. Multiple family members have heart disease and diabetes.

REVIEW OF SYSTEMS: Cardiovascular, respiratory, GI, and genitourinary systems were reviewed in the HPI, and there are no other pertinent findings. Musculoskeletal: No claudication. No arthritic deformities. Endocrine: He has a history of diabetes and thyroid disease. Psychiatric: No history of depression or any other psychiatric illness. No hallucinations.

PHYSICAL EXAMINATION: He is alert and oriented to place, time, and person. He is not in any obvious distress. Vital signs: Blood pressure: 121/73. Pulse: 75 per minute. Respiratory rate: 23 per minute. O_2 saturation 97%. Temperature: 36.4. Head: Normocephalic, atraumatic. No cervical lymphadenopathy. Neck is supple. Oropharynx is clear. Trachea is central. General: He is mildly pale, not jaundiced, not cyanosed. No peripheral lymphadenopathy. CVS: First and second heart sounds are normal. He has a metallic sound due to a mechanical aortic valve. No cardiac murmurs appreciated. Chest: Good air entry bilaterally; no crackles, no rhonchi. Breath sounds at the bases are somewhat coarse. Abdomen: He has a feeding tube in place in the left hypochondrium. The point of entrance of the tube is stained with a thin, purulent material. No abdominal tenderness. No guarding. Bowel sounds are present and normal. Genitourinary: Kidneys are not palpable. No costovertebral angle tenderness. No suprapubic tenderness. Musculoskeletal: No finger clubbing. No peripheral cyanosis. No pedal edema. Neurologic: No gross neurologic abnormality noted. Moves all extremities fully. Normal tone and power of all extremities. Psychiatric: He is not depressed. No delusions or hallucinations.

EKG: Normal sinus rhythm. No ST/T changes.

LABORATORY DATA: Hemoglobin 13.2, WBC 8.6, platelets 220, MCV 92.3. BUN 10, glucose 139, creatinine 0.9, potassium 4.7, sodium 137, chloride 102, bicarbonate 27.

ASSESSMENT AND PLAN:

1. Chest pain. The chest pain is of new onset in a patient who has risk factors for coronary artery disease. I will treat this as unstable angina. Will send two more sets of cardiac enzymes and also three sets EKG. Will also obtain a lipid panel. Will send a sample for PT/INR and a comprehensive metabolic panel. The patient has been given aspirin. Will continue with Lovenox 60 mg every 12 hours and continue with beta blocker, Lopressor 25 mg daily. I will maintain the patient on intravenous nitroglycerin 5 mcg/minute and oxygen by nasal cannula 2 liters per minute.

2. History of pulmonary embolism. This patient has been on anticoagulation, and that will be continued.

3. Diabetes mellitus. The patient states that his blood sugars have been adequately controlled, and he discontinued hypoglycemic agents himself. Will monitor Accu-Cheks and re-start oral hypoglycemics if indicated.

4. Hypertension. Blood pressure is well controlled at this time. Will administer antihypertensives.

5. Chronic renal insufficiency. His most recent creatinine was 0.9. Will continue to monitor renal function.

6. Mechanical aortic valve. Because of endoscopy that is planned for Friday, the patient has been off Coumadin and is currently on Lovenox. We will continue Lovenox and re-start Coumadin after the procedure.

7. Esophageal cancer. The patient is being followed by the Oncology team. No acute condition is related to the cancer at this time.

Code status was discussed with the patient and family, and he elects to be code I.

PROGRESS NOTE

SUBJECTIVE: The patient complains of abdominal pain, which has intensity of 5/10. It radiates to the back. He describes it as stabbing in character. He has associated nausea but no vomiting. No change in bowel or urinary habit. Denies chest pain, shortness of breath, paroxysmal nocturnal dyspnea, or orthopnea. Has not been having fever. No hematemesis, melena, or hematochezia.

REVIEW OF SYSTEMS: Cardiovascular, respiratory, and neurologic systems were reviewed, and there are no other pertinent findings.

OBJECTIVE: He is alert and oriented to place, time, and person. He is not in obvious distress. Vital signs: blood pressure 114/61, pulse 80 per minute, Respiratory rate 20 per minute, O_2 saturation 97%, temperature 36.5. Chest: Good air entry bilaterally, no crackles, no rhonchi. Chest: CVS: First and second heart sounds normal. He has a metallic sound due to mechanical aortic valve. No cardiac murmurs are appreciated. Abdomen is soft and nontender, no pulsatile mass noted. No hepatosplenomegaly and no ascites. He has a feeding tube on the left hypochondrium.

LABORATORY DATA: Cardiac enzymes negative. Blood sugar ranged from 94 to 235. Albumin is 2.7, creatinine 8.6. Otherwise, the comprehensive metabolic panel is normal. LDL of 83, HDL of 46, triglyceride of 143, cholesterol of 158. INR is 2.7.

ASSESSMENT AND PLAN:

1. Abdominal pain: Radiating to the back. Need to rule out aortic dissection. I will get a CT scan with contrast. Will continue to monitor the patient hemodynamically. I will increase the patient's Protonix to 40 mg b.i.d. and will start Reglan 5 mg with meals. I will also start the patient on Maalox 10 mL every 6 hours p.r.n. I will send sample for amylase and lipase.

2. Chest pain: The patient has not had chest pain since admission. He is scheduled for noninvasive adenosine Cardiolite this morning. He is currently on Lovenox 15 mg every 12 hours, Lopressor 25 mg, and intravenous nitroglycerin 5 mcg per minute.

3. History of pulmonary embolism.

4. Diabetes mellitus. We will continue with Accu-Cheks and will make adjustments as necessary.

5. Hypertension: Blood pressures have been within acceptable range.

6. Chronic renal insufficiency: The patient seems stable from this standpoint.

7. Mechanical aortic valve.

8. Esophageal cancer.

PHARMACOLOGIC NUCLEAR PERFUSION STRESS TEST

INDICATION: Chest pain

PAST MEDICAL HISTORY includes:

1. Aortic valve replacement in 1997.

2. Coronary artery disease, coronary artery bypass grafting surgery, supraventricular tachycardia, hypertension, angina, diabetes mellitus, myocardial infarction in 1997, chronic renal insufficiency, esophageal CA status post resection with pull-through, pulmonary embolism, hypernatremia, anemia of chronic disease, thrombocytopenia.

CURRENT MEDICATIONS:

1. Ambien.

2. Atropine.

3. Cardizem CD.

4. Coumadin.

5. Digoxin.

6. Folic acid.

7. K-Dur.

8. Lorazepam.

9. Metoprolol.

10. Protonix.

11. Reglan.

12. Synthroid.

13. Zocor.

14. Zoloft.

DISCHARGE SUMMARY

REASON FOR HOSPITALIZATION: Chest pain

SUMMARY OF HOSPITAL COURSE: The patient is a 65-year-old man with past medical history of diabetes mellitus, hypertension, chronic renal insufficiency, and advanced esophageal cancer status post resection with gastric pull-through. He also has a history of coronary artery disease and had CABG and aortic valve replacement about seven years ago. He was transferred from Anytown 5 days ago, because of chest pain that started at rest and was associated with nausea and some shortness of breath. The chest pain was relieved by sublingual nitroglycerin. At the time of evaluation in the emergency department, the patient was hemodynamically stable but was having another episode of mild chest pain. He was started on intravenous nitroglycerin, and Lovenox was continued at 60 mg every 12 hours. He had a stress test, which showed predominantly fixed decreased defect in the posterior/inferior wall. There was also suggestion of a possible small amount of reversibility around the basilar aspect of the posterior/inferior wall, which might have been due to technical difficulties. The findings were discussed with Dr. Green, who thought that they were insignificant to warrant any invasive procedures. The patient's chest pain was thought to be due to the advanced esophageal cancer. Because the chest pain was radiating to the back, a CT scan of the chest and abdomen was done, to rule out aortic dissection. In the scan, an incidental finding of soft tissue density in the lung was noted. Oncology consult was requested, and it was thought that the soft tissue densities were most likely due to metastasis from the esophageal cancer. The patient was informed of the findings and was started on analgesics for pain control. His symptoms have improved and he remains hemodynamically stable. Cardiac enzymes were not elevated. Amylase and lipase were normal. The only abnormality noted on comprehensive metabolic panel was albumin of 2.7 and total protein of 5.8.

PLAN: The patient is to be discharged home. Appointment will be scheduled with the primary care physician. He also has appointment tomorrow with the gastroenterology physician for an esophagogastroduodenoscopy.

FINAL DIAGNOSES:

1. Chest pain due to metastatic esophageal cancer.

2. Unstable angina ruled out.

3. Soft tissue density in the lung thought to be due to metastatic disease from esophageal carcinoma.

4. History of pulmonary embolism.

5. Aortic mechanical valve.

6. Anticoagulation with Lovenox.

7. Diabetes mellitus.

8. Hypertension.

9. Chronic renal insufficiency.

10. Dysphagia.

11. Hypoalbuminemia.

DISCHARGE MEDICATIONS:

1. Digoxin 0.125 mg daily.

2. Enoxaparin 18 mg subcutaneously daily.

3. Ferrous sulfate 324 mg daily.

4. Folic acid 1 mg daily.

5. Glyburide 5 mg daily.

6. Kytril.

7. Lovenox 0.1 mg daily.

8. Metoprolol 25 mg daily.

9. Multivitamin 1 tablet daily.

10. Oxycodone 1 tablet every 2–4 hours.

11. Pantoprazole 40 mg three times daily.

12. Potassium chloride 30 mEq twice daily with food.

13. Sertraline (Zoloft) 50 mg daily.

14. Zolpidem 5 mg at bedtime.

15. Lomotil 1 tablet four times a day as needed.

16. Lorazepam 0.5 mg p.r.n. every 8 hours.

CONSULTATIONS:

1. Oncology.

2. Telephone consultation with Cardiology.

CONDITION ON DISCHARGE: At the time of discharge, patient is hemodynamically stable. Vital signs are blood pressure 103/86. Pulse is 81 per minute. Respiratory rate 20 per minute. Oxygen saturation 94% on room air. Temperature 36.5°. His code status at the time of discharge is code I.

13. **CASE 13**

ADMISSION HISTORY

PATIENT IDENTIFICATION: The patient is a 4-year-old female with a history of asthma/previous pneumonias in the past who presents with cough, hypoxia, wheezing refractory to home treatment, and inability to intake orals.

CHIEF COMPLAINT: Inability to intake orals, cough, hypoxia, and wheezing

HISTORY OF PRESENT ILLNESS: The patient was in her prior normal state of health until approximately 4 AM, 20 hours prior to admission, when she woke up and had some increasing wheezing, refractory to treatment at home, including Pulmicort, Zyrtec, Albuterol, and Singulair.

Mother notes that the patient is unable to sit up with this. She has been vomiting all the liquids and oral intakes she has had today. Mom noted that the patient felt feverish and chilled today, but no objective temperatures were taken at home. The patient's mother notes that usually once a year the patient has some episode of either pneumonia/exacerbation of asthma. It seems like she had some allergic component to it with recent allergy test results that showed the patient is allergic to dust, molds, and cats. Of note, the patient was exposed to a cat in her grandmother's home during the night last night. Mother notes cough associated with this, but it is nonproductive in nature since 4 AM, and the wheezing is as described above, refractory to treatment.

PAST MEDICAL HISTORY:

1. Past history of asthma/pneumonia.

2. Allergic rhinitis, possible component involved with her asthma.

3. Allergy testing in the past to dust, molds, and cat.

4. The patient was born at full term. No neonatal complications or maternal complications.

ALLERGIES: No known drug allergies.

MEDICATIONS:

1. Pulmicort.

2. Albuterol.

3. Singulair, 5 mg, she believes.

4. Zyrtec.

5. Tylenol.

FAMILY HISTORY: Father with asthma and both sides of her family having asthma. No noted early deaths due to cardiopulmonary disease. No known cardiopulmonary disease in other family members.

SOCIAL HISTORY: The patient lives in Anytown with her mother and mother's roommate. She does attend day care with her grandmother. No noted sick contacts. She does attend school. No smoking around her. No pets, except with her grandmother as above.

REVIEW OF SYSTEMS: Fully reviewed and contributory only for decreased urination today, decreased oral intake with vomiting, and a rash that occurred about 5 days ago that did not seem to be pruritic in nature that they put some Neosporin on.

PHYSICAL EXAMINATION: Appearance: Four-year-old female in no obvious distress, breathing rapidly, somewhat timid. Temperature is 37, heart rate 160, respiratory rate 40, and O_2 sats are 88% on room air. HEENT: HEAD is atraumatic. EYES: EOMS intact and anicteric. PERRLA. Tympanic membranes: Left is clear, as well as right, with some cerumen impaction. No erythema, edema, or exudate. Nose: No obvious rhinitis or rhinorrhea with nasal cannula in. Throat: Oropharynx is clear without erythema, edema, or exudate. Neck: No obvious lymphadenopathy, thyromegaly, or tenderness appreciated. Oropharynx has sticky mucous membranes with little saliva. Lungs: Expiratory wheezes throughout, right greater than left. No crackles or rhonchi. Cardiovascular: Tachy S1 and S2. Regular rate and rhythm. No extra heart sounds, murmurs, rubs, or gallops. Abdomen: Soft. Nontender and nondistended. No organomegaly, pulsatile masses, or obvious tenderness. Bowel sounds are positive. Extremities: Right posterior leg behind the hamstrings: There seem to be some flush-colored domelike papules umbilicated in the center. No peripheral edema. Pulses are positive and symmetric bilaterally in the upper and lower extremities. Neurological: Intact cranial nerves II–XII as best I can tell with the child.

INVESTIGATIONS: White cell count 13.56 with 76% neutrophils. Hemoglobin is 15.3, platelets 310, sodium 138, chloride 99, potassium 4.6, bicarb 20.6, BUN 11, creatinine 0.5, calcium 10.5, and glucose 100.

Chest x-ray revealed a blunted right heart border with what appears to be some patchy-type infiltrates involving the right lung field. No obvious effusions or cardiomegaly noted.

ASSESSMENT AND PLAN:

1. Acute asthma exacerbation. The patient required nebulizers as well as oxygen in the emergency department. We will maintain her on her nebulizers and start steroids.

2. Hypoxia secondary to #1. O_2 sats on admission were 88% on room air.

3. Right-sided pneumonia. The patient will be started on antibiotics of Claforan 50 mg per kilogram IV every 6 hours, which is a gram every 6 hours.

4. Dehydration as evidenced by sticky mucous membranes and no oral intake today. We will start IV fluids tonight also.

The patient's case, impression, and plan will be discussed with Dr. Green and will be adjusted accordingly.

PEDIATRIC CONSULTATION

PATIENT IDENTIFICATION: The patient is a 4-year-old female who is hospital day 4 with an acute asthma exacerbation, hypoxia secondary to her asthma exacerbation, right-sided pneumonia, and dehydration.

HISTORY OF PRESENT ILLNESS: Mom reports that the patient has a history of asthma and an allergy problem. She does take Singulair 5 mg on a daily basis and has for the better part of 2 years. She has also been taking Zyrtec for the past 6 months, which was recommended by the allergist after her allergy testing. In the past, she has had one to two asthma exacerbations per year. At that time, Mom would give Albuterol and Pulmicort nebs on a p.r.n. basis. Mom said she has not had to use any nebulizers on the patient since sometime last fall, so it has been several months since her last nebulizer. When she started getting ill, Mom gave her three Albuterol nebulizers and two Pulmicort nebulizers at home with no improvement, and that is when she decided that they should come to the emergency department. She was also having coughing spells and would vomit anything that she took orally. The patient also has a history of allergies. She has had allergy testing, it sounds like with the allergist, and tested positive for dust, mold, and cats. The patient was exposed to a cat the day prior to admission at her grandmother's house.

PAST MEDICAL HISTORY: Significant for allergic rhinitis with allergy testing positive to dust, mold, and cats, and asthma is currently controlled with Singulair daily and Albuterol and Pulmicort p.r.n. The patient was a full-term delivery with no neonatal or maternal complications.

ALLERGIES: She has no known drug allergies.

CURRENT MEDICATIONS: While here in the hospital include:

1. Pulmicort nebulizer 0.5 mg b.i.d.

2. Albuterol/Atrovent nebulizers every 4 hours.

3. Albuterol nebulizer every 1 hour p.r.n.

4. Singulair 4 mg at bedtime.

5. Claforan 1 gram every 6 hours.

6. Solu-Medrol 20 mg every 6 hours, which is 1 mg per kilogram.

FAMILY HISTORY: The patient's father has asthma, as do several of her paternal relatives. Her maternal grandmother has allergies and asthma also. Nobody has any history of eczema as far as Mom knows.

SOCIAL HISTORY: The patient lives in town. She lives with her mother and her mother's roommate. She goes to Head Start for half days and then goes to her paternal grandmother's house. Her paternal grandmother runs a day care. No one at day care smokes. At home, the mother's roommate does smoke, although not in the presence of the patient. The patient has had no contact with other sick people, and has no exposure to pets, except for at maternal grandmother's house. The maternal grandmother does have a cat.

REVIEW OF SYSTEMS: Significant for improved appetite and urination since hospitalization. She does have a rash on the back of one leg, which was present on admit, and it has been improving.

PHYSICAL EXAMINATION: Appearance: This is a 4-year-old female who is in no distress. She interacts appropriately with me. Temperature is 36.2. T-maximum over the past 24 hours is 37.7. Blood pressure is 121/62 and pulse is 128. The pulse has typically been anywhere in the 1-teens to 140s. Respirations currently are at 32. She has run anywhere from 24 to 42. She is sating 91% on 3 liters; that was this morning. She is currently sating okay on 1 liter. HEENT examination: Head is atraumatic, normocephalic. Eyes: Extraocular movements are intact. Sclera non-icteric. Pupils are equal and reactive to light. Tympanic membranes: She has some cerumen in both external auditory canals, but the tympanic membranes appear normal bilaterally. External auditory ear canals are also normal in appearance bilaterally. Nose: Nasal cannula is in. She does have some nasal discharge that is clear. Throat: Moist and pink without erythema or exudate. Neck: She has no lymph nodes palpable in the anterior or posterior cervical triangles. Neck is nontender. Trachea is midline. Lungs show inspiratory and expiratory wheezes throughout all lung fields. She does have good air movement. There are no crackles or rhonchi. Heart is tachycardic with a normal S1 and S2. Regular rhythm. There is no murmur, rub, or gallop. Abdomen is soft, nontender, and nondistended. No organomegaly. Bowel sounds are active. Extremities: She has no peripheral edema. She has good peripheral pulses. She moves the extremities through a full range of motion times four. She does have a little bit of a rash that seems to be healing well on the back of her right leg.

LABORATORY: There has been no lab drawn since the day of admission.

IMAGING: She did have a chest x-ray done this morning, which showed a collapsed right upper lobe, as well as some perihilar opacities and opacities extending into the lower lung field medially. No pleural effusions.

ASSESSMENT AND PLAN:

1. Acute asthma exacerbation, status asthmaticus. The patient seems to be improving. I would recommend continuing the current treatment of Albuterol and Atrovent nebulizers, Pulmicort, and Solu-Medrol. Wean her off oxygen as able.

2. Right-sided pneumonia. The patient is doing well on Claforan right now. I would recommend checking a PPD in order to rule out any tuberculosis. Mom denied any tuberculosis exposure.

3. As long as the patient continues to improve, I would not alter the plan at all. On discharge, she will need to go home on the Pulmicort 0.5 mg nebulizer b.i.d. This may be able to be decreased as an outpatient.

The patient was discussed with Dr. Green, and she will see the patient after the clinic today.

DISCHARGE SUMMARY

REASON FOR HOSPITALIZATION: Exacerbation of asthma with pneumonia

SUMMARY OF HOSPITAL COURSE: The patient was admitted 6 days ago with an asthma exacerbation, known allergic rhinitis, and an acute pneumonia. She was started on IV steroids, IV fluids, nebulizer treatments with Albuterol, Atrovent, and Pulmicort, and IV antibiotics to cover her pneumonia. She was oxygen-dependent on admit. The patient continued to need oxygen for the first 3 days of her hospitalization up to 3 liters by nasal cannula. Her chest x-ray worsened and did show a collapse of the right upper lung lobe. At that time, pediatrics was consulted. No changes were made in her medications at that time, and the patient seemed to gradually start improving. A PPD test was placed. She was weaned off her oxygen and has been on room air since Friday morning. Medications were switched to oral antibiotics and oral prednisone on Friday morning, and the patient has done well. She is discharged home today, 6 days after admission.

INSTRUCTIONS TO PATIENT AND/OR FAMILY: Activity as tolerated. Diet also as tolerated.

MEDICATIONS: Include:

1. Albuterol unit dose nebulizer treatments q4h. while awake.

2. Pulmicort 0.5 nebulizer treatments b.i.d.

3. Azithromycin 100 mg orally for 3 more days.

4. Prednisolone 15 mg every 12 hours.

5. Singulair 4 mg q.h.s.

6. Zyrtec 1 mg daily.

FOLLOW-UP APPOINTMENT: Will be made next week.

CONDITION ON DISCHARGE AS COMPARED WITH CONDITION ON ADMISSION: The patient is doing much better following an acute asthma exacerbation associated with pneumonia.

DISCHARGE/FINAL DIAGNOSES: Include:

1. Acute asthma exacerbation.

2. Allergic rhinitis.

3. Pneumonia with collapse of right upper lung lobe.

4. Hypoxia and dehydration secondary to asthma exacerbation and pneumonia.

ICD-9-CM Official Guidelines for Coding and Reporting

Reprinted as released by the Centers for Medicare and Medicaid Services and the National Center for Health Statistics. See http://www.cdc.gov/nchs/datawh/ftpserv/ftpicd9/ftpicd9.htm#guidelines. You can also check the Evolve website for the latest updates at http://evolve.elsevier.com/Buck/ccs.

Effective October 1, 2007
Narrative changes appear in bold text
Items underlined have been moved within the guidelines since November 15, 2006
The guidelines include the updated V Code Table

The Centers for Medicare and Medicaid Services (CMS) and the National Center for Health Statistics (NCHS), two departments within the U.S. Federal Government's Department of Health and Human Services (DHHS) provide the following guidelines for coding and reporting using the International Classification of Diseases, 9th Revision, Clinical Modification (ICD-9-CM). These guidelines should be used as a companion document to the official version of the ICD-9-CM as published on CD-ROM by the U.S. Government Printing Office (GPO).

These guidelines have been approved by the four organizations that make up the Cooperating Parties for the ICD-9-CM: the American Hospital Association (AHA), the American Health Information Management Association (AHIMA), CMS, and NCHS. These guidelines are included on the official government version of the ICD-9-CM, and also appear in *"Coding Clinic for ICD-9-CM"* published by the AHA.

These guidelines are a set of rules that have been developed to accompany and complement the official conventions and instructions provided within the ICD-9-CM itself. These guidelines are based on the coding and sequencing instructions in Volumes I, II and III of ICD-9-CM, but provide additional instruction. Adherence to these guidelines when assigning ICD-9-CM diagnosis and procedure codes is required under the Health Insurance Portability and Accountability Act (HIPAA). The diagnosis codes (Volumes 1-2) have been adopted under HIPAA for all healthcare settings. Volume 3 procedure codes have been adopted for inpatient procedures reported by hospitals. A joint effort between the healthcare provider and the coder is essential to achieve complete and accurate documentation, code assignment, and reporting of diagnoses and procedures. These guidelines have been developed to assist both the healthcare provider and the coder in identifying those diagnoses and procedures that are to be reported. The importance of consistent, complete documentation in the medical record cannot be overemphasized. Without such documentation accurate coding cannot be achieved. The entire record should be reviewed to determine the specific reason for the encounter and the conditions treated.

The term encounter is used for all settings, including hospital admissions. In the context of these guidelines, the term provider is used throughout the guidelines to mean physician or any qualified health care practitioner who is legally accountable for establishing the patient's diagnosis. Only this set of guidelines, approved by the Cooperating Parties, is official.

The guidelines are organized into sections. Section I includes the structure and conventions of the classification and general guidelines that apply to the entire classification, and chapter-specific guidelines that correspond to the chapters as they are arranged in the classification. Section II includes guidelines for selection of principal diagnosis for non-outpatient settings. Section III includes guidelines for reporting additional diagnoses in non-outpatient settings. Section IV is for outpatient coding and reporting.

ICD-9-CM Official Guidelines for Coding and Reporting

Section I.   **Conventions, general coding guidelines and chapter specific guidelines**

A. Conventions for the ICD-9-CM

1. Format:

2. Abbreviations

   a. Index abbreviations

   b. Tabular abbreviations

3. Punctuation

4. Includes and Excludes Notes and Inclusion terms

5. Other and Unspecified codes

   a. "Other" codes

   b. "Unspecified" codes

6. Etiology/manifestation convention ("code first", "use additional code" and "in diseases classified elsewhere" notes)

7. "And"

8. "With"

9. "See" and "See Also"

B. General Coding Guidelines

1. Use of Both Alphabetic Index and Tabular List

2. Locate each term in the Alphabetic Index

3. Level of Detail in Coding

4. Code or codes from 001.0 through V84.8

5. Selection of codes 001.0 through 999.9

6. Signs and symptoms

7. Conditions that are an integral part of a disease process

8. Conditions that are not an integral part of a disease process

9. Multiple coding for a single condition

10. Acute and Chronic Conditions

11. Combination Code

12. Late Effects

13. Impending or Threatened Condition

14. **Reporting Same Diagnosis Code More Than Once**

15. **Admissions/Encounters for Rehabilitation**

16. **Documenting for BMI and Pressure Ulcer Stages**

C. Chapter-Specific Coding Guidelines

1. Chapter 1: Infectious and Parasitic Diseases (001-139)

   a. Human Immunodeficiency Virus (HIV) Infections

   b. Septicemia, Systemic Inflammatory Response Syndrome (SIRS), Sepsis, Severe Sepsis, and Septic Shock

   c. **Methicillin Resistant Staphylococcus aureus (MRSA) Conditions**

2. Chapter 2: Neoplasms (140-239)

   a. Treatment directed at the malignancy

   b. Treatment of secondary site

   c. Coding and sequencing of complications

   d. Primary malignancy previously excised

   e. Admissions/Encounters involving chemotherapy, immunotherapy and radiation therapy

   f. Admission/encounter to determine extent of malignancy

   g. Symptoms, signs, and ill-defined conditions listed in Chapter 16 associated with neoplasms

   h. Admission/encounter for pain control/management

   i. **Malignant neoplasm associated with transplanted organ**

3. Chapter 3: Endocrine, Nutritional, and Metabolic Diseases and Immunity Disorders (240-279)

   a. Diabetes mellitus

4. Chapter 4: Diseases of Blood and Blood Forming Organs (280-289)

   a. Anemia of chronic disease

5. Chapter 5: Mental Disorders (290-319)

   Reserved for future guideline expansion

6. Chapter 6: Diseases of Nervous System and Sense Organs (320-389)

   a. Pain – Category

7. Chapter 7: Diseases of Circulatory System (390-459)

   a. Hypertension

   b. Cerebral infarction/stroke/cerebrovascular accident (CVA)

    c. Postoperative cerebrovascular accident

    d. Late Effects of Cerebrovascular Disease

    e. Acute myocardial infarction (AMI)

8. Chapter 8: Diseases of Respiratory System (460-519)

    a. Chronic Obstructive Pulmonary Disease [COPD] and Asthma

    b. Chronic Obstructive Pulmonary Disease [COPD] and Bronchitis

    c. Acute Respiratory Failure

    d. Influenza due to identified avian influenza virus (avian influenza)

9. Chapter 9: Diseases of Digestive System (520-579)

    Reserved for future guideline expansion

10. Chapter 10: Diseases of Genitourinary System (580-629)

    a. Chronic kidney disease

11. Chapter 11: Complications of Pregnancy, Childbirth, and the Puerperium (630-679)

    a. General Rules for Obstetric Cases

    b. Selection of OB Principal or First-listed Diagnosis

    c. Fetal Conditions Affecting the Management of the Mother

    d. HIV Infection in Pregnancy, Childbirth and the Puerperium

    e. Current Conditions Complicating Pregnancy

    f. Diabetes mellitus in pregnancy

    g. Gestational diabetes

    h. Normal Delivery, Code 650

    i. The Postpartum and Peripartum Periods

    j. Code 677, Late effect of complication of pregnancy

    k. Abortions

12. Chapter 12: Diseases Skin and Subcutaneous Tissue (680-709)

    a. Pressure ulcer stage codes

13. Chapter 13: Diseases of Musculoskeletal and Connective Tissue (710-739)

    a. Coding of Pathologic Fractures

14. Chapter 14: Congenital Anomalies (740-759)

    a. Codes in categories 740-759, Congenital Anomalies

15. Chapter 15: Newborn (Perinatal) Guidelines (760-779)

    a. General Perinatal Rules

    b. Use of codes V30-V39

    c. Newborn transfers

    d. Use of category V29

    e. Use of other V codes on perinatal records

    f. Maternal Causes of Perinatal Morbidity

    g. Congenital Anomalies in Newborns

    h. Coding Additional Perinatal Diagnoses

    i. Prematurity and Fetal Growth Retardation

    j. Newborn sepsis

16. Chapter 16: Signs, Symptoms and Ill-Defined Conditions (780-799)

Reserved for future guideline expansion

17. Chapter 17: Injury and Poisoning (800-999)

    a. Coding of Injuries

    b. Coding of Traumatic Fractures

    c. Coding of Burns

    d. Coding of Debridement of Wound, Infection, or Burn

    e. Adverse Effects, Poisoning and Toxic Effects

    f. Complications of care

    g. SIRS due to Non-infectious Process

18. Classification of Factors Influencing Health Status and Contact with Health Service (Supplemental V01-V89)

    a. Introduction

    b. V codes use in any healthcare setting

    c. V Codes indicate a reason for an encounter

    d. Categories of V Codes

    e. V Code Table

19. Supplemental Classification of External Causes of Injury and Poisoning (E-codes, E800-E999)

    a. General E Code Coding Guidelines

    b. Place of Occurrence Guideline

    c. Adverse Effects of Drugs, Medicinal and Biological Substances Guidelines

    d. Multiple Cause E Code Coding Guidelines

    e. Child and Adult Abuse Guideline

    f. Unknown or Suspected Intent Guideline

    g. Undetermined Cause

    h. Late Effects of External Cause Guidelines

    i. Misadventures and Complications of Care Guidelines

    j. Terrorism Guidelines

Section II. Selection of Principal Diagnosis

    A. Codes for symptoms, signs, and ill-defined conditions

    B. Two or more interrelated conditions, each potentially meeting the definition for principal diagnosis

    C. Two or more diagnoses that equally meet the definition for principal diagnosis

    D. Two or more comparative or contrasting conditions

    E. A symptom(s) followed by contrasting/comparative diagnoses

    F. Original treatment plan not carried out

    G. Complications of surgery and other medical care

    H. Uncertain Diagnosis

    I. Admission from Observation Unit

      1. Admission Following Medical Observation

      2. Admission Following Post-Operative Observation

    J. Admission from Outpatient Surgery

Section III. Reporting Additional Diagnoses

    A. Previous conditions

    B. Abnormal findings

    C. Uncertain Diagnosis

Section IV. Diagnostic Coding and Reporting Guidelines for Outpatient Services

    A. Selection of first-listed condition

      1. Outpatient Surgery

      2. Observation Stay

    B. Codes from 001.0 through **V89.09**

    C. Accurate reporting of ICD-9-CM diagnosis codes

    D. Selection of codes 001.0 through 999.9

    E. Codes that describe symptoms and signs

    F. Encounters for circumstances other than a disease or injury

    G. Level of Detail in Coding

      1. ICD-9-CM codes with 3, 4, or 5 digits

      2. Use of full number of digits required for a code

    H. ICD-9-CM code for the diagnosis, condition, problem, or other reason for encounter/visit

    I. Uncertain diagnosis

    J. Chronic diseases

    K. Code all documented conditions that coexist

    L. Patients receiving diagnostic services only

M. Patients receiving therapeutic services only

N. Patients receiving preoperative evaluations only

O. Ambulatory surgery

P. Routine outpatient prenatal visits

Appendix I: Present on Admission Reporting Guidelines

SECTION I. CONVENTIONS, GENERAL CODING GUIDELINES AND CHAPTER SPECIFIC GUIDELINES

The conventions, general guidelines and chapter-specific guidelines are applicable to all health care settings unless otherwise indicated.

A. Conventions for the ICD-9-CM

The conventions for the ICD-9-CM are the general rules for use of the classification independent of the guidelines. These conventions are incorporated within the index and tabular of the ICD-9-CM as instructional notes. The conventions are as follows:

1. Format:

The ICD-9-CM uses an indented format for ease in reference

2. Abbreviations

a. Index abbreviations

NEC   "Not elsewhere classifiable" This abbreviation in the index represents "other specified" when a specific code is not available for a condition the index directs the coder to the "other specified" code in the tabular.

b. Tabular abbreviations

NEC   "Not elsewhere classifiable" This abbreviation in the tabular represents "other specified". When a specific code is not available for a condition the tabular includes an NEC entry under a code to identify the code as the "other specified" code.

(See Section I.A.5.a. "Other" codes").

NOS   "Not otherwise specified" This abbreviation is the equivalent of unspecified.

(See Section I.A.5.b., "Unspecified" codes)

3. Punctuation

[ ] Brackets are used in the tabular list to enclose synonyms, alternative wording or explanatory phrases. Brackets are used in the index to identify manifestation codes.

(See Section I.A.6. "Etiology/manifestations")

( ) Parentheses are used in both the index and tabular to enclose supplementary words that may be present or absent in the statement of a disease or procedure without affecting the code number to which it is assigned. The terms within the parentheses are referred to as nonessential modifiers.

: Colons are used in the Tabular list after an incomplete term which needs one or more of the modifiers following the colon to make it assignable to a given category.

4. Includes and Excludes Notes and Inclusion terms

Includes: This note appears immediately under a three-digit code title to further define, or give examples of, the content of the category.

Excludes: An excludes note under a code indicates that the terms excluded from the code are to be coded elsewhere. In some cases the codes for the excluded terms should not be used in conjunction with the code from which it is excluded. An example of this is a congenital condition excluded from an acquired form of the same condition. The congenital and acquired codes should not be used together. In other cases, the excluded terms may be used together with an excluded code. An example of this is when fractures of different bones are coded to different codes. Both codes may be used together if both types of fractures are present.

Inclusion terms: List of terms is included under certain four and five digit codes. These terms are the conditions for which that code number is to be used. The terms may be synonyms of the code title, or, in the case of "other specified" codes, the terms are a list of the various conditions assigned to that code. The inclusion terms are not necessarily exhaustive. Additional terms found only in the index may also be assigned to a code.

5. Other and Unspecified codes

a. "Other" codes

Codes titled "other" or "other specified" (usually a code with a 4th digit 8 or fifth-digit 9 for diagnosis codes) are for use when the information in the medical record provides detail for which a specific code does not exist. Index entries with NEC in the line designate "other" codes in the tabular. These index entries represent specific disease entities for which no specific code exists so the term is included within an "other" code.

b. "Unspecified" codes

Codes (usually a code with a 4th digit 9 or 5th digit 0 for diagnosis codes) titled "unspecified" are for use when the information in the medical record is insufficient to assign a more specific code.

6. Etiology/manifestation convention ("code first", "use additional code" and "in diseases classified elsewhere" notes)

Certain conditions have both an underlying etiology and multiple body system manifestations due to the underlying etiology. For such conditions, the ICD-9-CM has a coding convention that requires the underlying condition be sequenced first followed by the manifestation. Wherever such a combination exists, there is a "use additional code" note at the etiology code, and a "code first" note at the manifestation code. These instructional notes indicate the proper sequencing order of the codes, etiology followed by manifestation.

In most cases the manifestation codes will have in the code title, "in diseases classified elsewhere." Codes with this title are a component of the etiology/manifestation convention. The code title indicates that it is a manifestation code. "In diseases classified elsewhere" codes are never permitted to be used as first listed or principal diagnosis codes. They must be used in conjunction with an underlying condition code and they must be listed following the underlying condition.

There are manifestation codes that do not have "in diseases classified elsewhere" in the title. For such codes a "use additional code" note will still be present and the rules for sequencing apply.

In addition to the notes in the tabular, these conditions also have a specific index entry structure. In the index both conditions are listed together with the etiology code first followed by the manifestation codes in brackets. The code in brackets is always to be sequenced second.

The most commonly used etiology/manifestation combinations are the codes for Diabetes mellitus, category 250. For each code under category 250 there is a use additional code note for the manifestation that is specific for that particular diabetic manifestation. Should a patient have more than one manifestation of diabetes, more than one code from category 250 may be used with as many manifestation codes as are needed to fully describe the patient's complete diabetic condition. The category 250 diabetes codes should be sequenced first, followed by the manifestation codes.

"Code first" and "Use additional code" notes are also used as sequencing rules in the classification for certain codes that are not part of an etiology/manifestation combination.

See – Section I.B.9. "Multiple coding for a single condition".

7. "And"

The word "and" should be interpreted to mean either "and" or "or" when it appears in a title.

8. "With"

The word "with" in the alphabetic index is sequenced immediately following the main term, not in alphabetical order.

9. "See" and "See Also"

The "see" instruction following a main term in the index indicates that another term should be referenced. It is necessary to go to the main term referenced with the "see" note to locate the correct code.

A "see also" instruction following a main term in the index instructs that there is another main term that may also be referenced that may provide additional index entries that may be useful. It is not necessary to follow the "see also" note when the original main term provides the necessary code.

B. General Coding Guidelines

1. Use of Both Alphabetic Index and Tabular List

Use both the Alphabetic Index and the Tabular List when locating and assigning a code. Reliance on only the Alphabetic Index or the Tabular List leads to errors in code assignments and less specificity in code selection.

2. Locate each term in the Alphabetic Index

Locate each term in the Alphabetic Index and verify the code selected in the Tabular List. Read and be guided by instructional notations that appear in both the Alphabetic Index and the Tabular List.

3. Level of Detail in Coding

Diagnosis and procedure codes are to be used at their highest number of digits available.

ICD-9-CM diagnosis codes are composed of codes with 3, 4, or 5 digits. Codes with three digits are included in ICD-9-CM as the heading of a category of codes that may be further subdivided by the use of fourth and/or fifth digits, which provide greater detail.

A three-digit code is to be used only if it is not further subdivided. Where fourth-digit subcategories and/or fifth-digit subclassifications are provided, they must be assigned. A code is invalid if it has not been coded to the full number of digits required for that code. For example, Acute myocardial infarction, code 410, has fourth digits that describe the location of the infarction (e.g., 410.2, Of inferolateral wall), and fifth digits that identify the episode of care. It would be incorrect to report a code in category 410 without a fourth and fifth digit.

ICD-9-CM Volume 3 procedure codes are composed of codes with either 3 or 4 digits. Codes with two digits are included in ICD-9-CM as the heading of a category of codes that may be further subdivided by the use of third and/or fourth digits, which provide greater detail.

4. Code or codes from 001.0 through V89.09

The appropriate code or codes from 001.0 through **V89.09** must be used to identify diagnoses, symptoms, conditions, problems, complaints or other reason(s) for the encounter/visit.

5. Selection of codes 001.0 through 999.9

The selection of codes 001.0 through 999.9 will frequently be used to describe the reason for the admission/encounter. These codes are from the section of ICD-9-CM for the classification of diseases and injuries (e.g., infectious and parasitic diseases; neoplasms; symptoms, signs, and ill-defined conditions, etc.).

6. Signs and symptoms

Codes that describe symptoms and signs, as opposed to diagnoses, are acceptable for reporting purposes when a related definitive diagnosis has not been established (confirmed) by the provider. Chapter 16 of ICD-9-CM, Symptoms, Signs, and Ill-defined conditions (codes 780.0-799.9) contain many, but not all codes for symptoms.

7. Conditions that are an integral part of a disease process

Signs and symptoms that are **associated routinely with a** disease process should not be assigned as additional codes, unless otherwise instructed by the classification.

8. Conditions that are not an integral part of a disease process

Additional signs and symptoms that may not be associated routinely with a disease process should be coded when present.

9. Multiple coding for a single condition

In addition to the etiology/manifestation convention that requires two codes to fully describe a single condition that affects multiple body systems, there are other single conditions that also require more than one code. "Use additional code" notes are found in the tabular at codes that are not part of an etiology/manifestation pair where a secondary code is useful to fully describe a condition. The sequencing rule is the same as the etiology/manifestation pair – , "use additional code" indicates that a secondary code should be added.

For example, for infections that are not included in chapter 1, a secondary code from category 041, Bacterial infection in conditions classified elsewhere and of unspecified site, may be required to identify the bacterial organism causing the infection. A "use additional code" note will normally be found at the infectious disease code, indicating a need for the organism code to be added as a secondary code.

"Code first" notes are also under certain codes that are not specifically manifestation codes but may be due to an underlying cause. When a "code first" note is present and an underlying condition is present the underlying condition should be sequenced first.

"Code, if applicable, any causal condition first", notes indicate that this code may be assigned as a principal diagnosis when the causal condition is unknown or not applicable. If a causal condition is known, then the code for that condition should be sequenced as the principal or first-listed diagnosis.

Multiple codes may be needed for late effects, complication codes and obstetric codes to more fully describe a condition. See the specific guidelines for these conditions for further instruction.

10. Acute and Chronic Conditions

If the same condition is described as both acute (subacute) and chronic, and separate subentries exist in the Alphabetic Index at the same indentation level, code both and sequence the acute (subacute) code first.

11. Combination Code

A combination code is a single code used to classify:

Two diagnoses, or

A diagnosis with an associated secondary process (manifestation)

A diagnosis with an associated complication

Combination codes are identified by referring to subterm entries in the Alphabetic Index and by reading the inclusion and exclusion notes in the Tabular List.

Assign only the combination code when that code fully identifies the diagnostic conditions involved or when the Alphabetic Index so directs. Multiple coding should not be used when the classification provides a combination code that clearly identifies all of the elements documented in the diagnosis. When the combination code lacks necessary specificity in describing the manifestation or complication, an additional code should be used as a secondary code.

12. Late Effects

A late effect is the residual effect (condition produced) after the acute phase of an illness or injury has terminated. There is no time limit on when a late effect code can be used. The residual may be apparent early, such as in cerebrovascular accident cases, or it may occur months or years later, such as that due to a previous injury. Coding of late effects generally requires two codes sequenced in the following order: The condition or nature of the late effect is sequenced first. The late effect code is sequenced second.

An exception to the above guidelines are those instances where the code for late effect is followed by a manifestation code identified in the Tabular List and title, or the late effect code has been expanded (at the fourth and fifth-digit levels) to include the manifestation(s). The code for the acute phase of an illness or injury that led to the late effect is never used with a code for the late effect.

13. Impending or Threatened Condition

Code any condition described at the time of discharge as "impending" or "threatened" as follows:

If it did occur, code as confirmed diagnosis.

If it did not occur, reference the Alphabetic Index to determine if the condition has a subentry term for "impending" or "threatened" and also reference main term entries for "Impending" and for "Threatened."

If the subterms are listed, assign the given code.

If the subterms are not listed, code the existing underlying condition(s) and not the condition described as impending or threatened.

14. Reporting Same Diagnosis Code More than Once

Each unique ICD-9-CM diagnosis code may be reported only once for an encounter. This applies to bilateral conditions or two different conditions classified to the same ICD-9-CM diagnosis code.

15. Admissions/Encounters for Rehabilitation

When the purpose for the admission/encounter is rehabilitation, sequence the appropriate V code from category V57, Care involving use of rehabilitation procedures, as the principal/first-listed diagnosis. The code for the condition for which the service is being performed should be reported as an additional diagnosis.

Only one code from category V57 is required. Code V57.89, Other specified rehabilitation procedures, should be assigned if more than one type of rehabilitation is performed during a single encounter. A procedure code should be reported to identify each type of rehabilitation therapy actually performed.

16. Documentation for BMI and Pressure Ulcer Stages

For the Body Mass Index (BMI) and pressure ulcer stage codes, code assignment may be based on medical record documentation from clinicians who are not the patient's provider (i.e., physician or other qualified healthcare

practitioner legally accountable for establishing the patient's diagnosis), since this information is typically documented by other clinicians involved in the care of the patient (e.g., a dietitian often documents the BMI and nurses often documents the pressure ulcer stages). However, the associated diagnosis (such as overweight, obesity, or pressure ulcer) must be documented by the patient's provider. If there is conflicting medical record documentation, either from the same clinician or different clinicians, the patient's attending provider should be queried for clarification.

The BMI and pressure ulcer stage codes should only be reported as secondary diagnoses. As with all other secondary diagnosis codes, the BMI and pressure ulcer stage codes should only be assigned when they meet the definition of a reportable additional diagnosis (see Section III, Reporting Additional Diagnoses).

C. Chapter-Specific Coding Guidelines

In addition to general coding guidelines, there are guidelines for specific diagnoses and/or conditions in the classification. Unless otherwise indicated, these guidelines apply to all health care settings. Please refer to Section II for guidelines on the selection of principal diagnosis.

1. Chapter 1: Infectious and Parasitic Diseases (001-139)

a. Human Immunodeficiency Virus (HIV) Infections

1) Code only confirmed cases

Code only confirmed cases of HIV infection/illness. This is an exception to the hospital inpatient guideline Section II, H.

In this context, "confirmation" does not require documentation of positive serology or culture for HIV; the provider's diagnostic statement that the patient is HIV positive, or has an HIV-related illness is sufficient.

2) Selection and sequencing of HIV codes

(a) Patient admitted for HIV-related condition

If a patient is admitted for an HIV-related condition, the principal diagnosis should be 042, followed by additional diagnosis codes for all reported HIV-related conditions.

(b) Patient with HIV disease admitted for unrelated condition

If a patient with HIV disease is admitted for an unrelated condition (such as a traumatic injury), the code for the unrelated condition (e.g., the nature of injury code) should be the principal diagnosis. Other diagnoses would be 042 followed by additional diagnosis codes for all reported HIV-related conditions.

(c) Whether the patient is newly diagnosed

Whether the patient is newly diagnosed or has had previous admissions/encounters for HIV conditions is irrelevant to the sequencing decision.

(d) Asymptomatic human immunodeficiency virus

V08 Asymptomatic human immunodeficiency virus [HIV] infection, is to be applied when the patient without any documentation of symptoms is listed as being "HIV positive," "known HIV," "HIV test positive," or similar terminology. Do not use this code if the term "AIDS" is used or if the patient is treated for any HIV-related illness or is described as having any condition(s) resulting from his/her HIV positive status; use 042 in these cases.

(e) Patients with inconclusive HIV serology

Patients with inconclusive HIV serology, but no definitive diagnosis or manifestations of the illness, may be assigned code 795.71, Inconclusive serologic test for Human Immunodeficiency Virus [HIV].

(f) Previously diagnosed HIV-related illness

Patients with any known prior diagnosis of an HIV-related illness should be coded to 042. Once a patient has developed an HIV-related illness, the patient should always be assigned code 042 on every subsequent admission/encounter. Patients previously diagnosed with any HIV illness (042) should never be assigned to 795.71 or V08.

(g) HIV Infection in Pregnancy, Childbirth and the Puerperium

During pregnancy, childbirth or the puerperium, a patient admitted (or presenting for a health care encounter) because of an HIV-related illness should receive a principal diagnosis code of 647.6X, Other specified infectious and parasitic diseases in the mother classifiable elsewhere, but complicating the pregnancy, childbirth or the puerperium, followed by 042 and the code(s) for the HIV-related illness(es). Codes from Chapter 15 always take sequencing priority.

Patients with asymptomatic HIV infection status admitted (or presenting for a health care encounter) during pregnancy, childbirth, or the puerperium should receive codes of 647.6X and V08.

(h) Encounters for testing for HIV

If a patient is being seen to determine his/her HIV status, use code V73.89, Screening for other specified viral disease. Use code V69.8, Other problems related to lifestyle, as a secondary code if an asymptomatic patient is in a known high risk group for HIV. Should a patient with signs or symptoms or illness, or a confirmed HIV related diagnosis be tested for HIV, code the signs and symptoms or the diagnosis. An additional counseling code V65.44 may be used if counseling is provided during the encounter for the test.

When a patient returns to be informed of his/her HIV test results use code V65.44, HIV counseling, if the results of the test are negative.

If the results are positive but the patient is asymptomatic use code V08, Asymptomatic HIV infection. If the results are positive and the patient is symptomatic use code 042, HIV infection, with codes for the HIV related symptoms or diagnosis. The HIV counseling code may also be used if counseling is provided for patients with positive test results.

b. Septicemia, Systemic Inflammatory Response Syndrome (SIRS), Sepsis, Severe Sepsis, and Septic Shock

1) SIRS, Septicemia, and Sepsis

(a) The terms septicemia and sepsis are often used interchangeably by providers, however they are not considered synonymous terms. The following descriptions are provided for reference but do not preclude querying the provider for clarification about terms used in the documentation:

(i) Septicemia generally refers to a systemic disease associated with the presence of pathological microorganisms or toxins in the blood, which can include bacteria, viruses, fungi or other organisms.

(ii) Systemic inflammatory response syndrome (SIRS) generally refers to the systemic response to infection, trauma/burns, or other insult (such as cancer) with symptoms including fever, tachycardia, tachypnea, and leukocytosis.

(iii) Sepsis generally refers to SIRS due to infection.

(iv) Severe sepsis generally refers to sepsis with associated acute organ dysfunction.

(b) The Coding of SIRS, sepsis, and severe sepsis

The coding of SIRS, sepsis and severe sepsis requires a minimum of 2 codes: a code for the underlying cause (such as infection or trauma) and a code from subcategory 995.9 Systemic inflammatory response syndrome (SIRS).

(i) The code for the underlying cause (such as infection or trauma) must be sequenced before the code from subcategory 995.9 Systemic inflammatory response syndrome (SIRS).

(ii) Sepsis and severe sepsis require a code for the systemic infection (038.xx, 112.5, etc.) and either code 995.91, Sepsis, or 995.92, Severe sepsis. If the causal organism is not documented, assign code 038.9, Unspecified septicemia.

(iii) Severe sepsis requires additional code(s) for the associated acute organ dysfunction(s).

(iv) If a patient has sepsis with multiple organ dysfunctions, follow the instructions for coding severe sepsis.

(v) Either the term sepsis or SIRS must be documented to assign a code from subcategory 995.9.

(vi) *See Section I.C.17.g), Injury and poisoning, for information regarding systemic inflammatory response syndrome (SIRS) due to trauma/burns and other non-infectious processes.*

(c) Due to the complex nature of sepsis and severe sepsis, some cases may require querying the provider prior to assignment of the codes.

2) Sequencing sepsis and severe sepsis

(a) Sepsis and severe sepsis as principal diagnosis

If sepsis or severe sepsis is present on admission, and meets the definition of principal diagnosis, the systemic infection code (e.g., 038.xx, 112.5, etc) should be assigned as the principal diagnosis, followed by code 995.91, Sepsis, or 995.92, Severe sepsis, as required by the sequencing rules in the Tabular List. Codes from subcategory 995.9 can never be assigned as a principal diagnosis. A code should also be assigned for any localized infection, if present.

If the sepsis or severe sepsis is due to a postprocedural infection, see Section **I.C.1.6.10** for guidelines related to sepsis due to postprocedural infection.

(b) Sepsis and severe sepsis as secondary diagnoses

When sepsis or severe sepsis develops during the encounter (it was not present on admission), the systemic infection code and code 995.91 or 995.92 should be assigned as secondary diagnoses.

(c) Documentation unclear as to whether sepsis or severe sepsis is present on admission

Sepsis or severe sepsis may be present on admission but the diagnosis may not be confirmed until sometime after admission. If the documentation is not clear whether the sepsis or severe sepsis was present on admission, the provider should be queried.

3) Sepsis/SIRS with Localized Infection

If the reason for admission is both sepsis, severe sepsis, or SIRS and a localized infection, such as pneumonia or cellulitis, a code for the systemic infection (038.xx, 112.5, etc) should be assigned first, then code 995.91 or 995.92, followed by the code for the localized infection. If the patient is admitted with a localized infection, such as pneumonia, and sepsis/SIRS doesn't develop until after admission, see guideline I.C.1.b2.b).

If the localized infection is postprocedural, *see Section* **I.C.1.6.10** *for guidelines related to sepsis due to postprocedural infection.*

Note: The term urosepsis is a nonspecific term. If that is the only term documented then only code 599.0 should be assigned based on the default for the term in the ICD-9-CM index, in addition to the code for the causal organism if known.

4) Bacterial Sepsis and Septicemia

In most cases, it will be a code from category 038, Septicemia, that will be used in conjunction with a code from subcategory 995.9 such as the following:

(a) Streptococcal sepsis

If the documentation in the record states streptococcal sepsis, codes 038.0, Streptococcal septicemia, and code 995.91 should be used, in that sequence.

(b) Streptococcal septicemia

If the documentation states streptococcal septicemia, only code 038.0 should be assigned, however, the provider should be queried whether the patient has sepsis, an infection with SIRS.

5) Acute organ dysfunction that is not clearly associated with the sepsis

If a patient has sepsis and an acute organ dysfunction, but the medical record documentation indicates that the acute organ dysfunction is related to a medical condition other than the sepsis, do not assign code 995.92, Severe sepsis. An acute organ dysfunction must be associated with the sepsis in order to assign the severe sepsis code. If the documentation is not clear as to whether an acute organ dysfunction is related to the sepsis or another medical condition, query the provider.

6) Septic shock

(a) Sequencing of septic shock

Septic shock generally refers to circulatory failure associated with severe sepsis, and, therefore, it represents a type of acute organ dysfunction.

For all cases of septic shock, the code for the systemic infection should be sequenced first, followed by codes 995.92 and 785.52. Any additional codes for other acute organ dysfunctions should also be assigned. As noted in the sequencing instructions in the Tabular List, the code for septic shock cannot be assigned as a principal diagnosis.

(b) Septic Shock without documentation of severe sepsis

Septic shock indicates the presence of severe sepsis.

Code 995.92, Severe sepsis, must be assigned with code 785.52, Septic shock, even if the term severe sepsis is not documented in the record. The "use additional code" note and the "code first" note in the tabular support this guideline.

7) Sepsis and septic shock complicating abortion and pregnancy

Sepsis and septic shock **complicating** abortion, ectopic pregnancy, and molar pregnancy are classified to category codes in Chapter 11 (630-639).

See section I.C.11.

8) Negative or inconclusive blood cultures

Negative or inconclusive blood cultures do not preclude a diagnosis of septicemia or sepsis in patients with clinical evidence of the condition, however, the provider should be queried.

9) Newborn sepsis

See Section I.C.15.j for information on the coding of newborn sepsis.

10) Sepsis due to a Postprocedural Infection

(a) Documentation of causal relationship

As with all postprocedural complications, code assignment is based on the provider's documentation of the relationship between the infection and the procedure.

(b) Sepsis due to postprocedural infection

In cases of postprocedural sepsis, the complication code, such as code 998.59, Other postoperative infection, or 674.3x, Other complications of obstetrical surgical wounds, should be coded first followed by the appropriate sepsis codes (systemic infection code and either code 995.91or 995.92). An additional code(s) for any acute organ dysfunction should also be assigned for cases of severe sepsis.

11) External cause of injury codes with SIRS

Refer to Section I.C.19.a.7 for instruction on the use of external cause of injury codes with codes for SIRS resulting from trauma.

12) Sepsis and Severe Sepsis Associated with Non-infectious Process

In some cases, a non-infectious process, such as trauma, may lead to an infection which can result in sepsis or severe sepsis. If sepsis or severe sepsis is documented as associated with a non-infectious condition, such as a burn or serious injury, and this condition meets the definition for principal diagnosis, the code for the non-infectious condition should be sequenced first, followed by the code for the systemic infection and either code 995.91, Sepsis, or 995.92, Severe sepsis. Additional codes for any associated acute organ dysfunction(s) should also be assigned for cases of severe sepsis. If the sepsis or severe sepsis meets the definition of principal diagnosis, the systemic infection and sepsis codes should be sequenced before the non-infectious condition. When both the associated non-infectious condition and the sepsis or severe sepsis meet the definition of principal diagnosis, either may be assigned as principal diagnosis.

See Section I.C.1.b.2)(a) for guidelines pertaining to sepsis or severe sepsis as the principal diagnosis.

(b) Only one SIRS (subcategory 995.9) code should be assigned

Only one code from subcategory 995.9 should be assigned. Therefore, when a non-infectious condition leads to an infection resulting in sepsis or severe sepsis, assign either code 995.91 or 995.92. Do not additionally assign code 995.93, Systemic inflammatory response syndrome due to non-infectious process without acute organ dysfunction, or 995.94, Systemic inflammatory response syndrome with acute organ dysfunction.

See Section I.C.17.g for information on the coding of SIRS due to trauma/burns or other non-infectious disease processes.

c. **Methicillin Resistant *Staphylococcus aureus* (MRSA) Conditions**

   1) **Selection and sequencing of MRSA codes**

      (a) **Combination codes for MRSA infection**

      When a patient is diagnosed with an infection that is due to methicillin resistant *Staphylococcus aureus* (MRSA), and that infection has a combination code that includes the causal organism (e.g., septicemia, pneumonia) assign the appropriate code for the condition (e.g., code 038.12, Methicillin resistant Staphylococcus aureus septicemia or code 482.42, Methicillin resistant pneumonia due to Staphylococcus aureus). Do not assign code 041.12, Methicillin resistant Staphylococcus aureus, as an additional code because the code includes the type of infection and the MRSA organism. Do not assign a code from subcategory V09.0, Infection with microorganisms resistant to penicillins, as an additional diagnosis.

      See Section C.1.b.1 for instructions on coding and sequencing of septicemia.

      (b) **Other codes for MRSA infection**

      When there is documentation of a current infection (e.g., wound infection, stitch abscess, urinary tract infection) due to MRSA, and that infection does not have a combination code that includes the causal organism, select the appropriate code to identify the condition along with code 041.12, Methicillin resistant Staphylococcus aureus, for the MRSA infection. Do not assign a code from subcategory V09.0, Infection with microorganisms resistant to penicillins.

      (c) **Methicillin susceptible Staphylococcus aureus (MSSA) and MRSA colonization**

      The condition or state of being colonized or carrying MSSA or MRSA is called colonization or carriage, while an individual person is described as being colonized or being a carrier. Colonization means that MSSA or MSRA is present on or in the body without necessarily causing illness. A positive MRSA colonization test might be documented by the provider as "MRSA screen positive" or "MRSA nasal swab positive".

Assign code V02.54, Carrier or suspected carrier, Methicillin resistant Staphylococcus aureus, for patients documented as having MRSA colonization. Assign code V02.53, Carrier or suspected carrier, Methicillin susceptible Staphylococcus aureus, for patient documented as having MSSA colonization. Colonization is not necessarily indicative of a disease process or as the cause of a specific condition the patient may have unless documented as such by the provider.

Code V02.59, Other specified bacterial diseases, should be assigned for other types of staphylococcal colonization (e.g., *S. epidermidis, S. saprophyticus*). Code V02.59 should not be assigned for colonization with any type of *Staphylococcus aureus* (MRSA, MSSA).

(d) MRSA colonization and infection

If a patient is documented as having both MRSA colonization and infection during a hospital admission, code V02.54, Carrier or suspected carrier, Methicillin resistant *Staphylococcus aureus*, and a code for the MRSA infection may both be assigned.

2. **Chapter 2: Neoplasms (140-239)**

   <u>**General guidelines**</u>

   Chapter 2 of the ICD-9-CM contains the codes for most benign and all malignant neoplasms. Certain benign neoplasms, such as prostatic adenomas, may be found in the specific body system chapters. To properly code a neoplasm it is necessary to determine from the record if the neoplasm is benign, in-situ, malignant, or of uncertain histologic behavior. If malignant, any secondary (metastatic) sites should also be determined.

   The neoplasm table in the Alphabetic Index should be referenced first. However, if the histological term is documented, that term should be referenced first, rather than going immediately to the Neoplasm Table, in order to determine which column in the Neoplasm Table is appropriate. For example, if the documentation indicates "adenoma," refer to the term in the Alphabetic Index to review the entries under this term and the instructional note to "see also neoplasm, by site, benign." The table provides the proper code based on the type of neoplasm and the site. It is important to select the proper column in the table that corresponds to the type of neoplasm. The tabular should then be referenced to verify that the correct code has been selected from the table and that a more specific site code does not exist.

   See Section I. C. 18.d.4. for information regarding V codes for genetic susceptibility to cancer.

   a. **Treatment directed at the malignancy**

      If the treatment is directed at the malignancy, designate the malignancy as the principal diagnosis.

      The only exception to this guideline is if a patient admission/encounter is solely for the administration of chemotherapy, immunotherapy or radiation therapy, assign the appropriate V58.x code as the first-listed or principal

diagnosis, and the diagnosis or problem for which the service is being performed as a secondary diagnosis.

b. Treatment of secondary site

When a patient is admitted because of a primary neoplasm with metastasis and treatment is directed toward the secondary site only, the secondary neoplasm is designated as the principal diagnosis even though the primary malignancy is still present.

c. Coding and sequencing of complications

Coding and sequencing of complications associated with the malignancies or with the therapy thereof are subject to the following guidelines:

1) Anemia associated with malignancy

When admission/encounter is for management of an anemia associated with the malignancy, and the treatment is only for anemia, the appropriate anemia code (such as code 285.22, Anemia in neoplastic disease) is designated as the principal diagnosis and is followed by the appropriate code(s) for the malignancy.

Code 285.22 may also be used as a secondary code if the patient suffers from anemia and is being treated for the malignancy.

2) Anemia associated with chemotherapy, immunotherapy and radiation therapy

When the admission/encounter is for management of an anemia associated with chemotherapy, immunotherapy or radiotherapy and the only treatment is for the anemia, the anemia is sequenced first followed by code E933.1. The appropriate neoplasm code should be assigned as an additional code.

3) Management of dehydration due to the malignancy

When the admission/encounter is for management of dehydration due to the malignancy or the therapy, or a combination of both, and only the dehydration is being treated (intravenous rehydration), the dehydration is sequenced first, followed by the code(s) for the malignancy.

4) Treatment of a complication resulting from a surgical procedure

When the admission/encounter is for treatment of a complication resulting from a surgical procedure, designate the complication as the principal or first-listed diagnosis if treatment is directed at resolving the complication.

d. Primary malignancy previously excised

When a primary malignancy has been previously excised or eradicated from its site and there is no further treatment directed to that site and there is no evidence of any existing primary malignancy, a code from category V10, Personal history of malignant neoplasm, should be used to indicate the former site of the malignancy. Any mention of extension, invasion, or metastasis to another site is coded as a secondary malignant neoplasm to that site.

The secondary site may be the principal or first-listed with the V10 code used as a secondary code.

e. Admissions/Encounters involving chemotherapy, immunotherapy and radiation therapy

1) Episode of care involves surgical removal of neoplasm

When an episode of care involves the surgical removal of a neoplasm, primary or secondary site, followed by adjunct chemotherapy or radiation treatment during the same episode of care, the neoplasm code should be assigned as principal or first-listed diagnosis, using codes in the 140-198 series or where appropriate in the 200-203 series.

2) Patient admission/encounter solely for administration of chemotherapy, immunotherapy and radiation therapy

If a patient admission/encounter is solely for the administration of chemotherapy, immunotherapy or radiation therapy assign code V58.0, Encounter for radiation therapy, or V58.11, Encounter for antineoplastic chemotherapy, or V58.12, Encounter for antineoplastic immunotherapy as the first-listed or principal diagnosis. If a patient receives more than one of these therapies during the same admission more than one of these codes may be assigned, in any sequence.

The malignancy for which the therapy is being administered should be assigned as a secondary diagnosis.

3) Patient admitted for radiotherapy/chemotherapy and immunotherapy and develops complications

When a patient is admitted for the purpose of radiotherapy, immunotherapy or chemotherapy and develops complications such as uncontrolled nausea and vomiting or dehydration, the principal or first-listed diagnosis is V58.0, Encounter for radiotherapy, or V58.11, Encounter for antineoplastic chemotherapy, or V58.12, Encounter for antineoplastic immunotherapy followed by any codes for the complications.

f. Admission/encounter to determine extent of malignancy

When the reason for admission/encounter is to determine the extent of the malignancy, or for a procedure such as paracentesis or thoracentesis, the primary malignancy or appropriate metastatic site is designated as the principal or first-listed diagnosis, even though chemotherapy or radiotherapy is administered.

g. Symptoms, signs, and ill-defined conditions listed in Chapter 16 <u>associated with neoplasms</u>

Symptoms, signs, and ill-defined conditions listed in Chapter 16 characteristic of, or associated with, an existing primary or secondary site malignancy cannot be used to replace the malignancy as principal or first-listed diagnosis, regardless of the number of admissions or encounters for treatment and care of the neoplasm.

See section I.C.18.d.14, Encounter for prophylactic organ removal.

h. Admission/encounter for pain control/management

See Section I.C.6.a.5 for information on coding admission/encounter for pain control/management.

i. Malignant neoplasm associated with transplanted organ

A malignant neoplasm of a transplanted organ should be coded as a transplant complication. Assign first the appropriate code from subcategory 996.8, Complications of transplanted organ, followed by code 199.2, Malignant neoplasm associated with transplanted organ. Use an additional code for the specific malignancy.

3. Chapter 3: Endocrine, Nutritional, and Metabolic Diseases and Immunity Disorders (240-279)

a. Diabetes mellitus

Codes under category 250, Diabetes mellitus, identify complications/manifestations associated with diabetes mellitus. A fifth-digit is required for all category 250 codes to identify the type of diabetes mellitus and whether the diabetes is controlled or uncontrolled.

See I.C.3.a.7 for secondary diabetes.

1) Fifth-digits for category 250:

The following are the fifth-digits for the codes under category 250:

0   type II or unspecified type, not stated as uncontrolled

1   type I, [juvenile type], not stated as uncontrolled

2   type II or unspecified type, uncontrolled

3   type I, [juvenile type], uncontrolled

The age of a patient is not the sole determining factor, though most type I diabetics develop the condition before reaching puberty. For this reason type I diabetes mellitus is also referred to as juvenile diabetes.

2) Type of diabetes mellitus not documented

If the type of diabetes mellitus is not documented in the medical record the default is type II.

3) Diabetes mellitus and the use of insulin

All type I diabetics must use insulin to replace what their bodies do not produce. However, the use of insulin does not mean that a patient is a type I diabetic. Some patients with type II diabetes mellitus are unable to control their blood sugar through diet and oral medication alone and do require insulin. If the documentation in a medical record does not indicate the type of diabetes but does indicate that the patient uses insulin, the appropriate fifth-digit for type II must be used. For type II patients who routinely use insulin, code V58.67, Long-term (current) use of insulin, should also be assigned to indicate that the patient uses insulin. Code V58.67 should not be assigned if insulin is given temporarily to bring a type II patient's blood sugar under control during an encounter.

4) Assigning and sequencing diabetes codes and associated conditions

When assigning codes for diabetes and its associated conditions, the code(s) from category 250 must be sequenced before the codes for the associated conditions. The diabetes codes and the secondary codes that correspond to them are paired codes that follow the etiology/manifestation convention of the classification *(See Section I.A.6., Etiology/manifestation convention)*. Assign as many codes from category 250 as needed to identify all of the associated conditions that the patient has. The corresponding secondary codes are listed under each of the diabetes codes.

(a) Diabetic retinopathy/diabetic macular edema

Diabetic macular edema, code 362.07, is only present with diabetic retinopathy. Another code from subcategory 362.0, Diabetic retinopathy, must be used with code 362.07. Codes under subcategory 362.0 are diabetes manifestation codes, so they must be used following the appropriate diabetes code.

5) Diabetes mellitus in pregnancy and gestational diabetes

(a) For diabetes mellitus complicating pregnancy, see Section I.C.11.f., Diabetes mellitus in pregnancy.

(b) For gestational diabetes, see Section I.C.11, g., Gestational diabetes.

6) Insulin pump malfunction

(a) Underdose of insulin due insulin pump failure

An underdose of insulin due to an insulin pump failure should be assigned 996.57, Mechanical complication due to insulin pump, as the principal or first listed code, followed by the appropriate diabetes mellitus code based on documentation.

(b) Overdose of insulin due to insulin pump failure

The principal or first listed code for an encounter due to an insulin pump malfunction resulting in an overdose of insulin, should also be 996.57, Mechanical complication due to insulin pump, followed by code 962.3, Poisoning by insulins and antidiabetic agents, and the appropriate diabetes mellitus code based on documentation.

7) Secondary Diabetes Mellitus

Codes under category 249, Secondary diabetes mellitus, identify complications/manifestations associated with secondary diabetes mellitus. Secondary diabetes is always caused by another condition or event (e.g., cystic fibrosis, malignant neoplasm of pancreas, pancreatectomy, adverse effect of drug, or poisoning).

(a) Fifth-digits for category 249:

A fifth-digit is required for all category 249 codes to identify whether the diabetes is controlled or uncontrolled.

(b) **Secondary diabetes mellitus and the use of insulin**

For patients who routinely use insulin, code V58.67, Long-term (current) use of insulin, should also be assigned. Code V58.67 should not be assigned if insulin is given temporarily to bring a patient's blood sugar under control during an encounter.

(c) **Assigning and sequencing secondary diabetes codes and associated conditions**

When assigning codes for secondary diabetes and its associated conditions (e.g. renal manifestations), the code(s) from category 249 must be sequenced before the codes for the associated conditions. The secondary diabetes codes and the diabetic manifestation codes that correspond to them are paired codes that follow the etiology/manifestation convention of the classification. Assign as many codes from category 249 as needed to identify all of the associated conditions that the patient has. The corresponding codes for the associated conditions are listed under each of the secondary diabetes codes. For example, secondary diabetes with diabetic nephrosis is assigned to code 249.40, followed by 581.81.

(d) **Assigning and sequencing secondary diabetes codes and its causes**

The sequencing of the secondary diabetes codes in relationship to codes for the cause of the diabetes is based on the reason for the encounter, applicable ICD-9-CM sequencing conventions, and chapter-specific guidelines.

If a patient is seen for treatment of the secondary diabetes or one of its associated conditions, a code from category 249 is sequenced as the principal or first-listed diagnosis, with the cause of the secondary diabetes (e.g. cystic fibrosis) sequenced as an additional diagnosis.

If, however, the patient is seen for the treatment of the condition causing the secondary diabetes (e.g., malignant neoplasm of pancreas), the code for the cause of the secondary diabetes should be sequenced as the principal or first-listed diagnosis followed by a code from category 249.

(i) **Secondary diabetes mellitus due to pancreatectomy**

For postpancreatectomy diabetes mellitus (lack of insulin due to the surgical removal of all or part of the pancreas), assign code 251.3, Postsurgical hypoinsulinemia. A code from subcategory 249 should not be assigned for secondary diabetes mellitus due to pancreatectomy. Code also any diabetic manifestations (e.g. diabetic nephrosis 581.81).

(ii) Secondary diabetes due to drugs

Secondary diabetes may be caused by an adverse effect of correctly administered medications, poisoning or late effect of poisoning.

See section I.C.17.e for coding of adverse effects and poisoning, and section I.C.19 for E code reporting.

4. Chapter 4: Diseases of Blood and Blood Forming Organs (280-289)

a. Anemia of chronic disease

Subcategory 285.2, Anemia in chronic illness, has codes for anemia in chronic kidney disease, code 285.21; anemia in neoplastic disease, code 285.22; and anemia in other chronic illness, code 285.29. These codes can be used as the principal/first listed code if the reason for the encounter is to treat the anemia. They may also be used as secondary codes if treatment of the anemia is a component of an encounter, but not the primary reason for the encounter. When using a code from subcategory 285 it is also necessary to use the code for the chronic condition causing the anemia.

1) Anemia in chronic kidney disease

When assigning code 285.21, Anemia in chronic kidney disease, it is also necessary to assign a code from category 585, Chronic kidney disease, to indicate the stage of chronic kidney disease.

See I.C.10.a. Chronic kidney disease (CKD).

2) Anemia in neoplastic disease

When assigning code 285.22, Anemia in neoplastic disease, it is also necessary to assign the neoplasm code that is responsible for the anemia. Code 285.22 is for use for anemia that is due to the malignancy, not for anemia due to antineoplastic chemotherapy drugs, which is an adverse effect.

See I.C.2.c.1 Anemia associated with malignancy.

See I.C.2.c.2 Anemia associated with chemotherapy, immunotherapy and radiation therapy.

See I.C.17.e.1. Adverse effects.

5. Chapter 5: Mental Disorders (290-319)

Reserved for future guideline expansion

6. Chapter 6: Diseases of Nervous System and Sense Organs (320-389)

a. Pain – Category 338

1) General coding information

Codes in category 338 may be used in conjunction with codes from other categories and chapters to provide more detail about acute or chronic pain and neoplasm-related pain, unless otherwise indicated below.

If the pain is not specified as acute or chronic, do not assign codes from category 338, except for post-thoracotomy pain, postoperative pain or neoplasm related pain, or central pain syndrome.

A code from subcategories 338.1 and 338.2 should not be assigned if the underlying (definitive) diagnosis is known, unless the reason for the encounter is pain control/management and not management of the underlying condition.

(a) Category 338 Codes as Principal or First-Listed Diagnosis

Category 338 codes are acceptable as principal diagnosis or the first-listed code:

- When pain control or pain management is the reason for the admission/encounter (e.g., a patient with displaced intervertebral disc, nerve impingement and severe back pain presents for injection of steroid into the spinal canal). The underlying cause of the pain should be reported as an additional diagnosis, if known.

- When an admission or encounter is for a procedure aimed at treating the underlying condition (e.g., spinal fusion, kyphoplasty), a code for the underlying condition (e.g., vertebral fracture, spinal stenosis) should be assigned as the principal diagnosis. No code from category 338 should be assigned.

- When a patient is admitted for the insertion of a neurostimulator for pain control, assign the appropriate pain code as the principal of first listed diagnosis. When an admission or encounter is for a procedure aimed at treating the underlying condition and a neurostimulator is inserted for pain control during the same admission/encounter, a code for the underlying condition should be assigned as the principal diagnosis and the appropriate pain code should be assigned as a secondary diagnosis.

(b) Use of Category 338 Codes in Conjunction with Site Specific Pain Codes

(i) Assigning Category 338 Codes and Site-Specific Pain Codes

Codes from category 338 may be used in conjunction with codes that identify the site of pain (including codes from chapter 16) if the category 338 code provides additional information. For example, if the code describes the site of the pain, but does not fully describe whether the pain is acute or chronic, then both codes should be assigned.

(ii) Sequencing of Category 338 Codes with Site-Specific Pain Codes

The sequencing of category 338 codes with site-specific pain codes (including chapter 16 codes), is dependent on the circumstances of the encounter/admission as follows:

- If the encounter is for pain control or pain management, assign the code from category 338 followed by the code identifying the specific site of pain (e.g., encounter for pain management for acute neck pain from trauma is assigned code 338.11, Acute pain due to trauma, followed by code 723.1, Cervicalgia, to identify the site of pain).

- If the encounter is for any other reason except pain control or pain management, and a related definitive diagnosis has not been established (confirmed) by the provider, assign the code for the specific site of pain first, followed by the appropriate code from category 338.

2) **Pain due to devices, <u>implants and grafts</u>**

Pain associated with devices, implants or grafts left in a surgical site (for example painful hip prothesis) is assigned to the appropriate code(s) found in Chapter 17, Injury and Poisoning. Use additional code(s) from category 338 to identify acute or chronic pain due to presence of the device, implant or graft (338.18-338.19 or 338.28-338.29).

3) **Postoperative Pain**

Post-thoracotomy pain and other postoperative pain are classified to subcategories 338.1 and 338.2, depending on whether the pain is acute or chronic. The default for post-thoracotomy and other postoperative pain not specified as acute or chronic is the code for the acute form.

<u>Routine or expected postoperative pain immediately after surgery should not be coded.</u>

(a) **Postoperative pain not associated with specific postoperative complication**

Postoperative pain not associated with a specific postoperative complication is assigned to the appropriate postoperative pain code in category 338.

(b) **Postoperative pain associated with specific postoperative complication**

Postoperative pain associated with a specific postoperative complication (such as painful suture wires) is assigned to the appropriate code(s) found in Chapter 17, Injury and Poisoning. If appropriate, use additional code(s) from category 338 to identify acute or chronic pain (338.18 or 338.28). If pain control/management is the reason for the encounter, a code from category 338 should be assigned as the principal or first-listed diagnosis in accordance with *Section I.C.6.a.1.a above.*

(c) **Postoperative pain as principal or first-listed diagnosis**

Postoperative pain may be reported as the principal or first-listed diagnosis when the stated reason for the admission/encounter is documented as postoperative pain control/management.

(d) Postoperative pain as secondary diagnosis

Postoperative pain may be reported as a secondary diagnosis code when a patient presents for outpatient surgery and develops an unusual or inordinate amount of postoperative pain.

Routine or expected postoperative pain immediately after surgery should not be coded.

The provider's documentation should be used to guide the coding of postoperative pain, as well as *Section III. Reporting Additional Diagnoses* and *Section IV. Diagnostic Coding and Reporting in the Outpatient Setting.*

See Section II.I.2 for information on sequencing of diagnoses for patients admitted to hospital inpatient care following post-operative observation.

See Section II.J for information on sequencing of diagnoses for patients admitted to hospital inpatient care from outpatient surgery.

See Section IV.A.2 for information on sequencing of diagnoses for patients admitted for observation.

4) Chronic pain

Chronic pain is classified to subcategory 338.2. There is no time frame defining when pain becomes chronic pain. The provider's documentation should be used to guide use of these codes.

5) Neoplasm Related Pain

Code 338.3 is assigned to pain documented as being related, associated or due to cancer, primary or secondary malignancy, or tumor. This code is assigned regardless of whether the pain is acute or chronic.

This code may be assigned as the principal or first-listed code when the stated reason for the admission/encounter is documented as pain control/pain management. The underlying neoplasm should be reported as an additional diagnosis.

When the reason for the admission/encounter is management of the neoplasm and the pain associated with the neoplasm is also documented, code 338.3 may be assigned as an additional diagnosis.

See Section I.C.2 for instructions on the sequencing of neoplasms for all other stated reasons for the admission/encounter (except for pain control/pain management).

6) Chronic pain syndrome

This condition is different than the term "chronic pain," and therefore this code should only be used when the provider has specifically documented this condition.

7. Chapter 7: Diseases of Circulatory System (390-459)

a. Hypertension

Hypertension Table

The Hypertension Table, found under the main term, "Hypertension", in the Alphabetic Index, contains a complete listing of all conditions due to or associated with hypertension and classifies them according to malignant, benign, and unspecified.

1) Hypertension, Essential, or NOS

Assign hypertension (arterial) (essential) (primary) (systemic) (NOS) to category code 401 with the appropriate fourth digit to indicate malignant (.0), benign (.1), or unspecified (.9). Do not use either .0 malignant or .1 benign unless medical record documentation supports such a designation.

2) Hypertension with Heart Disease

Heart conditions (425.8, 429.0-429.3, 429.8, 429.9) are assigned to a code from category 402 when a causal relationship is stated (due to hypertension) or implied (hypertensive). Use an additional code from category 428 to identify the type of heart failure in those patients with heart failure. More than one code from category 428 may be assigned if the patient has systolic or diastolic failure and congestive heart failure.

The same heart conditions (425.8, 429.0-429.3, 429.8, 429.9) with hypertension, but without a stated causal relationship, are coded separately. Sequence according to the circumstances of the admission/encounter.

3) Hypertensive Chronic Kidney Disease

Assign codes from category 403, Hypertensive chronic kidney disease, when conditions classified to **category** 585 are present. Unlike hypertension with heart disease, ICD-9-CM presumes a cause-and-effect relationship and classifies chronic kidney disease (CKD) with hypertension as hypertensive chronic kidney disease.

Fifth digits for category 403 should be assigned as follows:

* 0 with CKD stage I through stage IV, or unspecified.

* 1 with CKD stage V or end stage renal disease. The appropriate code from category 585, Chronic kidney disease, should be used as a secondary code with a code from category 403 to identify the stage of chronic kidney disease.

See Section I.C.10.a for information on the coding of chronic kidney disease.

4) Hypertensive Heart and Chronic Kidney Disease

Assign codes from combination category 404, Hypertensive heart and chronic kidney disease, when both hypertensive kidney disease and hypertensive heart disease are stated in the diagnosis. Assume a relationship between the hypertension and the chronic kidney disease, whether or not the condition is so designated. Assign an additional code from category 428, to identify the type of heart failure. More than one code from category 428 may be assigned if the patient has systolic or diastolic failure and congestive heart failure.

Fifth digits for category 404 should be assigned as follows:

- 0 without heart failure and with chronic kidney disease (CKD) stage I through stage IV, or unspecified

- 1 with heart failure and with CKD stage I through stage IV, or unspecified

- 2 without heart failure and with CKD stage V or end stage renal disease

- 3 with heart failure and with CKD stage V or end stage renal disease

The appropriate code from category 585, Chronic kidney disease, should be used as a secondary code with a code from category 404 to identify the stage of kidney disease.

See Section I.C.10.a for information on the coding of chronic kidney disease.

5) Hypertensive Cerebrovascular Disease

First assign codes from 430-438, Cerebrovascular disease, then the appropriate hypertension code from categories 401-405.

6) Hypertensive Retinopathy

Two codes are necessary to identify the condition. First assign the code from subcategory 362.11, Hypertensive retinopathy, then the appropriate code from categories 401-405 to indicate the type of hypertension.

7) Hypertension, Secondary

Two codes are required: one to identify the underlying etiology and one from category 405 to identify the hypertension.

Sequencing of codes is determined by the reason for dmission/encounter.

8) Hypertension, Transient

Assign code 796.2, Elevated blood pressure reading without diagnosis of hypertension, unless patient has an established diagnosis of hypertension. Assign code 642.3x for transient hypertension of pregnancy.

9) Hypertension, Controlled

Assign appropriate code from categories 401-405. This diagnostic statement usually refers to an existing state of hypertension under control by therapy.

10) Hypertension, Uncontrolled

Uncontrolled hypertension may refer to untreated hypertension or hypertension not responding to current therapeutic regimen.

In either case, assign the appropriate code from categories 401-405 to designate the stage and type of hypertension. Code to the type of hypertension.

11) Elevated Blood Pressure

For a statement of elevated blood pressure without further specificity, assign code 796.2, Elevated blood pressure reading without diagnosis of hypertension, rather than a code from category 401.

b. Cerebral infarction/stroke/cerebrovascular accident (CVA)

The terms stroke and CVA are often used interchangeably to refer to a cerebral infarction. The terms stroke, CVA, and cerebral infarction NOS are all indexed to the default code 434.91, Cerebral artery occlusion, unspecified, with infarction. Code 436, Acute, but ill-defined, cerebrovascular disease, should not be used when the documentation states stroke or CVA.

See section I.C.18.d.3 for information on coding status post administration of tPA in a different facility within the last 24 hours.

c. Postoperative cerebrovascular accident

A cerebrovascular hemorrhage or infarction that occurs as a result of medical intervention is coded to 997.02, Iatrogenic cerebrovascular infarction or hemorrhage. Medical record documentation should clearly specify the cause- and-effect relationship between the medical intervention and the cerebrovascular accident in order to assign this code. A secondary code from the code range 430-432 or from a code from subcategories 433 or 434 with a fifth digit of "1" should also be used to identify the type of hemorrhage or infarct.

This guideline conforms to the use additional code note instruction at category 997. Code 436, Acute, but ill-defined, cerebrovascular disease, should not be used as a secondary code with code 997.02.

d. Late Effects of Cerebrovascular Disease

1) Category 438, Late Effects of Cerebrovascular disease

Category 438 is used to indicate conditions classifiable to categories 430-437 as the causes of late effects (neurologic deficits), themselves classified elsewhere. These "late effects" include neurologic deficits that persist after initial onset of conditions classifiable to 430-437. The neurologic deficits caused by cerebrovascular disease may be present from the onset or may arise at any time after the onset of the condition classifiable to 430-437.

2) Codes from category 438 with codes from 430-437

Codes from category 438 may be assigned on a health care record with codes from 430-437, if the patient has a current cerebrovascular accident (CVA) and deficits from an old CVA.

3) Code V12.54

Assign code V12.**54, Transient ischemic attack (TIA), and cerebral infarction without residual deficits** (and not a code from category 438) as an additional code for history of cerebrovascular disease when no neurologic deficits are present.

e. **Acute myocardial infarction (AMI)**

1) **ST elevation myocardial infarction (STEMI) and non ST elevation myocardial infarction (NSTEMI)**

The ICD-9-CM codes for acute myocardial infarction (AMI) identify the site, such as anterolateral wall or true posterior wall. Subcategories 410.0-410.6 and 410.8 are used for ST elevation myocardial infarction (STEMI). Subcategory 410.7, Subendocardial infarction, is used for non ST elevation myocardial infarction (NSTEMI) and nontransmural MIs.

2) **Acute myocardial infarction, unspecified**

Subcategory 410.9 is the default for the unspecified term acute myocardial infarction. If only STEMI or transmural MI without the site is documented, query the provider as to the site, or assign a code from subcategory 410.9.

3) **AMI documented as nontransmural or subendocardial but site provided**

If an AMI is documented as nontransmural or subendocardial, but the site is provided, it is still coded as a subendocardial AMI. If NSTEMI evolves to STEMI, assign the STEMI code. If STEMI converts to NSTEMI due to thrombolytic therapy, it is still coded as STEMI.

See section I.C.18.d.3 for information on coding status post administration of tPA in a different facility within the last 24 hours.

8. **Chapter 8: Diseases of Respiratory System (460-519)**

a. **Chronic Obstructive Pulmonary Disease [COPD] and Asthma**

See I.C.17.f ventilator-associated pneumonia.

1) **Conditions that comprise COPD and Asthma**

The conditions that comprise COPD are obstructive chronic bronchitis, subcategory 491.2, and emphysema, category 492. All asthma codes are under category 493, Asthma. Code 496, Chronic airway obstruction, not elsewhere classified, is a nonspecific code that should only be used when the documentation in a medical record does not specify the type of COPD being treated.

2) **Acute exacerbation of chronic obstructive bronchitis and asthma**

The codes for chronic obstructive bronchitis and asthma distinguish between uncomplicated cases and those in acute exacerbation. An acute exacerbation is a worsening or a decompensation of a chronic condition. An acute exacerbation is not equivalent to an infection superimposed on a chronic condition, though an exacerbation may be triggered by an infection.

3) **Overlapping nature of the conditions that comprise COPD and asthma**

Due to the overlapping nature of the conditions that make up COPD and asthma, there are many variations in the way these conditions are documented. Code selection must be based on the terms as documented. When selecting the correct code for the documented type of COPD and asthma, it is essential to first review the index, and then verify the code in the tabular list. There are many instructional notes under the different COPD subcategories and codes. It is important that all such notes be reviewed to assure correct code assignment.

4) Acute exacerbation of asthma and status asthmaticus

An acute exacerbation of asthma is an increased severity of the asthma symptoms, such as wheezing and shortness of breath. Status asthmaticus refers to a patient's failure to respond to therapy administered during an asthmatic episode and is a life threatening complication that requires emergency care. If status asthmaticus is documented by the provider with any type of COPD or with acute bronchitis, the status asthmaticus should be sequenced first. It supersedes any type of COPD including that with acute exacerbation or acute bronchitis. It is inappropriate to assign an asthma code with 5th digit 2, with acute exacerbation, together with an asthma code with 5th digit 1, with status asthmatics. Only the 5th digit 1 should be assigned.

b. Chronic Obstructive Pulmonary Disease [COPD] and Bronchitis

1) Acute bronchitis with COPD

Acute bronchitis, code 466.0, is due to an infectious organism. When acute bronchitis is documented with COPD, code 491.22, Obstructive chronic bronchitis with acute bronchitis, should be assigned. It is not necessary to also assign code 466.0. If a medical record documents acute bronchitis with COPD with acute exacerbation, only code 491.22 should be assigned. The acute bronchitis included in code 491.22 supersedes the acute exacerbation. If a medical record documents COPD with acute exacerbation without mention of acute bronchitis, only code 491.21 should be assigned.

c. Acute Respiratory Failure

1) Acute respiratory failure as principal diagnosis

Code 518.81, Acute respiratory failure, may be assigned as a principal diagnosis when it is the condition established after study to be chiefly responsible for occasioning the admission to the hospital, and the selection is supported by the Alphabetic Index and Tabular List. However, chapter-specific coding guidelines (such as obstetrics, poisoning, HIV, newborn) that provide sequencing direction take precedence.

2) Acute respiratory failure as secondary diagnosis

Respiratory failure may be listed as a secondary diagnosis if it occurs after admission, or if it is present on admission, but does not meet the definition of principal diagnosis.

3) Sequencing of acute respiratory failure and another acute condition

When a patient is admitted with respiratory failure and another acute condition, (e.g., myocardial infarction, cerebrovascular accident, aspiration pneumonia), the principal diagnosis will not be the same in every situation. **This applies whether the other acute condition is a respiratory or nonrespiratory condition.** Selection of the principal diagnosis will be dependent on the circumstances of admission. If both the respiratory failure and the other acute condition are equally responsible for occasioning the admission to the hospital, and there are no chapter-specific sequencing rules, the guideline regarding two or more diagnoses that equally meet the definition for principal diagnosis *(Section II, C.)* may be applied in these situations.

If the documentation is not clear as to whether acute respiratory failure and another condition are equally responsible for occasioning the admission, query the provider for clarification.

d. **Influenza due to identified avian influenza virus (avian influenza)**

Code only confirmed cases of avian influenza. This is an exception to the hospital inpatient guideline Section II, H. (Uncertain Diagnosis).

In this context, "confirmation" does not require documentation of positive laboratory testing specific for avian influenza. However, coding should be based on the provider's diagnostic statement that the patient has avian influenza.

If the provider records "suspected or possible or probable avian influenza," the appropriate influenza code from category 487 should be assigned. Code 488, Influenza due to identified avian influenza virus, should not be assigned.

9. **Chapter 9: Diseases of Digestive System (520-579)**

Reserved for future guideline expansion

10. **Chapter 10: Diseases of Genitourinary System (580-629)**

a. **Chronic kidney disease**

1) **Stages of chronic kidney disease (CKD)**

The ICD-9-CM classifies CKD based on severity. The severity of CKD is designated by stages I–V. Stage II, code 585.2, equates to mild CKD; stage III, code 585.3, equates to moderate CKD; and stage IV, code 585.4, equates to severe CKD. Code 585.6, End stage renal disease (ESRD), is assigned when the provider has documented end-stage-renal disease (ESRD).

If both a stage of CKD and ESRD are documented, assign code 585.6 only.

2) **Chronic kidney disease and kidney transplant status**

Patients who have undergone kidney transplant may still have some form of CKD, because the kidney transplant may not fully restore kidney function. Therefore, the presence of CKD alone does not constitute a transplant complication. Assign the appropriate 585 code for the patient's stage of CKD and code V42.0. If a transplant complication such as failure or rejection is documented, see section I.C.17.f.**2**.b for information on coding complications of a kidney transplant. If the documentation is unclear as to whether the patient has a complication of the transplant, query the provider.

3) Chronic kidney disease with other conditions

Patients with CKD may also suffer from other serious conditions, most commonly diabetes mellitus and hypertension. The sequencing of the CKD code in relationship to codes for other contributing conditions is based on the conventions in the tabular list.

See I.C.3.a.4 for sequencing instructions for diabetes.

See I.C.4.a.1 for anemia in CKD.

See I.C.7.a.3 for hypertensive chronic kidney disease.

See I.C.17.f.2.b, Kidney transplant complications, for instructions on coding of documented rejection or failure.

11. Chapter 11: Complications of Pregnancy, Childbirth, and the Puerperium (630-679)

a. General Rules for Obstetric Cases

1) Codes from chapter 11 and sequencing priority

Obstetric cases require codes from chapter 11, codes in the range 630-679, Complications of Pregnancy, Childbirth, and the Puerperium. Chapter 11 codes have sequencing priority over codes from other chapters. Additional codes from other chapters may be used in conjunction with chapter 11 codes to further specify conditions. Should the provider document that the pregnancy is incidental to the encounter, then code V22.2 should be used in place of any chapter 11 codes. It is the provider's responsibility to state that the condition being treated is not affecting the pregnancy.

2) Chapter 11 codes used only on the maternal record

Chapter 11 codes are to be used only on the maternal record, never on the record of the newborn.

3) Chapter 11 fifth-digits

Categories 640-648, 651-676 have required fifth-digits, which indicate whether the encounter is antepartum, postpartum and whether a delivery has also occurred.

4) Fifth-digits, appropriate for each code

The fifth-digits, which are appropriate for each code number, are listed in brackets under each code. The fifth-digits on each code should all be consistent with each other. That is, should a delivery occur all of the fifth-digits should indicate the delivery.

b. Selection of OB Principal or First-listed Diagnosis

1) Routine outpatient prenatal visits

For routine outpatient prenatal visits when no complications are present codes V22.0, Supervision of normal first pregnancy, and V22.1, Supervision of other normal pregnancy, should be used as the first-listed diagnoses. These codes should not be used in conjunction with chapter 11 codes.

2) Prenatal outpatient visits for high-risk patients

For prenatal outpatient visits for patients with high-risk pregnancies, a code from category V23, Supervision of high-risk pregnancy, should be used as the principal or first-listed diagnosis. Secondary chapter 11 codes may be used in conjunction with these codes if appropriate.

3) Episodes when no delivery occurs

In episodes when no delivery occurs, the principal diagnosis should correspond to the principal complication of the pregnancy, which necessitated the encounter. Should more than one complication exist, all of which are treated or monitored, any of the complications codes may be sequenced first.

4) When a delivery occurs

When a delivery occurs, the principal diagnosis should correspond to the main circumstances or complication of the delivery. In cases of cesarean delivery, the selection of the principal diagnosis should correspond to the reason the cesarean delivery was performed unless the reason for admission/encounter was unrelated to the condition resulting in the cesarean delivery.

5) Outcome of delivery

An outcome of delivery code, V27.0-V27.9, should be included on every maternal record when a delivery has occurred. These codes are not to be used on subsequent records or on the newborn record.

c. Fetal Conditions Affecting the Management of the Mother

1) Codes from category 655

Known or suspected fetal abnormality affecting management of the mother, and category 656, Other fetal and placental problems affecting the management of the mother, are assigned only when the fetal condition is actually responsible for modifying the management of the mother, i.e., by requiring diagnostic studies, additional observation, special care, or termination of pregnancy. The fact that the fetal condition exists does not justify assigning a code from this series to the mother's record.

See I.C.18.d for suspected maternal and fetal conditions not found.

2) In utero surgery

In cases when surgery is performed on the fetus, a diagnosis code from category 655, Known or suspected fetal abnormalities affecting management of the mother, should be assigned identifying the fetal condition. Procedure code 75.36, Correction of fetal defect, should be assigned on the hospital inpatient record.

No code from Chapter 15, the perinatal codes, should be used on the mother's record to identify fetal conditions. Surgery performed in utero on a fetus is still to be coded as an obstetric encounter.

d. HIV Infection in Pregnancy, Childbirth and the Puerperium

During pregnancy, childbirth or the puerperium, a patient admitted because of an HIV-related illness should receive a principal diagnosis of 647.6X, Other specified infectious and parasitic diseases in the mother classifiable elsewhere, but complicating the pregnancy, childbirth or the puerperium, followed by 042 and the code(s) for the HIV-related illness(es).

Patients with asymptomatic HIV infection status admitted during pregnancy, childbirth, or the puerperium should receive codes of 647.6X and V08.

e. Current Conditions Complicating Pregnancy

Assign a code from subcategory 648.x for patients that have current conditions when the condition affects the management of the pregnancy, childbirth, or the puerperium. Use additional secondary codes from other chapters to identify the conditions, as appropriate.

f. Diabetes mellitus in pregnancy

Diabetes mellitus is a significant complicating factor in pregnancy. Pregnant women who are diabetic should be assigned code 648.0x, Diabetes mellitus complicating pregnancy, and a secondary code from category 250, Diabetes mellitus, **or category 249, Secondary diabetes** to identify the type of diabetes.

Code V58.67, Long-term (current) use of insulin, should also be assigned if the diabetes mellitus is being treated with insulin.

g. Gestational diabetes

Gestational diabetes can occur during the second and third trimester of pregnancy in women who were not diabetic prior to pregnancy. Gestational diabetes can cause complications in the pregnancy similar to those of pre-existing diabetes mellitus. It also puts the woman at greater risk of developing diabetes after the pregnancy. Gestational diabetes is coded to 648.8x, Abnormal glucose tolerance. Codes 648.0x and 648.8x should never be used together on the same record.

Code V58.67, Long-term (current) use of insulin, should also be assigned if the gestational diabetes is being treated with insulin.

h. Normal Delivery, Code 650

1) Normal delivery

Code 650 is for use in cases when a woman is admitted for a full-term normal delivery and delivers a single, healthy infant without any complications antepartum, during the delivery, or postpartum during the delivery episode. Code 650 is always a principal diagnosis. It is not to be used if any other code from chapter 11 is needed to describe a current complication of the antenatal, delivery, or perinatal period. Additional codes from other chapters may be used with code 650 if they are not related to or are in any way complicating the pregnancy.

2) Normal delivery with resolved antepartum complication

Code 650 may be used if the patient had a complication at some point during her pregnancy, but the complication is not present at the time of the admission for delivery.

3) V27.0, Single liveborn, outcome of delivery

V27.0, Single liveborn, is the only outcome of delivery code appropriate for use with 650.

i. The Postpartum and Peripartum Periods

1) Postpartum and peripartum periods

The postpartum period begins immediately after delivery and continues for six weeks following delivery. The peripartum period is defined as the last month of pregnancy to five months postpartum.

2) Postpartum complication

A postpartum complication is any complication occurring within the six-week period.

3) Pregnancy-related complications after 6 week period

Chapter 11 codes may also be used to describe pregnancy-related complications after the six-week period should the provider document that a condition is pregnancy related.

4) Postpartum complications occurring during the same admission as delivery

Postpartum complications that occur during the same admission as the delivery are identified with a fifth digit of "2." Subsequent admissions/encounters for postpartum complications should be identified with a fifth digit of "4."

5) Admission for routine postpartum care following delivery outside hospital

When the mother delivers outside the hospital prior to admission and is admitted for routine postpartum care and no complications are noted, code V24.0, Postpartum care and examination immediately after delivery, should be assigned as the principal diagnosis.

6) Admission following delivery outside hospital with postpartum conditions

A delivery diagnosis code should not be used for a woman who has delivered prior to admission to the hospital. Any postpartum conditions and/or postpartum procedures should be coded.

j. Code 677, Late effect of complication of pregnancy

1) Code 677

Code 677, Late effect of complication of pregnancy, childbirth, and the puerperium is for use in those cases when an initial complication of a pregnancy develops a sequelae requiring care or treatment at a future date.

2) After the initial postpartum period

This code may be used at any time after the initial postpartum period.

3) Sequencing of Code 677

This code, like all late effect codes, is to be sequenced following the code describing the sequelae of the complication.

k. Abortions

1) Fifth-digits required for abortion categories

Fifth-digits are required for abortion categories 634-637. Fifth-digit 1, incomplete, indicates that all of the products of conception have not been expelled from the uterus. Fifth-digit 2, complete, indicates that all products of conception have been expelled from the uterus.

2) Code from categories 640-648 and 651-659

A code from categories 640-648 and 651-659 may be used as additional codes with an abortion code to indicate the complication leading to the abortion.

Fifth digit 3 is assigned with codes from these categories when used with an abortion code because the other fifth digits will not apply. Codes from the 660-669 series are not to be used for complications of abortion.

3) Code 639 for complications

Code 639 is to be used for all complications following abortion. Code 639 cannot be assigned with codes from categories 634-638.

4) Abortion with Liveborn Fetus

When an attempted termination of pregnancy results in a liveborn fetus assign code 644.21, Early onset of delivery, with an appropriate code from category V27, Outcome of Delivery. The procedure code for the attempted termination of pregnancy should also be assigned.

5) Retained Products of Conception following an abortion

Subsequent admissions for retained products of conception following a spontaneous or legally induced abortion are assigned the appropriate code from category 634, Spontaneous abortion, or 635 Legally induced abortion, with a fifth digit of "1" (incomplete). This advice is appropriate even when the patient was discharged previously with a discharge diagnosis of complete abortion.

12. Chapter 12: Diseases Skin and Subcutaneous Tissue (680-709)

a. Pressure ulcer stage codes

1) Pressure ulcer stages

Two codes are needed to completely describe a pressure ulcer: A code from subcategory 707.0, Pressure ulcer, to identify the site of the pressure ulcer and a code from subcategory 707.2, Pressure ulcer stages.

The codes in subcategory 707.2, Pressure ulcer stages, are to be used as an additional diagnosis with a code(s) from subcategory 707.0, Pressure Ulcer. Codes from 707.2, Pressure ulcer stages, may not be assigned as a principal or first-listed diagnosis. The pressure ulcer stage codes should only be used with pressure ulcers and not with other types of ulcers (e.g., stasis ulcer).

The ICD-9-CM classifies pressure ulcer stages based on severity, which is designated by stages I-IV and unstageable.

2) **Unstageable pressure ulcers**

Assignment of code 707.25, Pressure ulcer, unstageable, should be based on the clinical documentation. Code 707.25 is used for pressure ulcers whose stage cannot be clinically determined (e.g., the ulcer is covered by eschar or has been treated with a skin or muscle graft) and pressure ulcers that are documented as deep tissue injury but not documented as due to trauma. This code should not be confused with code 707.20, Pressure ulcer, stage unspecified. Code 707.20 should be assigned when there is no documentation regarding the stage of the pressure ulcer.

3) **Documented pressure ulcer stage**

Assignment of the pressure ulcer stage code should be guided by clinical documentation of the stage or documentation of the terms found in the index. For clinical terms describing the stage that are not found in the index, and there is no documentation of the stage, the provider should be queried.

4) **Bilateral pressure ulcers with same stage**

When a patient has bilateral pressure ulcers (e.g., both buttocks) and both pressure ulcers are documented as being the same stage, only the code for the site and one code for the stage should be reported.

5) **Bilateral pressure ulcers with different stages**

When a patient has bilateral pressure ulcers at the same site (e.g., both buttocks) and each pressure ulcer is documented as being at a different stage, assign one code for the site and the appropriate codes for the pressure ulcer stage.

6) **Multiple pressure ulcers of different sites and stages**

When a patient has multiple pressure ulcers at different sites (e.g., buttock, heel, shoulder) and each pressure ulcer is documented as being at different stages (e.g., stage 3 and stage 4), assign the appropriate codes for each different site and a code for each different pressure ulcer stage.

7) **Patients admitted with pressure ulcers documented as healed**

No code is assigned if the documentation states that the pressure ulcer is completely healed.

8) **Patients admitted with pressure ulcers documented as healing**

Pressure ulcers described as healing should be assigned the appropriate pressure ulcer stage code based on the

A-41

documentation in the medical record. If the documentation does not provide information about the stage of the healing pressure ulcer, assign code 707.20, Pressure ulcer stage, unspecified.

If the documentation is unclear as to whether the patient has a current (new) pressure ulcer or if the patient is being treated for a healing pressure ulcer, query the provider.

9) **Patient admitted with pressure ulcer evolving into another stage during the admission**

If a patient is admitted with a pressure ulcer at one stage and it progresses to a higher stage, assign the code for highest stage reported for that site.

13. **Chapter 13: Diseases of Musculoskeletal and Connective Tissue (710-739)**

a. **Coding of Pathologic Fractures**

1) **Acute Fractures vs. Aftercare**

Pathologic fractures are reported using subcategory 733.1, when the fracture is newly diagnosed. Subcategory 733.1 may be used while the patient is receiving active treatment for the fracture. Examples of active treatment are: surgical treatment, emergency department encounter, evaluation and treatment by a new physician.

Fractures are coded using the aftercare codes (subcategories V54.0, V54.2, V54.8 or V54.9) for encounters after the patient has completed active treatment of the fracture and is receiving routine care for the fracture during the healing or recovery phase. Examples of fracture aftercare are: cast change or removal, removal of external or internal fixation device, medication adjustment, and follow up visits following fracture treatment.

Care for complications of surgical treatment for fracture repairs during the healing or recovery phase should be coded with the appropriate complication codes.

Care of complications of fractures, such as malunion and nonunion, should be reported with the appropriate codes.

See Section I. C. 17.b for information on the coding of traumatic fractures.

14. **Chapter 14: Congenital Anomalies (740-759)**

a. **Codes in categories 740-759, Congenital Anomalies**

Assign an appropriate code(s) from categories 740-759, Congenital Anomalies, when an anomaly is documented. A congenital anomaly may be the principal/first listed diagnosis on a record or a secondary diagnosis.

When a congenital anomaly does not have a unique code assignment, assign additional code(s) for any manifestations that may be present. When the code assignment specifically identifies the congenital anomaly, manifestations that are an inherent component of the anomaly should not be coded separately. Additional codes should be assigned for manifestations that are not an inherent component.

Codes from Chapter 14 may be used throughout the life of the patient. If a congenital anomaly has been corrected, a personal history code should be used to identify the history of the anomaly. Although present at birth, a congenital anomaly may not be identified until later in life. Whenever the condition is diagnosed by the physician, it is appropriate to assign a code from codes 740-759.

For the birth admission, the appropriate code from category V30, Liveborn infants, according to type of birth should be sequenced as the principal diagnosis, followed by any congenital anomaly codes, 740759.

15. Chapter 15: Newborn (Perinatal) Guidelines (760-779)

For coding and reporting purposes the perinatal period is defined as before birth through the 28th day following birth. The following guidelines are provided for reporting purposes. Hospitals may record other diagnoses as needed for internal data use.

a. General Perinatal Rules

1) Chapter 15 Codes

They are never for use on the maternal record. Codes from Chapter 11, the obstetric chapter, are never permitted on the newborn record. Chapter 15 code may be used throughout the life of the patient if the condition is still present.

2) Sequencing of perinatal codes

Generally, codes from Chapter 15 should be sequenced as the principal/first-listed diagnosis on the newborn record, with the exception of the appropriate V30 code for the birth episode, followed by codes from any other chapter that provide additional detail. The "use additional code" note at the beginning of the chapter supports this guideline. If the index does not provide a specific code for a perinatal condition, assign code 779.89, Other specified conditions originating in the perinatal period, followed by the code from another chapter that specifies the condition. Codes for signs and symptoms may be assigned when a definitive diagnosis has not been established.

3) Birth process or community acquired conditions

If a newborn has a condition that may be either due to the birth process or community acquired and the documentation does not indicate which it is, the default is due to the birth process and the code from Chapter 15 should be used. If the condition is community-acquired, a code from Chapter 15 should not be assigned.

4) Code all clinically significant conditions

All clinically significant conditions noted on routine newborn examination should be coded. A condition is clinically significant if it requires:

- clinical evaluation; or
- therapeutic treatment; or

- diagnostic procedures; or

- extended length of hospital stay; or

- increased nursing care and/or monitoring; or

- has implications for future health care needs

Note: The perinatal guidelines listed above are the same as the general coding guidelines for "additional diagnoses", except for the final point regarding implications for future health care needs. Codes should be assigned for conditions that have been specified by the provider as having implications for future health care needs. Codes from the perinatal chapter should not be assigned unless the provider has established a definitive diagnosis.

b. **Use of codes V30-V39**

When coding the birth of an infant, assign a code from categories V30-V39, according to the type of birth. A code from this series is assigned as a principal diagnosis, and assigned only once to a newborn at the time of birth.

c. **Newborn transfers**

If the newborn is transferred to another institution, the V30 series is not used at the receiving hospital.

d. **Use of category V29**

1) **Assigning a code from category V29**

Assign a code from category V29, Observation and evaluation of newborns and infants for suspected conditions not found, to identify those instances when a healthy newborn is evaluated for a suspected condition that is determined after study not to be present. Do not use a code from category V29 when the patient has identified signs or symptoms of a suspected problem; in such cases, code the sign or symptom.

A code from category V29 may also be assigned as a principal code for readmissions or encounters when the V30 code no longer applies. Codes from category V29 are for use only for healthy newborns and infants for which no condition after study is found to be present.

2) **V29 code on a birth record**

A V29 code is to be used as a secondary code after the V30, Outcome of delivery, code.

e. **Use of other V codes on perinatal records**

V codes other than V30 and V29 may be assigned on a perinatal or newborn record code. The codes may be used as a principal or first-listed diagnosis for specific types of encounters or for readmissions or encounters when the V30 code no longer applies.

See Section I.C.18 for information regarding the assignment of V codes.

f. **Maternal Causes of Perinatal Morbidity**

Codes from categories 760-763, Maternal causes of perinatal morbidity and mortality, are assigned only when the maternal condition has actually affected the fetus or newborn. The fact that the mother has an associated medical condition or experiences some complication of pregnancy, labor or delivery does not justify the routine assignment of codes from these categories to the newborn record.

g. Congenital Anomalies in Newborns

For the birth admission, the appropriate code from category V30, Liveborn infants according to type of birth, should be used, followed by any congenital anomaly codes, categories 740-759. Use additional secondary codes from other chapters to specify conditions associated with the anomaly, if applicable.

Also, see Section I.C.14 for information on the coding of congenital anomalies.

h. Coding Additional Perinatal Diagnoses

1) Assigning codes for conditions that require treatment

Assign codes for conditions that require treatment or further investigation, prolong the length of stay, or require resource utilization.

2) Codes for conditions specified as having implications for future health care needs

Assign codes for conditions that have been specified by the provider as having implications for future health care needs.

Note: This guideline should not be used for adult patients.

3) Codes for newborn conditions originating in the perinatal period

Assign a code for newborn conditions originating in the perinatal period (categories 760-779), as well as complications arising during the current episode of care classified in other chapters, only if the diagnoses have been documented by the responsible provider at the time of transfer or discharge as having affected the fetus or newborn.

i. Prematurity and Fetal Growth Retardation

Providers utilize different criteria in determining prematurity. A code for prematurity should not be assigned unless it is documented. The 5th digit assignment for codes from category 764 and subcategories 765.0 and 765.1 should be based on the recorded birth weight and estimated gestational age.

A code from subcategory 765.2, Weeks of gestation, should be assigned as an additional code with category 764 and codes from 765.0 and 765.1 to specify weeks of gestation as documented by the provider in the record.

j. Newborn sepsis

Code 771.81, Septicemia [sepsis] of newborn, should be assigned with a secondary code from category 041, Bacterial infections in conditions classified elsewhere and of unspecified site, to identify the organism. A code from category 038, Septicemia, should not be used on a newborn record. **Do not assign code 995.91, Sepsis, as c**ode 771.81 describes the sepsis. **If applicable, use additional codes**

to identify severe sepsis (995.92) and any associated acute organ dysfunction.

16. Chapter 16: Signs, Symptoms and Ill-Defined Conditions (780-799)

Reserved for future guideline expansion

17. Chapter 17: Injury and Poisoning (800-999)

a. Coding of Injuries

When coding injuries, assign separate codes for each injury unless a combination code is provided, in which case the combination code is assigned. Multiple injury codes are provided in ICD-9-CM, but should not be assigned unless information for a more specific code is not available. These codes are not to be used for normal, healing surgical wounds or to identify complications of surgical wounds.

The code for the most serious injury, as determined by the provider and the focus of treatment, is sequenced first.

1) Superficial injuries

Superficial injuries such as abrasions or contusions are not coded when associated with more severe injuries of the same site.

2) Primary injury with damage to nerves/blood vessels

When a primary injury results in minor damage to peripheral nerves or blood vessels, the primary injury is sequenced first with additional code(s) from categories 950-957, Injury to nerves and spinal cord, and/or 900-904, Injury to blood vessels. When the primary injury is to the blood vessels or nerves, that injury should be sequenced first.

b. Coding of Traumatic Fractures

The principles of multiple coding of injuries should be followed in coding fractures. Fractures of specified sites are coded individually by site in accordance with both the provisions within categories 800-829 and the level of detail furnished by medical record content. Combination categories for multiple fractures are provided for use when there is insufficient detail in the medical record (such as trauma cases transferred to another hospital), when the reporting form limits the number of codes that can be used in reporting pertinent clinical data, or when there is insufficient specificity at the fourth-digit or fifth-digit level. More specific guidelines are as follows:

1) Acute Fractures vs. Aftercare

Traumatic fractures are coded using the acute fracture codes (800-829) while the patient is receiving active treatment for the fracture. Examples of active treatment are: surgical treatment, emergency department encounter, and evaluation and treatment by a new physician.

Fractures are coded using the aftercare codes (subcategories V54.0, V54.1, V54.8, or V54.9) for encounters after the patient has completed active treatment of the fracture and is receiving routine care for the fracture during the healing or recovery phase. Examples of fracture aftercare are: cast change or removal,

removal of external or internal fixation device, medication adjustment, and follow up visits following fracture treatment.

Care for complications of surgical treatment for fracture repairs during the healing or recovery phase should be coded with the appropriate complication codes.

Care of complications of fractures, such as malunion and nonunion, should be reported with the appropriate codes.

Pathologic fractures are not coded in the 800-829 range, but instead are assigned to subcategory 733.1. *See Section I.C.13.a for additional information.*

2) Multiple fractures of same limb

Multiple fractures of same limb classifiable to the same three-digit or four-digit category are coded to that category.

3) Multiple unilateral or bilateral fractures of same bone

Multiple unilateral or bilateral fractures of same bone(s) but classified to different fourth-digit subdivisions (bone part) within the same three-digit category are coded individually by site.

4) Multiple fracture categories 819 and 828

Multiple fracture categories 819 and 828 classify bilateral fractures of both upper limbs (819) and both lower limbs (828), but without any detail at the fourth-digit level other than open and closed type of fractures.

5) Multiple fractures sequencing

Multiple fractures are sequenced in accordance with the severity of the fracture. The provider should be asked to list the fracture diagnoses in the order of severity.

c. Coding of Burns

Current burns (940-948) are classified by depth, extent and by agent (E code). Burns are classified by depth as first degree (erythema), second degree (blistering), and third degree (full-thickness involvement).

1) Sequencing of burn and related condition codes

Sequence first the code that reflects the highest degree of burn when more than one burn is present.

a. When the reason for the admission or encounter is for treatment of external multiple burns, sequence first the code that reflects the burn of the highest degree.

b. When a patient has both internal and external burns, the circumstances of admission govern the selection of the principal diagnosis or first-listed diagnosis.

c. When a patient is admitted for burn injuries and other related conditions such as smoke inhalation and/or respiratory failure, the circumstances of admission govern the selection of the principal or first-listed diagnosis.

2) Burns of the same local site

Classify burns of the same local site (three-digit category level, 940-947) but of different degrees to the subcategory identifying the highest degree recorded in the diagnosis.

3) Non-healing burns

Non-healing burns are coded as acute burns.

Necrosis of burned skin should be coded as a non-healed burn.

4) Code 958.3, Posttraumatic wound infection

Assign code 958.3, Posttraumatic wound infection, not elsewhere classified, as an additional code for any documented infected burn site.

5) Assign separate codes for each burn site

When coding burns, assign separate codes for each burn site. Category 946 Burns of Multiple specified sites, should only be used if the location of the burns are not documented. Category 949, Burn, unspecified, is extremely vague and should rarely be used.

6) Assign codes from category 948, Burns

Burns classified according to extent of body surface involved, when the site of the burn is not specified or when there is a need for additional data. It is advisable to use category 948 as additional coding when needed to provide data for evaluating burn mortality, such as that needed by burn units. It is also advisable to use category 948 as an additional code for reporting purposes when there is mention of a third-degree burn involving 20 percent or more of the body surface.

In assigning a code from category 948:

Fourth-digit codes are used to identify the percentage of total body surface involved in a burn (all degree).

Fifth-digits are assigned to identify the percentage of body surface involved in third-degree burn.

Fifth-digit zero (0) is assigned when less than 10 percent or when no body surface is involved in a third-degree burn.

Category 948 is based on the classic "rule of nines" in estimating body surface involved: head and neck are assigned nine percent, each arm nine percent, each leg 18 percent, the anterior trunk 18 percent, posterior trunk 18 percent, and genitalia one percent. Providers may change these percentage assignments where necessary to accommodate infants and children who have proportionately larger heads than adults and patients who have large buttocks, thighs, or abdomen that involve burns.

7) Encounters for treatment of late effects of burns

Encounters for the treatment of the late effects of burns (i.e., scars or joint contractures) should be coded to the residual condition (sequelae) followed by the appropriate late effect code (906.5-906.9). A late effect E code may also be used, if desired.

8) Sequelae with a late effect code and current burn

When appropriate, both a sequelae with a late effect code, and a current burn code may be assigned on the same record (when both a current burn and sequelae of an old burn exist).

d. Coding of Debridement of Wound, Infection, or Burn

Excisional debridement involves surgical removal or cutting away, as opposed to a mechanical (brushing, scrubbing, washing) debridement.

For coding purposes, excisional debridement is assigned to code 86.22.

Nonexcisional debridement is assigned to code 86.28.

e. Adverse Effects, Poisoning and Toxic Effects

The properties of certain drugs, medicinal and biological substances or combinations of such substances, may cause toxic reactions. The occurrence of drug toxicity is classified in ICD-9-CM as follows:

1) Adverse Effect

When the drug was correctly prescribed and properly administered, code the reaction plus the appropriate code from the E930-E949 series. Codes from the E930-E949 series must be used to identify the causative substance for an adverse effect of drug, medicinal and biological substances, correctly prescribed and properly administered. The effect, such as tachycardia, delirium, gastrointestinal hemorrhaging, vomiting, hypokalemia, hepatitis, renal failure, or respiratory failure, is coded and followed by the appropriate code from the E930-E949 series.

Adverse effects of therapeutic substances correctly prescribed and properly administered (toxicity, synergistic reaction, side effect, and idiosyncratic reaction) may be due to (1) differences among patients, such as age, sex, disease, and genetic factors, and (2) drug-related factors, such as type of drug, route of administration, duration of therapy, dosage, and bioavailability.

2) Poisoning

(a) Error was made in drug prescription

Errors made in drug prescription or in the administration of the drug by provider, nurse, patient, or other person, use the appropriate poisoning code from the 960-979 series.

(b) Overdose of a drug intentionally taken

If an overdose of a drug was intentionally taken or administered and resulted in drug toxicity, it would be coded as a poisoning (960-979 series).

(c) Nonprescribed drug taken with correctly prescribed and properly administered drug

If a nonprescribed drug or medicinal agent was taken in combination with a correctly prescribed and properly administered drug, any drug toxicity or other reaction resulting from the interaction of the two drugs would be classified as a poisoning.

(d) Interaction of drug(s) and alcohol

When a reaction results from the interaction of a drug(s) and alcohol, this would be classified as poisoning.

(e) Sequencing of poisoning

When coding a poisoning or reaction to the improper use of a medication (e.g., wrong dose, wrong substance, wrong route of administration) the poisoning code is sequenced first, followed by a code for the manifestation. If there is also a diagnosis of drug abuse or dependence to the substance, the abuse or dependence is coded as an additional code.

See Section I.C.3.a.6.b. if poisoning is the result of insulin pump malfunctions and Section I.C.19 for general use of E-codes.

3) Toxic Effects

(a) Toxic effect codes

When a harmful substance is ingested or comes in contact with a person, this is classified as a toxic effect. The toxic effect codes are in categories 980-989.

(b) Sequencing toxic effect codes

A toxic effect code should be sequenced first, followed by the code(s) that identify the result of the toxic effect.

(c) External cause codes for toxic effects

An external cause code from categories E860-E869 for accidental exposure, codes E950.6 or E950.7 for intentional self-harm, category E962 for assault, or categories E980-E982, for undetermined, should also be assigned to indicate intent.

f. Complications of care

1) Complications of care

(a) Documentation of complications of care

As with all procedural or postprocedural complications, code assignment is based on the provider's documentation of the relationship between the condition and the procedure.

2) Transplant complications

(a) Transplant complications other than kidney

Codes under subcategory 996.8, Complications of transplanted organ, are for use for both complications and rejection of transplanted organs. A transplant complication code is only assigned if the complication affects the function of the transplanted organ. Two codes are required to fully describe a transplant complication, the appropriate code from subcategory 996.8 and a secondary code that identifies the complication.

Pre-existing conditions or conditions that develop after the transplant are not coded as complications unless they affect the function of the transplanted organs.

See I.C.18.d.3) for transplant organ removal status.

See I.C.2.c for malignant neoplasm associated with transplanted organ.

(b) Chronic kidney disease and kidney transplant complications

Patients who have undergone kidney transplant may still have some form of chronic kidney disease (CKD) because the kidney transplant may not fully restore kidney function. Code 996.81 should be assigned for documented complications of a kidney transplant, such as transplant failure or rejection **or other transplant complication**. Code 996.81 should not be assigned for post kidney transplant patients who have chronic kidney (CKD) unless a transplant complication such as transplant failure or rejection is documented. If the documentation is unclear as to whether the patient has a complication of the transplant, query the provider.

For patients with CKD following a kidney transplant, but who do not have a complication such as failure or rejection, *see section I.C.10.a.2, Chronic kidney disease and kidney transplant status.*

3) Ventilator associated pneumonia

(a) Documentation of Ventilator associated Pneumonia

As with all procedural or postprocedural complications, code assignment is based on the provider's documentation of the relationship between the condition and the procedure.

Code 997.31, Ventilator associated pneumonia, should be assigned only when the provider has documented ventilator associated pneumonia (VAP). An additional code to identify the organism (e.g., Pseudomonas aeruginosa, code 041.7) should also be assigned. Do not assign an additional code from categories 480-484 to identify the type of pneumonia.

Code 997.31 should not be assigned for cases where the patient has pneumonia and is on a mechanical ventilator but the provider has not specifically stated that the pneumonia is ventilator-associated pneumonia.

If the documentation is unclear as to whether the patient has a pneumonia that is a complication attributable to the mechanical ventilator, query the provider.

(b) Patient admitted with pneumonia and develops VAP

A patient may be admitted with one type of pneumonia (e.g., code 481, Pneumococcal pneumonia) and subsequently develop VAP. In this instance, the principal diagnosis would be the

appropriate code from categories 480-484 for the pneumonia diagnosed at the time of admission. Code 997.31, Ventilator associated pneumonia, would be assigned as an additional diagnosis when the provider has also documented the presence of ventilator associated pneumonia.

g. **SIRS due to Non-infectious Process**

The systemic inflammatory response syndrome (SIRS) can develop as a result of certain non-infectious disease processes, such as trauma, malignant neoplasm, or pancreatitis. When SIRS is documented with a noninfectious condition, and no subsequent infection is documented, the code for the underlying condition, such as an injury, should be assigned, followed by code 995.93, Systemic inflammatory response syndrome due to noninfectious process without acute organ dysfunction, or 995.94, Systemic inflammatory response syndrome due to non-infectious process with acute organ dysfunction. If an acute organ dysfunction is documented, the appropriate code(s) for the associated acute organ dysfunction(s) should be assigned in addition to code 995.94. If acute organ dysfunction is documented, but it cannot be determined if the acute organ dysfunction is associated with SIRS or due to another condition (e.g., directly due to the trauma), the provider should be queried.

When the non-infectious condition has led to an infection that results in SIRS, *see Section I.C.1.b.**12** for the guideline for sepsis and severe sepsis associated with a non-infectious process.*

18. **Classification of Factors Influencing Health Status and Contact with Health Service (Supplemental V01-V84)**

Note: The chapter specific guidelines provide additional information about the use of V codes for specified encounters.

a. **Introduction**

ICD-9-CM provides codes to deal with encounters for circumstances other than a disease or injury. The Supplementary Classification of Factors Influencing Health Status and Contact with Health Services (V01.0-V84.8) is provided to deal with occasions when circumstances other than a disease or injury (codes 001-999) are recorded as a diagnosis or problem.

There are four primary circumstances for the use of V codes:

1) A person who is not currently sick encounters the health services for some specific reason, such as to act as an organ donor, to receive prophylactic care, such as inoculations or health screenings, or to receive counseling on health related issues.

2) A person with a resolving disease or injury, or a chronic, long-term condition requiring continuous care, encounters the health care system for specific aftercare of that disease or injury (e.g., dialysis for renal disease; chemotherapy for malignancy; cast change). A diagnosis/symptom code should be used whenever a current, acute, diagnosis is being treated or a sign or symptom is being studied.

3) Circumstances or problems influence a person's health status but are not in themselves a current illness or injury.

4) Newborns, to indicate birth status

b. V codes use in any healthcare setting

V codes are for use in any healthcare setting. V codes may be used as either a first listed (principal diagnosis code in the inpatient setting) or secondary code, depending on the circumstances of the encounter. Certain V codes may only be used as first listed, others only as secondary codes.

See Section I.C.18.e, V Code Table.

c. V Codes indicate a reason for an encounter

They are not procedure codes. A corresponding procedure code must accompany a V code to describe the procedure performed.

d. Categories of V Codes

1) Contact/Exposure

Category V01 indicates contact with or exposure to communicable diseases. These codes are for patients who do not show any sign or symptom of a disease but have been exposed to it by close personal contact with an infected individual or are in an area where a disease is epidemic. These codes may be used as a first listed code to explain an encounter for testing, or, more commonly, as a secondary code to identify a potential risk.

2) Inoculations and vaccinations

Categories V03-V06 are for encounters for inoculations and vaccinations. They indicate that a patient is being seen to receive a prophylactic inoculation against a disease. The injection itself must be represented by the appropriate procedure code. A code from V03-V06 may be used as a secondary code if the inoculation is given as a routine part of preventive health care, such as a well-baby visit.

3) Status

Status codes indicate that a patient is either a carrier of a disease or has the sequelae or residual of a past disease or condition. This includes such things as the presence of prosthetic or mechanical devices resulting from past treatment. A status code is informative, because the status may affect the course of treatment and its outcome. A status code is distinct from a history code. The history code indicates that the patient no longer has the condition.

A status code should not be used with a diagnosis code from one of the body system chapters, if the diagnosis code includes the information provided by the status code. For example, code V42.1, Heart transplant status, should not be used with code 996.83, Complications of transplanted heart. The status code does not provide additional information. The complication code indicates that the patient is a heart transplant patient.

The status V codes/categories are:

V02   Carrier or suspected carrier of infectious diseases

Carrier status indicates that a person harbors the specific organisms of a disease without manifest symptoms and is capable of transmitting the infection.

V07.5X   **Prophylactic use of agents affecting estrogen receptors and estrogen level**

This code indicates when a patient is receiving a drug that affects estrogen receptors and estrogen levels for prevention of cancer.

V08   Asymptomatic HIV infection status

This code indicates that a patient has tested positive for HIV but has manifested no signs or symptoms of the disease.

V09   Infection with drug-resistant microorganisms

This category indicates that a patient has an infection that is resistant to drug treatment.

Sequence the infection code first.

V21   Constitutional states in development

V22.2   Pregnant state, incidental

This code is a secondary code only for use when the pregnancy is in no way complicating the reason for visit. Otherwise, a code from the obstetric chapter is required.

V26.5x Sterilization status

V42   Organ or tissue replaced by transplant

V43   Organ or tissue replaced by other means

V44   Artificial opening status

V45   Other postsurgical states

Assign code V45.87, Transplant organ removal status, to indicate that a transplanted organ has been previously removed. This code should not be assigned for the encounter in which the transplanted organ is removed. The complication necessitating removal of the transplant organ should be assigned for that encounter.

See section I.C17.f.2. for information on the coding of organ transplant complications.

Assign code V45.88, Status post administration of tPA (rtPA) in a different facility within the last 24 hours prior to admission to the current facility, as a secondary diagnosis when a patient is received by transfer into a facility and documentation indicates they were administered

tissue plasminogen activator (tPA) within the last 24 hours prior to admission to the current facility.

This guideline applies even if the patient is still receiving the tPA at the time they are received into the current facility.

The appropriate code for the condition for which the tPA was administered (such as cerebrovascular disease or myocardial infarction) should be assigned first.

Code V45.88 is only applicable to the receiving facility record and not to the transferring facility record.

V46   Other dependence on machines

V49.6   Upper limb amputation status

V49.7   Lower limb amputation status

> **Note**: Categories V42-V46, and subcategories V49.6, V49.7 are for use only if there are no complications or malfunctions of the organ or tissue replaced, the amputation site or the equipment on which the patient is dependent.

V49.81   Postmenopausal status

V49.82   Dental sealant status

V49.83   Awaiting organ transplant status

V58.6x   Long-term (current) drug use

> Codes from this subcategory indicates a patient's continuous use of a prescribed drug (including such things as aspirin therapy) for the long-term treatment of a condition or for prophylactic use. It is not for use for patients who have addictions to drugs. **This subcategory is not for use of medications for detoxification or maintenance programs to prevent withdrawal symptoms in patients with drug dependence (e.g., methadone maintenance for opiate dependence). Assign the appropriate code for the drug dependence instead.**
>
> Assign a code from subcategory V58.6, Long-term (current) drug use, if the patient is receiving a medication for an extended period as a prophylactic **measure (such as for the prevention of deep vein thrombosis) or as treatment of a chronic condition (such as arthritis) or a disease requiring a lengthy course of treatment (such as cancer). Do not assign a code from subcategory V58.6 for medication being administered for a brief period of time to treat an acute illness or injury (such as a course of antibiotics to treat acute bronchitis).**

V83   Genetic carrier status

Genetic carrier status indicates that a person carries a gene, associated with a particular disease, which may be passed to offspring who may develop that disease. The person does not have the disease and is not at risk of developing the disease.

V84   Genetic susceptibility status

Genetic susceptibility indicates that a person has a gene that increases the risk of that person developing the disease.

Codes from category V84, Genetic susceptibility to disease, should not be used as principal or first-listed codes. If the patient has the condition to which he/she is susceptible, and that condition is the reason for the encounter, the code for the current condition should be sequenced first. If the patient is being seen for follow-up after completed treatment for this condition, and the condition no longer exists, a follow-up code should be sequenced first, followed by the appropriate personal history and genetic susceptibility codes. If the purpose of the encounter is genetic counseling associated with procreative management, a code from subcategory V26.3, Genetic counseling and testing, should be assigned as the first-listed code, followed by a code from category V84. Additional codes should be assigned for any applicable family or personal history.

See Section I.C. 18.d.14 for information on prophylactic organ removal due to a genetic susceptibility.

V86   Estrogen receptor status

V88   Acquired absence of other organs and tissue

4) History (of)

There are two types of history V codes, personal and family. Personal history codes explain a patient's past medical condition that no longer exists and is not receiving any treatment, but that has the potential for recurrence, and therefore may require continued monitoring. The exceptions to this general rule are category V14, Personal history of allergy to medicinal agents, and subcategory V15.0, Allergy, other than to medicinal agents. A person who has had an allergic episode to a substance or food in the past should always be considered allergic to the substance.

Family history codes are for use when a patient has a family member(s) who has had a particular disease that causes the patient to be at higher risk of also contracting the disease.

Personal history codes may be used in conjunction with follow-up codes and family history codes may be used in conjunction with screening codes to explain the need for a test or procedure. History codes are also acceptable on any medical record regardless of the reason for visit. A history of an illness, even if no longer present, is important information that may alter the type of treatment ordered.

The history V code categories are:

V10   Personal history of malignant neoplasm

V12   Personal history of certain other diseases

V13   Personal history of other diseases

Except: V13.4, Personal history of arthritis, and V13.6, Personal history of congenital malformations. These conditions are life-long so are not true history codes.

V14   Personal history of allergy to medicinal agents

V15   Other personal history presenting hazards to health

Except: V15.7, Personal history of contraception.

V16   Family history of malignant neoplasm

V17   Family history of certain chronic disabling diseases

V18   Family history of certain other specific diseases

V19   Family history of other conditions

V87   Other specified personal exposures and history presenting hazards to health

5) **Screening**

Screening is the testing for disease or disease precursors in seemingly well individuals so that early detection and treatment can be provided for those who test positive for the disease. Screenings that are recommended for many subgroups in a population include: routine mammograms for women over 40, a fecal occult blood test for everyone over 50, an amniocentesis to rule out a fetal anomaly for pregnant women over 35, because the incidence of breast cancer and colon cancer in these subgroups is higher than in the general population, as is the incidence of Down's syndrome in older mothers.

The testing of a person to rule out or confirm a suspected diagnosis because the patient has some sign or symptom is a diagnostic examination, not a screening. In these cases, the sign or symptom is used to explain the reason for the test.

A screening code may be a first listed code if the reason for the visit is specifically the screening exam. It may also be used as an additional code if the screening is done during an office visit for other health problems. A screening code is not necessary if the screening is inherent to a routine examination, such as a pap smear done during a routine pelvic examination.

Should a condition be discovered during the screening then the code for the condition may be assigned as an additional diagnosis.

The V code indicates that a screening exam is planned. A procedure code is required to confirm that the screening was performed.

The screening V code categories:

V28   Antenatal screening

V73-V82   Special screening examinations

6) Observation

There are **three** observation V code categories. They are for use in very limited circumstances when a person is being observed for a suspected condition that is ruled out. The observation codes are not for use if an injury or illness or any signs or symptoms related to the suspected condition are present. In such cases the diagnosis/symptom code is used with the corresponding E code to identify any external cause.

The observation codes are to be used as principal diagnosis only. The only exception to this is when the principal diagnosis is required to be a code from the V30, Live born infant, category. Then the V29 observation code is sequenced after the V30 code. Additional codes may be used in addition to the observation code but only if they are unrelated to the suspected condition being observed.

Codes from subcategory V89.0, Suspected maternal and fetal conditions not found, may either be used as a first listed or as an additional code assignment depending on the case. They are for use in very limited circumstances on a maternal record when an encounter is for a suspected maternal or fetal condition that is ruled out during that encounter (for example, a maternal or fetal condition may be suspected due to an abnormal test result). These codes should not be used when the condition is confirmed. In those cases, the confirmed condition should be coded. In addition, these codes are not for use if an illness or any signs or symptoms related to the suspected condition or problem are present. In such cases the diagnosis/symptom code is used.

Additional codes may be used in addition to the code from subcategory V89.0, but only if they are unrelated to the suspected condition being evaluated.

Codes from subcategory V89.0 may not be used for encounters for antenatal screening of mother. *See Section I.C.18.d., Screening).*

For encounters for suspected fetal condition that are inconclusive following testing and evaluation, assign the appropriate code from category 655, 656, 657 or 658.

The observation V code categories:

V29   Observation and evaluation of newborns for suspected condition not found

For the birth encounter, a code from category V30 should be sequenced before the V29 code.

V71   Observation and evaluation for suspected condition not found

V89   Suspected maternal and fetal conditions not found

7) Aftercare

Aftercare visit codes cover situations when the initial treatment of a disease or injury has been performed and the patient requires continued care during the healing or recovery phase, or for the long-term consequences of the disease. The aftercare V code should not be used if treatment is directed at a current, acute disease or injury. The diagnosis code is to be used in these cases. Exceptions to this rule are codes V58.0, Radiotherapy, and codes from subcategory V58.1, Encounter for chemotherapy and immunotherapy for neoplastic conditions. These codes are to be first listed, followed by the diagnosis code when a patient's encounter is solely to receive radiation therapy or chemotherapy for the treatment of a neoplasm. Should a patient receive both chemotherapy and radiation therapy during the same encounter code V58.0 and V58.1 may be used together on a record with either one being sequenced first.

The aftercare codes are generally first listed to explain the specific reason for the encounter. An aftercare code may be used as an additional code when some type of aftercare is provided in addition to the reason for admission and no diagnosis code is applicable. An example of this would be the closure of a colostomy during an encounter for treatment of another condition.

Aftercare codes should be used in conjunction with any other aftercare codes or other diagnosis codes to provide better detail on the specifics of an aftercare encounter visit, unless otherwise directed by the classification. The sequencing of multiple aftercare codes is discretionary.

Certain aftercare V code categories need a secondary diagnosis code to describe the resolving condition or sequelae, for others, the condition is inherent in the code title.

Additional V code aftercare category terms include, fitting and adjustment, and attention to artificial openings.

Status V codes may be used with aftercare V codes to indicate the nature of the aftercare. For example code V45.81, Aortocoronary bypass status, may be used with code V58.73, Aftercare following surgery of the circulatory system, NEC, to indicate the surgery for which the aftercare is being performed. Also, a transplant status code may be used following code V58.44, Aftercare following organ transplant, to identify the organ transplanted. A status code should not be used when the aftercare code indicates the type of status, such as using V55.0, Attention to tracheostomy with V44.0, Tracheostomy status.

See Section I. B.16 Admissions/Encounter for Rehabilitation

The aftercare V category/codes:

V51   **Encounter for breast reconstruction following mastectomy**

V52   Fitting and adjustment of prosthetic device and implant

V53	Fitting and adjustment of other device
V54	Other orthopedic aftercare
V55	Attention to artificial openings
V56	Encounter for dialysis and dialysis catheter care
V57	Care involving the use of rehabilitation procedures
V58.0	Radiotherapy
V58.11	Encounter for antineoplastic chemotherapy
V58.12	Encounter for antineoplastic immunotherapy
V58.3x	Attention to dressings and sutures
V58.41	Encounter for planned post-operative wound closure
V58.42	Aftercare, surgery, neoplasm
V58.43	Aftercare, surgery, trauma
V58.44	Aftercare involving organ transplant
V58.49	Other specified aftercare following surgery
V58.7x	Aftercare following surgery
V58.81	Fitting and adjustment of vascular catheter
V58.82	Fitting and adjustment of non-vascular catheter
V58.83	Monitoring therapeutic drug
V58.89	Other specified aftercare

8) Follow-up

The follow-up codes are used to explain continuing surveillance following completed treatment of a disease, condition, or injury. They imply that the condition has been fully treated and no longer exists. They should not be confused with aftercare codes that explain current treatment for a healing condition or its sequelae. Follow-up codes may be used in conjunction with history codes to provide the full picture of the healed condition and its treatment. The follow-up code is sequenced first, followed by the history code.

A follow-up code may be used to explain repeated visits. Should a condition be found to have recurred on the follow-up visit, then the diagnosis code should be used in place of the follow-up code.

The follow-up V code categories:

V24	Postpartum care and evaluation
V67	Follow-up examination

9) Donor

Category V59 is the donor codes. They are used for living individuals who are donating blood or other body tissue. These codes are only for individuals donating for others, not for self donations. They are not for use to identify cadaveric donations.

10) Counseling

Counseling V codes are used when a patient or family member receives assistance in the aftermath of an illness or injury, or when support is required in coping with family or social problems. They are not necessary for use in conjunction with a diagnosis code when the counseling component of care is considered integral to standard treatment.

The counseling V categories/codes:

V25.0   General counseling and advice for contraceptive management

V26.3   Genetic counseling

V26.4   General counseling and advice for procreative management

V61.**X**   Other family circumstances

V65.1   Person consulted on behalf of another person

V65.3   Dietary surveillance and counseling

V65.4   Other counseling, not elsewhere classified

11) Obstetrics and related conditions

See Section I.C.11., the Obstetrics guidelines for further instruction on the use of these codes.

V codes for pregnancy are for use in those circumstances when none of the problems or complications included in the codes from the Obstetrics chapter exist (a routine prenatal visit or postpartum care). Codes V22.0, Supervision of normal first pregnancy, and V22.1, Supervision of other normal pregnancy, are always first listed and are not to be used with any other code from the OB chapter.

The outcome of delivery, category V27, should be included on all maternal delivery records. It is always a secondary code.

V codes for family planning (contraceptive) or procreative management and counseling should be included on an obstetric record either during the pregnancy or the postpartum stage, if applicable.

Obstetrics and related conditions V code categories:

V22   Normal pregnancy

V23   Supervision of high-risk pregnancy

Except: V23.2, Pregnancy with history of abortion. Code 646.3, Habitual aborter, from the OB chapter is required to indicate a history of abortion during a pregnancy.

V24   Postpartum care and evaluation

V25   Encounter for contraceptive management

Except V25.0x

(See Section I.C.18.d.11, Counseling)

V26   Procreative management Except V26.5x, Sterilization status, V26.3 and V26.4

(See Section I.C.18.d.11., Counseling)

V27   Outcome of delivery

V28   Antenatal screening

(See Section I.C.18.d.6., Screening)

12) Newborn, infant and child

See Section I.C.15, the Newborn guidelines for further instruction on the use of these codes.

Newborn   V code categories:

V20   Health supervision of infant or child

V29   Observation and evaluation of newborns for suspected condition not found

(See Section I.C.18.d.7, Observation)

V30-V39   Liveborn infant according to type of birth

13) Routine and administrative examinations

The V codes allow for the description of encounters for routine examinations, such as, a general check-up, or, examinations for administrative purposes, such as, a pre-employment physical. The codes are not to be used if the examination is for diagnosis of a suspected condition or for treatment purposes. In such cases the diagnosis code is used. During a routine exam, should a diagnosis or condition be discovered, it should be coded as an additional code. Pre-existing and chronic conditions and history codes may also be included as additional codes as long as the examination is for administrative purposes and not focused on any particular condition.

Pre-operative examination V codes are for use only in those situations when a patient is being cleared for surgery and no treatment is given.

The V codes categories/code for routine and administrative examinations:

V20.2   Routine infant or child health check

Any injections given should have a corresponding procedure code.

V70   General medical examination

V72   Special investigations and examinations

Codes V72.5 and V72.6 may be used if the reason for the patient encounter is for routine laboratory/radiology testing in the absence of any signs, symptoms, or associated diagnosis. If routine testing is performed during the same encounter as a test to evaluate a sign, symptom, or diagnosis, it is appropriate to assign both the V code and the code describing the reason for the non-routine test.

14) Miscellaneous V codes

The miscellaneous V codes capture a number of other health care encounters that do not fall into one of the other categories. Certain of these codes identify the reason for the encounter, others are for use as additional codes that provide useful information on circumstances that may affect a patient's care and treatment.

Prophylactic Organ Removal

For encounters specifically for prophylactic removal of breasts, ovaries, or another organ due to a genetic susceptibility to cancer or a family history of cancer, the principal or first listed code should be a code from subcategory V50.4, Prophylactic organ removal, followed by the appropriate genetic susceptibility code and the appropriate family history code.

If the patient has a malignancy of one site and is having prophylactic removal at another site to prevent either a new primary malignancy or metastatic disease, a code for the malignancy should also be assigned in addition to a code from subcategory V50.4. A V50.4 code should not be assigned if the patient is having organ removal for treatment of a malignancy, such as the removal of the testes for the treatment of prostate cancer.

Miscellaneous V code categories/codes:

V07   Need for isolation and other prophylactic measures

   Except for V07.5, Prophylactic use of agents affecting estrogen receptors and estrogen levels

V50   Elective surgery for purposes other than remedying health states

V58.5   Orthodontics

V60   Housing, household, and economic circumstances

V62   Other psychosocial circumstances

V63   Unavailability of other medical facilities for care

V64   Persons encountering health services for specific procedures, not carried out

V66   Convalescence and Palliative Care

V68   Encounters for administrative purposes

V69   Problems related to lifestyle

V85   Body Mass Index

15) Nonspecific V codes

Certain V codes are so non-specific, or potentially redundant with other codes in the classification, that there can be little justification for their use in the inpatient setting. Their use in the outpatient setting should be limited to those instances when there is no further documentation to permit more precise coding. Otherwise, any sign or symptom or any other reason for visit that is captured in another code should be used.

Nonspecific V code categories/codes:

V11	Personal history of mental disorder A code from the mental disorders chapter, with an in remission fifth-digit, should be used.
V13.4	Personal history of arthritis
V13.6	Personal history of congenital malformations
V15.7	Personal history of contraception
V23.2	Pregnancy with history of abortion
V40	Mental and behavioral problems
V41	Problems with special senses and other special functions
V47	Other problems with internal organs
V48	Problems with head, neck, and trunk
V49	Problems with limbs and other problems

Exceptions:

V49.6	Upper limb amputation status
V49.7	Lower limb amputation status
V49.81	Postmenopausal status
V49.82	Dental sealant status
V49.83	Awaiting organ transplant status

V51.**8**	**Other a**ftercare involving the use of plastic surgery
V58.2	Blood transfusion, without reported diagnosis
V58.9	Unspecified aftercare

See Section IV.K. and Section IV.L. of the Outpatient guidelines.

V CODE TABLE

October 1, 2008 (FY2009)

Items in bold indicate a new entry or change from the October 2007 table Items underlined have been moved within the table since November 2006

The V code table below contains columns for 1st listed, 1st or additional, additional only, and non-specific. Each code or category is listed in the left hand column and the allowable sequencing of the code or codes within the category is noted under the appropriate column.

As indicated by the footnote in the "1st Dx Only" column, the V codes designated as first-listed only are generally intended to be limited for use as a first-listed only diagnosis, but may be reported as an additional diagnosis in those situations when the patient has more than one encounter on a single day and the codes for the multiple encounters are combined, or when there is more than one V code that meets the definition of principal diagnosis (e.g., a patient is admitted to home healthcare for both aftercare and rehabilitation and they equally meet the definition of principal diagnosis). The V codes designated as first-listed only should not be reported if they do not meet the definition of principal or first-listed diagnosis.

See Section II and Section IV.A for information on selection of principal and first-listed diagnosis.

See Section II.C for information on two or more diagnoses that equally meet the definition for principal diagnosis.

Code(s)	Description	1st Dx Only[1]	1st or Add'l Dx[2]	Add'l Dx Only[3]	Non-Specific Diagnosis[4]
V01.X	Contact with or exposure to communicable diseases		X		
V02.X	Carrier or suspected carrier of infectious diseases		X		
V03.X	Need for prophylactic vaccination and inoculation against bacterial diseases		X		
V04.X	Need for prophylactic vaccination and inoculation against certain diseases		X		
V05.X	Need for prophylactic vaccination and inoculation against single diseases		X		
V06.X	Need for prophylactic vaccination and inoculation against combinations of diseases		X		
V07.0	**Isolation**		X		
V07.1	**Desensitization to allergens**		X		
V07.2	**Prophylactic immunotherapy**		X		
V07.3X	**Other prophylactic chemotherapy**		X		
V07.4	**Hormone replacement therapy (postmenopausal)**			X	
V07.5X	**Prophylactic use of agents affecting estrogen receptors and estrogen levels**			X	
V07.8	**Other specified prophylactic measure**		X		
V07.9	**Unspecified prophylactic measure**				X
V08	Asymptomatic HIV infection status		X		
V09.X	Infection with drug resistant organisms			X	
V10.X	Personal history of malignant neoplasm		X		

[1]Generally for use as first listed only but may be used as additional if patient has more than one encounter on one day or there is more than one reason for the encounter

[2]These codes may be used as first listed or additional codes

[3]These codes are only for use as additional codes

[4]These codes are primarily for use in the nonacute setting and should be limited to encounters for which no sign or symptom or reason for visit is documented in the record. Their use may be as either a first listed or additional code.

Code(s)	Description	1st Dx Only[1]	1st or Add'l Dx[2]	Add'l Dx Only[3]	Non-Specific Diagnosis[4]
V11.X	Personal history of mental disorder				X
V12.X	Personal history of certain other diseases		X		
V13.0X	Personal history of other disorders of urinary system		X		
V13.1	Personal history of trophoblastic disease		X		
V13.2X	Personal history of other genital system and obstetric disorders		X		
V13.3	Personal history of diseases of skin and subcutaneous tissue		X		
V13.4	Personal history of arthritis				X
V13.5**X**	Personal history of other musculoskeletal disorders		X		
V13.61	Personal history of hypospadias			X	
V13.69	Personal history of congenital malformations				X
V13.7	Personal history of perinatal problems		X		
V13.8	Personal history of other specified diseases		X		
V13.9	Personal history of unspecified disease				X
V14.X	Personal history of allergy to medicinal agents			X	
V15.0X	Personal history of allergy, other than to medicinal agents			X	
V15.1	Personal history of surgery to heart and great vessels			X	
V15.2X	**Personal history of surgery to other organs**			**X**	
V15.3	Personal history of irradiation			X	
V15.4X	Personal history of psychological trauma			X	
V15.5X	Personal history of injury			X	
V15.6	Personal history of poisoning			X	
V15.7	Personal history of contraception				X
V15.81	Personal history of noncompliance with medical treatment			X	
V15.82	Personal history of tobacco use			X	
V15.84	Personal history of exposure to asbestos			X	
V15.85	Personal history of exposure to potentially hazardous body fluids			X	
V15.86	Personal history of exposure to lead			X	
V15.87	Personal history of extracorporeal membrane oxygenation [ECMO]			X	
V15.88	History of fall		X		
V15.89	Other specified personal history presenting hazards to health			X	
V16.X	Family history of malignant neoplasm		X		
V17.X	Family history of certain chronic disabling diseases		X		
V18.X	Family history of certain other specific conditions		X		
V19.X	Family history of other conditions		X		
V20.X	Health supervision of infant or child	X			
V21.X	Constitutional states in development			X	
V22.0	Supervision of normal first pregnancy	X			
V22.1	Supervision of other normal pregnancy	X			
V22.2	Pregnancy state, incidental			X	
V23.X	Supervision of high-risk pregnancy		X		
V24.X	Postpartum care and examination	X			
V25.X	Encounter for contraceptive management		X		
V26.0	Tuboplasty or vasoplasty after previous sterilization		X		

[1]Generally for use as first listed only but may be used as additional if patient has more than one encounter on one day or there is more than one reason for the encounter

[2]These codes may be used as first listed or additional codes

[3]These codes are only for use as additional codes

[4]These codes are primarily for use in the nonacute setting and should be limited to encounters for which no sign or symptom or reason for visit is documented in the record. Their use may be as either a first listed or additional code.

Code(s)	Description	1st Dx Only[1]	1st or Add'l Dx[2]	Add'l Dx Only[3]	Non-Specific Diagnosis[4]
V26.1	Artificial insemination		X		
V26.2X	Procreative management investigation and testing		X		
V26.3X	Procreative management, genetic counseling and testing		X		
V26.4X	Procreative management, genetic counseling and advice		X		
V26.5X	Procreative management, sterilization status			X	
V26.81	Encounter for assisted reproductive fertility procedure cycle	X			
V26.89	Other specified procreative management		X		
V26.9	Unspecified procreative management		X		
V27.X	Outcome of delivery			X	
V28.X	Encounter for antenatal screening of mother		X		
V29.X	Observation and evaluation of newborns for suspected condition not found		X		
V30.X	Single liveborn	X			
V31.X	Twin, mate liveborn	X			
V32.X	Twin, mate stillborn	X			
V33.X	Twin, unspecified	X			
V34.X	Other multiple, mates all liveborn	X			
V35.X	Other multiple, mates all stillborn	X			
V36.X	Other multiple, mates live- and stillborn	X			
V37.X	Other multiple, unspecified	X			
V39.X	Unspecified	X			
V40.X	Mental and behavioral problems				X
V41.X	Problems with special senses and other special functions				X
V42.X	Organ or tissue replaced by transplant			X	
V43.0	Organ or tissue replaced by other means, eye globe			X	
V43.1	Organ or tissue replaced by other means, lens			X	
V43.21	Organ or tissue replaced by other means, heart assist device			X	
V43.22	Fully implantable artificial heart status		X		
V43.3	Organ or tissue replaced by other means, heart valve			X	
V43.4	Organ or tissue replaced by other means, blood vessel			X	
V43.5	Organ or tissue replaced by other means, bladder			X	
V43.6X	Organ or tissue replaced by other means, joint			X	
V43.7	Organ or tissue replaced by other means, limb			X	
V43.8X	Other organ or tissue replaced by other means			X	
V44.X	Artificial opening status			X	
V45.0X	Cardiac device in situ			X	
V45.1X	Renal dialysis status			X	
V45.2	Presence of cerebrospinal fluid drainage device			X	
V45.3	Intestinal bypass or anastomosis status			X	
V45.4	Arthrodesis status			X	
V45.5X	Presence of contraceptive device			X	
V45.6X	States following surgery of eye and adnexa			X	

[1]Generally for use as first listed only but may be used as additional if patient has more than one encounter on one day or there is more than one reason for the encounter

[2]These codes may be used as first listed or additional codes

[3]These codes are only for use as additional codes

[4]These codes are primarily for use in the nonacute setting and should be limited to encounters for which no sign or symptom or reason for visit is documented in the record. Their use may be as either a first listed or additional code.

Code(s)	Description	1st Dx Only[1]	1st or Add'l Dx[2]	Add'l Dx Only[3]	Non-Specific Diagnosis[4]
V45.7X	Acquired absence of organ		X		
V45.8X	Other postprocedural status			X	
V46.0	Other dependence on machines, aspirator			X	
V46.11	Dependence on respiratory, status			X	
V46.12	Encounter for respirator dependence during power failure	X			
V46.13	Encounter for weaning from respirator [ventilator]	X			
V46.14	Mechanical complication of respirator [ventilator]		X		
V46.2	Other dependence on machines, supplemental oxygen			X	
V46.3	**Wheelchair dependence**			**X**	
V46.8	Other dependence on other enabling machines			X	
V46.9	Unspecified machine dependence				X
V47.X	Other problems with internal organs				X
V48.X	Problems with head, neck and trunk				X
V49.0	Deficiencies of limbs				X
V49.1	Mechanical problems with limbs				X
V49.2	Motor problems with limbs				X
V49.3	Sensory problems with limbs				X
V49.4	Disfigurements of limbs				X
V49.5	Other problems with limbs				X
V49.6X	Upper limb amputation status		X		
V49.7X	Lower limb amputation status		X		
V49.81	Asymptomatic postmenopausal status (age-related) (natural)		X		
V49.82	Dental sealant status			X	
V49.83	Awaiting organ transplant status			X	
V49.84	Bed confinement status		X		
V49.85	Dual sensory impairment			X	
V49.89	Other specified conditions influencing health status		X		
V49.9	Unspecified condition influencing health status				X
V50.X	Elective surgery for purposes other than remedying health states		X		
V51.0	**Encounter for breast reconstruction following mastectomy**	**X**			
V51.8	**Other aftercare involving the use of plastic surgery**				**X**
V52.X	Fitting and adjustment of prosthetic device and implant		X		
V53.X	Fitting and adjustment of other device		X		
V54.X	Other orthopedic aftercare		X		
V55.X	Attention to artificial openings		X		
V56.0	Extracorporeal dialysis	X			
V56.1	Encounter for fitting and adjustment of extracorporeal dialysis catheter		X		
V56.2	Encounter for fitting and adjustment of peritoneal dialysis catheter		X		
V56.3X	Encounter for adequacy testing for dialysis		X		
V56.8	Encounter for other dialysis and dialysis catheter care		X		

[1]Generally for use as first listed only but may be used as additional if patient has more than one encounter on one day or there is more than one reason for the encounter
[2]These codes may be used as first listed or additional codes
[3]These codes are only for use as additional codes
[4]These codes are primarily for use in the nonacute setting and should be limited to encounters for which no sign or symptom or reason for visit is documented in the record. Their use may be as either a first listed or additional code.

Code(s)	Description	1st Dx Only[1]	1st or Add'l Dx[2]	Add'l Dx Only[3]	Non-Specific Diagnosis[4]
V57.X	Care involving use of rehabilitation procedures	X			
V58.0	Radiotherapy	X			
V58.11	Encounter for antineoplastic chemotherapy	X			
V58.12	Encounter for antineoplastic immunotherapy	X			
V58.2	Blood transfusion without reported diagnosis				X
V58.3X	Attention to dressings and sutures		X		
V58.4X	Other aftercare following surgery		X		
V58.5	Encounter for orthodontics				X
V58.6X	Long term (current) drug use			X	
V58.7X	Aftercare following surgery to specified body systems, not elsewhere classified		X		
V58.8X	Other specified procedures and aftercare		X		
V58.9	Unspecified aftercare				X
V59.X	Donors	X			
V60.X	Housing, household, and economic circumstances			X	
V61.X	Other family circumstances		X		
V62.X	Other psychosocial circumstances			X	
V63.X	Unavailability of other medical facilities for care		X		
V64.X	Persons encountering health services for specified procedure, not carried out			X	
V65.X	Other persons seeking consultation without complaint or sickness		X		
V66.0	Convalescence and palliative care following surgery	X			
V66.1	Convalescence and palliative care following radiotherapy	X			
V66.2	Convalescence and palliative care following chemotherapy	X			
V66.3	Convalescence and palliative care following psychotherapy and other treatment for mental disorder	X			
V66.4	Convalescence and palliative care following treatment of fracture	X			
V66.5	Convalescence and palliative care following other treatment	X			
V66.6	Convalescence and palliative care following combined treatment	X			
V66.7	Encounter for palliative care			X	
V66.9	Unspecified convalescence	X			
V67.X	Follow-up examination		X		
V68.X	Encounters for administrative purposes	X			
V69.X	Problems related to lifestyle		X		
V70.0	Routine general medical examination at a health care facility	X			
V70.1	General psychiatric examination, requestedby the authority	X			
V70.2	General psychiatric examination, other and unspecified	X			
V70.3	Other medical examination for administrative purposes	X			

[1]Generally for use as first listed only but may be used as additional if patient has more than one encounter on one day or there is more than one reason for the encounter
[2]These codes may be used as first listed or additional codes
[3]These codes are only for use as additional codes
[4]These codes are primarily for use in the nonacute setting and should be limited to encounters for which no sign or symptom or reason for visit is documented in the record. Their use may be as either a first listed or additional code.

Code(s)	Description	1st Dx Only[1]	1st or Add'l Dx[2]	Add'l Dx Only[3]	Non-Specific Diagnosis[4]
V70.4	Examination for medicolegal reasons	X			
V70.5	Health examination of defined subpopulations	X			
V70.6	Health examination in population surveys	X			
V70.7	Examination of participant in clinical trial		X		
V70.8	Other specified general medical examinations	X			
V70.9	Unspecified general medical examination	X			
V71.X	Observation and evaluation for suspected conditions not found	X			
V72.0	Examination of eyes and vision		X		
V72.1X	Examination of ears and hearing		X		
V72.2	Dental examination		X		
V72.3X	Gynecological examination		X		
V72.4X	Pregnancy examination or test		X		
V72.5	Radiological examination, NEC		X		
V72.6	Laboratory examination		X		
V72.7	Diagnostic skin and sensitization tests		X		
V72.81	Preoperative cardiovascular examination		X		
V72.82	Preoperative respiratory examination		X		
V72.83	Other specified preoperative examination		X		
V72.84	Preoperative examination, unspecified		X		
V72.85	Other specified examination		X		
V72.86	Encounter for blood typing		X		
V72.9	Unspecified examination				X
V73.X	Special screening examination for viral and chlamydial diseases		X		
V74.X	Special screening examination for bacterial and spirochetal diseases		X		
V75.X	Special screening examination for other infectious diseases		X		
V76.X	Special screening examination for malignant neoplasms		X		
V77.X	Special screening examination for endocrine, nutritional, metabolic and immunity disorders		X		
V78.X	Special screening examination for disorders of blood and blood-forming organs		X		
V79.X	Special screening examination for mental disorders and developmental handicaps		X		
V80.X	Special screening examination for neurological, eye, and ear diseases		X		
V81.X	Special screening examination for cardiovascular, respiratory, and genitourinary diseases		X		
V82.X	Special screening examination for other conditions		X		
V83.X	Genetic carrier status		X		
V84.X	Genetic susceptibility to disease			X	
V85	Body mass index			X	
V86	Estrogen receptor status			X	
V87.0X	**Contact with and (suspected) exposure to hazardous metals**		**X**		

[1]Generally for use as first listed only but may be used as additional if patient has more than one encounter on one day or there is more than one reason for the encounter

[2]These codes may be used as first listed or additional codes

[3]These codes are only for use as additional codes

[4]These codes are primarily for use in the nonacute setting and should be limited to encounters for which no sign or symptom or reason for visit is documented in the record. Their use may be as either a first listed or additional code.

Code(s)	Description	1st Dx Only[1]	1st or Add'l Dx[2]	Add'l Dx Only[3]	Non-Specific Diagnosis[4]
V87.1X	Contact with and (suspected) exposure to hazardous aromatic compounds		X		
V87.2	Contact with and (suspected) exposure to other potentially hazardous chemicals		X		
V87.3X	Contact with and (suspected) exposure to other potentially hazardous substances		X		
V87.4X	Personal history of drug therapy			X	
V88.0X	Acquired absence of cervix and uterus			X	
V89.0X	Suspected maternal and fetal anomalies not found		X		

[1]Generally for use as first listed only but may be used as additional if patient has more than one encounter on one day or there is more than one reason for the encounter

[2]These codes may be used as first listed or additional codes

[3]These codes are only for use as additional codes

[4]These codes are primarily for use in the nonacute setting and should be limited to encounters for which no sign or symptom or reason for visit is documented in the record. Their use may be as either a first listed or additional code.

19. Supplemental Classification of External Causes of Injury and Poisoning (E-codes, E800-E999)

Introduction: These guidelines are provided for those who are currently collecting E codes in order that there will be standardization in the process. If your institution plans to begin collecting E codes, these guidelines are to be applied. The use of E codes is supplemental to the application of ICD-9-CM diagnosis codes. E codes are never to be recorded as principal diagnoses (first-listed in non-inpatient setting) and are not required for reporting to CMS.

External causes of injury and poisoning codes (E codes) are intended to provide data for injury research and evaluation of injury prevention strategies. E codes capture how the injury or poisoning happened (cause), the intent (unintentional or accidental; or intentional, such as suicide or assault), and the place where the event occurred.

Some major categories of E codes include:

transport accidents

poisoning and adverse effects of drugs, medicinal substances and biologicals

accidental falls

accidents caused by fire and flames

accidents due to natural and environmental factors

late effects of accidents, assaults or self injury

assaults or purposely inflicted injury

suicide or self inflicted injury

These guidelines apply for the coding and collection of E codes from records in hospitals, outpatient clinics, emergency departments, other ambulatory care settings and provider offices, and nonacute care settings, except when other specific guidelines apply.

a. General E Code Coding Guidelines

1) Used with any code in the range of 001-V89

An E code may be used with any code in the range of 001-**V89**, which indicates an injury, poisoning, or adverse effect due to an external cause.

2) Assign the appropriate E code for all initial treatments

Assign the appropriate E code for the initial encounter of an injury, poisoning, or adverse effect of drugs, not for subsequent treatment.

External cause of injury codes (E-codes) may be assigned while the acute fracture codes are still applicable. *See Section I.C.17.b.1 for coding of acute fractures.*

3) Use the full range of E codes

Use the full range of E codes to completely describe the cause, the intent and the place of occurrence, if applicable, for all injuries, poisonings, and adverse effects of drugs.

4) Assign as many E codes as necessary

Assign as many E codes as necessary to fully explain each cause. If only one E code can be recorded, assign the E code most related to the principal diagnosis.

5) The selection of the appropriate E code

The selection of the appropriate E code is guided by the Index to External Causes, which is located after the alphabetical index to diseases and by Inclusion and Exclusion notes in the Tabular List.

6) E code can never be a principal diagnosis

An E code can never be a principal (first listed) diagnosis.

7) External cause code(s) with systemic inflammatory response syndrome (SIRS)

An external cause code is not appropriate with a code from subcategory 995.9, unless the patient also has an injury, poisoning, or adverse effect of drugs.

b. Place of Occurrence Guideline

Use an additional code from category E849 to indicate the Place of Occurrence for injuries and poisonings. The Place of Occurrence describes the place where the event occurred and not the patient's activity at the time of the event.

Do not use E849.9 if the place of occurrence is not stated.

c. Adverse Effects of Drugs, Medicinal and Biological Substances Guidelines

1) Do not code directly from the Table of Drugs

Do not code directly from the Table of Drugs and Chemicals.

Always refer back to the Tabular List.

2) Use as many codes as necessary to describe

Use as many codes as necessary to describe completely all drugs, medicinal or biological substances.

3)   If the same E code would describe the causative agent

If the same E code would describe the causative agent for more than one adverse reaction, assign the code only once.

4)   If two or more drugs, medicinal or biological substances

If two or more drugs, medicinal or biological substances are reported, code each individually unless the combination code is listed in the Table of Drugs and Chemicals. In that case, assign the E code for the combination.

5)   When a reaction results from the interaction of a drug(s)

When a reaction results from the interaction of a drug(s) and alcohol, use poisoning codes and E codes for both.

6)   If the reporting format limits the number of E codes

If the reporting format limits the number of E codes that can be used in reporting clinical data, code the one most related to the principal diagnosis. Include at least one from each category (cause, intent, place) if possible.

If there are different fourth digit codes in the same three digit category, use the code for "Other specified" of that category. If there is no "Other specified" code in that category, use the appropriate "Unspecified" code in that category.

If the codes are in different three digit categories, assign the appropriate E code for other multiple drugs and medicinal substances.

7)   Codes from the E930-E949 series

Codes from the E930-E949 series must be used to identify the causative substance for an adverse effect of drug, medicinal and biological substances, correctly prescribed and properly administered. The effect, such as tachycardia, delirium, gastrointestinal hemorrhaging, vomiting, hypokalemia, hepatitis, renal failure, or respiratory failure, is coded and followed by the appropriate code from the E930-E949 series.

d. Multiple Cause E Code Coding Guidelines

If two or more events cause separate injuries, an E code should be assigned for each cause. The first listed E code will be selected in the following order:

E codes for child and adult abuse take priority over all other E codes.

See Section I.C.19.e., Child and Adult abuse guidelines.

E codes for terrorism events take priority over all other E codes except child and adult abuse

E codes for cataclysmic events take priority over all other E codes except child and adult abuse and terrorism.

E codes for transport accidents take priority over all other E codes except cataclysmic events and child and adult abuse and terrorism.

The first-listed E code should correspond to the cause of the most serious diagnosis due to an assault, accident, or self-harm, following the order of hierarchy listed above.

e. Child and Adult Abuse Guideline

1) Intentional injury

When the cause of an injury or neglect is intentional child or adult abuse, the first listed E code should be assigned from categories E960-E968, Homicide and injury purposely inflicted by other persons, (except category E967). An E code from category E967, Child and adult battering and other maltreatment, should be added as an additional code to identify the perpetrator, if known.

2) Accidental intent

In cases of neglect when the intent is determined to be accidental E code E904.0, Abandonment or neglect of infant and helpless person, should be the first listed E code.

f. Unknown or Suspected Intent Guideline

1) If the intent (accident, self-harm, assault) of the cause of an injury or poisoning is unknown

If the intent (accident, self-harm, assault) of the cause of an injury or poisoning is unknown or unspecified, code the intent as undetermined E980-E989.

2) If the intent (accident, self-harm, assault) of the cause of an injury or poisoning is questionable

If the intent (accident, self-harm, assault) of the cause of an injury or poisoning is questionable, probable or suspected, code the intent as undetermined E980-E989.

g. Undetermined Cause

When the intent of an injury or poisoning is known, but the cause is unknown, use codes: E928.9, Unspecified accident, E958.9, Suicide and self-inflicted injury by unspecified means, and E968.9, Assault by unspecified means.

These E codes should rarely be used, as the documentation in the medical record, in both the inpatient outpatient and other settings, should normally provide sufficient detail to determine the cause of the injury.

h. Late Effects of External Cause Guidelines

1) Late effect E codes

Late effect E codes exist for injuries and poisonings but not for adverse effects of drugs, misadventures and surgical complications.

2) Late effect E codes (E929, E959, E969, E977, E989, or E999.1)

A late effect E code (E929, E959, E969, E977, E989, or E999.1) should be used with any report of a late effect or sequela resulting from a previous injury or poisoning (905-909).

3) Late effect E code with a related current injury

A late effect E code should never be used with a related current nature of injury code.

4) Use of late effect E codes for subsequent visits

Use a late effect E code for subsequent visits when a late effect of the initial injury or poisoning is being treated. There is no late effect E code for adverse effects of drugs. Do not use a late effect E code for subsequent visits for follow-up care (e.g., to assess healing, to receive rehabilitative therapy) of the injury or poisoning when no late effect of the injury has been documented.

i. Misadventures and Complications of Care Guidelines

1) Code range E870-E876

Assign a code in the range of E870-E876 if misadventures are stated by the provider.

2) Code range E878-E879

Assign a code in the range of E878-E879 if the provider attributes an abnormal reaction or later complication to a surgical or medical procedure, but does not mention misadventure at the time of the procedure as the cause of the reaction.

j. Terrorism Guidelines

1) Cause of injury identified by the Federal Government (FBI) as terrorism

When the cause of an injury is identified by the Federal Government (FBI) as terrorism, the first-listed E-code should be a code from category E979, Terrorism. The definition of terrorism employed by the FBI is found at the inclusion note at E979. The terrorism E-code is the only E-code that should be assigned. Additional E codes from the assault categories should not be assigned.

2) Cause of an injury is suspected to be the result of terrorism

When the cause of an injury is suspected to be the result of terrorism a code from category E979 should not be assigned. Assign a code in the range of E codes based circumstances on the documentation of intent and mechanism.

3) Code E979.9, Terrorism, secondary effects

Assign code E979.9, Terrorism, secondary effects, for conditions occurring subsequent to the terrorist event. This code should not be assigned for conditions that are due to the initial terrorist act.

4) Statistical tabulation of terrorism codes

For statistical purposes these codes will be tabulated within the category for assault, expanding the current category from E960-E969 to include E979 and E999.1.

SECTION II. SELECTION OF PRINCIPAL DIAGNOSIS

The circumstances of inpatient admission always govern the selection of principal diagnosis. The principal diagnosis is defined in the Uniform Hospital Discharge Data Set (UHDDS) as "that condition established after study to be chiefly responsible for occasioning the admission of the patient to the hospital for care."

The UHDDS definitions are used by hospitals to report inpatient data elements in a standardized manner. These data elements and their definitions can be found in the July 31, 1985, Federal Register (Vol. 50, No, 147), pp. 31038-40.

Since that time the application of the UHDDS definitions has been expanded to include all non-outpatient settings (acute care, short term, long term care and psychiatric hospitals; home health agencies; rehab facilities; nursing homes, etc).

In determining principal diagnosis the coding conventions in the ICD-9-CM, Volumes I and II take precedence over these official coding guidelines.

(See Section I.A., Conventions for the ICD-9-CM)

The importance of consistent, complete documentation in the medical record cannot be overemphasized. Without such documentation the application of all coding guidelines is a difficult, if not impossible, task.

A. Codes for symptoms, signs, and ill-defined conditions

Codes for symptoms, signs, and ill-defined conditions from Chapter 16 are not to be used as principal diagnosis when a related definitive diagnosis has been established.

B. Two or more interrelated conditions, each potentially meeting the definition for principal diagnosis.

When there are two or more interrelated conditions (such as diseases in the same ICD-9-CM chapter or manifestations characteristically associated with a certain disease) potentially meeting the definition of principal diagnosis, either condition may be sequenced first, unless the circumstances of the admission, the therapy provided, the Tabular List, or the Alphabetic Index indicate otherwise.

C. Two or more diagnoses that equally meet the definition for principal diagnosis

In the unusual instance when two or more diagnoses equally meet the criteria for principal diagnosis as determined by the circumstances of admission, diagnostic workup and/or therapy provided, and the Alphabetic Index, Tabular List, or another coding guidelines does not provide sequencing direction, any one of the diagnoses may be sequenced first.

D. Two or more comparative or contrasting conditions.

In those rare instances when two or more contrasting or comparative diagnoses are documented as "either/or" (or similar terminology), they are coded as if the diagnoses were confirmed and the diagnoses are sequenced according to the circumstances of the admission. If no further determination can be made as to which diagnosis should be principal, either diagnosis may be sequenced first.

E. A symptom(s) followed by contrasting/comparative diagnoses

When a symptom(s) is followed by contrasting/comparative diagnoses, the symptom code is sequenced first. All the contrasting/comparative diagnoses should be coded as additional diagnoses.

F. Original treatment plan not carried out

Sequence as the principal diagnosis the condition, which after study occasioned the admission to the hospital, even though treatment may not have been carried out due to unforeseen circumstances.

G. Complications of surgery and other medical care

When the admission is for treatment of a complication resulting from surgery or other medical care, the complication code is sequenced as the principal diagnosis. If the complication is classified to the 996-999 series and the code lacks the necessary specificity in describing the complication, an additional code for the specific complication should be assigned.

H. Uncertain Diagnosis

If the diagnosis documented at the time of discharge is qualified as "probable", "suspected", "likely", "questionable", "possible", or "still to be ruled out", or other similar terms indicating uncertainty, code the condition as if it existed or was established. The bases for these guidelines are the diagnostic workup, arrangements for further workup or observation, and initial therapeutic approach that correspond most closely with the established diagnosis.

Note: This guideline is applicable only to <u>inpatient admissions to</u> short-term, acute, long-term care and psychiatric hospitals.

I. Admission from Observation Unit

1. Admission Following Medical Observation

When a patient is admitted to an observation unit for a medical condition, which either worsens or does not improve, and is subsequently admitted as an inpatient of the same hospital for this same medical condition, the principal diagnosis would be the medical condition which led to the hospital admission.

2. Admission Following Post-Operative Observation

When a patient is admitted to an observation unit to monitor a condition (or complication) that develops following outpatient surgery, and then is subsequently admitted as an inpatient of the same hospital, hospitals should apply the Uniform Hospital Discharge Data Set (UHDDS) definition of principal diagnosis as "that condition established after study to be chiefly responsible for occasioning the admission of the patient to the hospital for care."

J. Admission from Outpatient Surgery

When a patient receives surgery in the hospital's outpatient surgery department and is subsequently admitted for continuing inpatient care at the same hospital, the following guidelines should be followed in selecting the principal diagnosis for the inpatient admission:

- If the reason for the inpatient admission is a complication, assign the complication as the principal diagnosis.

- If no complication, or other condition, is documented as the reason for the inpatient admission, assign the reason for the outpatient surgery as the principal diagnosis.

- If the reason for the inpatient admission is another condition unrelated to the surgery, assign the unrelated condition as the principal diagnosis.

SECTION III. REPORTING ADDITIONAL DIAGNOSES

GENERAL RULES FOR OTHER (ADDITIONAL) DIAGNOSES
For reporting purposes the definition for "other diagnoses" is interpreted as additional conditions that affect patient care in terms of requiring:

clinical evaluation; or
therapeutic treatment; or
diagnostic procedures; or
extended length of hospital stay; or
increased nursing care and/or monitoring.

The UHDDS item #11-b defines Other Diagnoses as "all conditions that coexist at the time of admission, that develop subsequently, or that affect the treatment received and/or the length of stay. Diagnoses that relate to an earlier episode which have no bearing on the current hospital stay are to be excluded." UHDDS definitions apply to inpatients in acute care, short-term, long term care and psychiatric hospital setting. The UHDDS definitions are used by acute care short-term hospitals to report inpatient data elements in a standardized manner. These data elements and their definitions can be found in the July 31, 1985, Federal Register (Vol. 50, No, 147), pp. 31038-40.

Since that time the application of the UHDDS definitions has been expanded to include all non-outpatient settings (acute care, short term, long term care and psychiatric hospitals; home health agencies; rehab facilities; nursing homes, etc).

The following guidelines are to be applied in designating "other diagnoses" when neither the Alphabetic Index nor the Tabular List in ICD-9-CM provide direction. The listing of the diagnoses in the patient record is the responsibility of the attending provider.

A. Previous conditions

If the provider has included a diagnosis in the final diagnostic statement, such as the discharge summary or the face sheet, it should ordinarily be coded. Some providers include in the diagnostic statement resolved conditions or diagnoses and status-post procedures from previous admission that have no bearing on the current stay. Such conditions are not to be reported and are coded only if required by hospital policy.

However, history codes (V10-V19) may be used as secondary codes if the historical condition or family history has an impact on current care or influences treatment.

B. Abnormal findings

Abnormal findings (laboratory, x-ray, pathologic, and other diagnostic results) are not coded and reported unless the provider indicates their clinical significance. If the findings are outside the normal range and the attending provider has ordered other tests to evaluate the condition or prescribed treatment, it is appropriate to ask the provider whether the abnormal finding should be added.

Please note: This differs from the coding practices in the outpatient setting for coding encounters for diagnostic tests that have been interpreted by a provider.

C. Uncertain Diagnosis

If the diagnosis documented at the time of discharge is qualified as "probable", "suspected", "likely", "questionable", "possible", or "still to be ruled out" or other similar terms indicating uncertainty, code the condition as if it existed or was established. The bases for these guidelines are the diagnostic workup, arrangements for further workup or observation, and initial therapeutic approach that correspond most closely with the established diagnosis.

Note: This guideline is applicable only to <u>inpatient admissions to</u> short-term, acute, long-term care and psychiatric hospitals.

SECTION IV. DIAGNOSTIC CODING AND REPORTING GUIDELINES FOR OUTPATIENT SERVICES

These coding guidelines for outpatient diagnoses have been approved for use by hospitals/providers in coding and reporting hospital-based outpatient services and provider-based office visits.

Information about the use of certain abbreviations, punctuation, symbols, and other conventions used in the ICD-9-CM Tabular List (code numbers and titles), can be found in Section IA of these guidelines, under "Conventions Used in the Tabular List." Information about the correct sequence to use in finding a code is also described in Section I.

The terms encounter and visit are often used interchangeably in describing outpatient service contacts and, therefore, appear together in these guidelines without distinguishing one from the other.

Though the conventions and general guidelines apply to all settings, coding guidelines for outpatient and provider reporting of diagnoses will vary in a number of instances from those for inpatient diagnoses, recognizing that:

The Uniform Hospital Discharge Data Set (UHDDS) definition of principal diagnosis applies only to inpatients in acute, short-term, long-term care and psychiatric hospitals.

Coding guidelines for inconclusive diagnoses (probable, suspected, rule out, etc.) were developed for inpatient reporting and do not apply to outpatients.

A. Selection of first-listed condition

In the outpatient setting, the term first-listed diagnosis is used in lieu of principal diagnosis.

In determining the first-listed diagnosis the coding conventions of ICD-9-CM, as well as the general and disease specific guidelines take precedence over the outpatient guidelines.

Diagnoses often are not established at the time of the initial encounter/visit. It may take two or more visits before the diagnosis is confirmed.

The most critical rule involves beginning the search for the correct code assignment through the Alphabetic Index. Never begin searching initially in the Tabular List as this will lead to coding errors.

1. Outpatient Surgery

When a patient presents for outpatient surgery, code the reason for the surgery as the first-listed diagnosis (reason for the encounter), even if the surgery is not performed due to a contraindication.

2. Observation Stay

When a patient is admitted for observation for a medical condition, assign a code for the medical condition as the first-listed diagnosis.

When a patient presents for outpatient surgery and develops complications requiring admission to observation, code the reason for the surgery as the first reported diagnosis (reason for the encounter), followed by codes for the complications as secondary diagnoses.

B. Codes from 001.0 through V89

The appropriate code or codes from 001.0 through **V89** must be used to identify diagnoses, symptoms, conditions, problems, complaints, or other reason(s) for the encounter/visit.

C. Accurate reporting of ICD-9-CM diagnosis codes

For accurate reporting of ICD-9-CM diagnosis codes, the documentation should describe the patient's condition, using terminology which includes specific diagnoses as well as symptoms, problems, or reasons for the encounter. There are ICD-9-CM codes to describe all of these.

D. Selection of codes 001.0 through 999.9

The selection of codes 001.0 through 999.9 will frequently be used to describe the reason for the encounter. These codes are from the section of ICD-9-CM for the classification of diseases and injuries (e.g. infectious and parasitic diseases; neoplasms; symptoms, signs, and ill-defined conditions, etc.).

E. Codes that describe symptoms and signs

Codes that describe symptoms and signs, as opposed to diagnoses, are acceptable for reporting purposes when a diagnosis has not been established (confirmed) by the provider. Chapter 16 of ICD-9-CM, Symptoms, Signs, and Ill-defined conditions (codes 780.0-799.9) contain many, but not all codes for symptoms.

F. Encounters for circumstances other than a disease or injury

ICD-9-CM provides codes to deal with encounters for circumstances other than a disease or injury. The Supplementary Classification of factors Influencing Health Status and Contact with Health Services (V01.0-**V89**) is provided to deal with occasions when circumstances other than a disease or injury are recorded as diagnosis or problems. ***See Section I.C. 18 for information on V-codes***

G. Level of Detail in Coding

1. ICD-9-CM codes with 3, 4, or 5 digits

ICD-9-CM is composed of codes with either 3, 4, or 5 digits. Codes with three digits are included in ICD-9-CM as the heading of a category of codes that may be further subdivided by the use of fourth and/or fifth digits, which provide greater specificity.

2. Use of full number of digits required for a code

A three-digit code is to be used only if it is not further subdivided. Where fourth-digit subcategories and/or fifth-digit subclassifications are provided, they must be assigned. A code is invalid if it has not been coded to the full number of digits required for that code.

See also discussion under Section I.b.3., General Coding Guidelines, Level of Detail in Coding.

H. ICD-9-CM code for the diagnosis, condition, problem, or other reason for encounter/visit

List first the ICD-9-CM code for the diagnosis, condition, problem, or other reason for encounter/visit shown in the medical record to be chiefly responsible for the services provided. List additional codes that describe any coexisting conditions. In some cases the first-listed diagnosis may be a symptom when a diagnosis has not been established (confirmed) by the physician.

I. Uncertain diagnosis

Do not code diagnoses documented as "probable", "suspected," "questionable," "rule out," or "working diagnosis" or other similar terms indicating uncertainty. Rather, code the condition(s) to the highest degree of certainty for that encounter/visit, such as symptoms, signs, abnormal test results, or other reason for the visit. **Please note:** This differs from the coding practices used by short-term, acute care, long-term care and psychiatric hospitals.

J. Chronic diseases

Chronic diseases treated on an ongoing basis may be coded and reported as many times as the patient receives treatment and care for the condition(s)

K. Code all documented conditions that coexist

Code all documented conditions that coexist at the time of the encounter/visit, and require or affect patient care treatment or management. Do not code conditions that were previously treated and no longer exist. However, history codes (V10-V19) may be used as secondary codes if the historical condition or family history has an impact on current care or influences treatment.

L. Patients receiving diagnostic services only

For patients receiving diagnostic services only during an encounter/visit, sequence first the diagnosis, condition, problem, or other reason for encounter/visit shown in the medical record to be chiefly responsible for the outpatient services provided during the encounter/visit. Codes for other diagnoses (e.g., chronic conditions) may be sequenced as additional diagnoses.

For encounters for routine laboratory/radiology testing in the absence of any signs, symptoms, or associated diagnosis, assign V72.5 and V72.6. If routine testing is performed during the same encounter as a test to evaluate a sign, symptom, or diagnosis, it is appropriate to assign both the V code and the code describing the reason for the non-routine test.

For outpatient encounters for diagnostic tests that have been interpreted by a physician, and the final report is available at the time of coding, code any confirmed or definitive diagnosis(es) documented in the interpretation. Do not code related signs and symptoms as additional diagnoses.

Please note: This differs from the coding practice in the hospital inpatient setting regarding abnormal findings on test results.

M. Patients receiving therapeutic services only

For patients receiving therapeutic services only during an encounter/visit, sequence first the diagnosis, condition, problem, or other reason for encounter/visit shown in the medical record to be chiefly responsible for the outpatient services provided during the encounter/visit. Codes for other diagnoses (e.g., chronic conditions) may be sequenced as additional diagnoses.

The only exception to this rule is that when the primary reason for the admission/encounter is chemotherapy, radiation therapy, or rehabilitation, the appropriate V code for the service is listed first, and the diagnosis or problem for which the service is being performed listed second.

N. Patients receiving preoperative evaluations only

For patients receiving preoperative evaluations only, sequence **first** a code from category V72.8, Other specified examinations, to describe the pre-op consultations. Assign a code for the condition to describe the reason for the surgery as an additional diagnosis. Code also any findings related to the pre-op evaluation.

O. Ambulatory surgery

For ambulatory surgery, code the diagnosis for which the surgery was performed. If the postoperative diagnosis is known to be different from the preoperative diagnosis at the time the diagnosis is confirmed, select the postoperative diagnosis for coding, since it is the most definitive.

P. Routine outpatient prenatal visits

For routine outpatient prenatal visits when no complications are present, codes V22.0, Supervision of normal first pregnancy, or V22.1, Supervision of other normal pregnancy, should be used as the principal diagnosis. These codes should not be used in conjunction with chapter 11 codes.

APPENDIX I PRESENT ON ADMISSION REPORTING GUIDELINES

Introduction

These guidelines are to be used as a supplement to the *ICD-9-CM Official Guidelines for Coding and Reporting* to facilitate the assignment of the Present on Admission (POA) indicator for each diagnosis and external cause of injury code reported on claim forms (UB-04 and 837 Institutional).

These guidelines are not intended to replace any guidelines in the main body of the *ICD-9-CM Official Guidelines for Coding and Reporting*. The POA guidelines are not intended to provide guidance on when a condition should be coded, but rather, how to apply the POA indicator to the final set of diagnosis codes that have been assigned in accordance with Sections I, II, and III of the official coding guidelines. Subsequent to the assignment of the ICD-9-CM codes, the POA indicator should then be assigned to those conditions that have been coded.

As stated in the Introduction to the ICD-9-CM Official Guidelines for Coding and Reporting, a joint effort between the healthcare provider and the coder is essential to achieve complete and accurate documentation, code assignment, and reporting of diagnoses and procedures. The importance of consistent, complete documentation in the medical record cannot be overemphasized. Medical record documentation from any provider involved in the care and treatment of the patient may be used to support the determination of whether a condition was present on admission or not. In the context of the official coding guidelines, the term "provider" means a physician or any qualified healthcare practitioner who is legally accountable for establishing the patient's diagnosis. **These guidelines are not a substitute for the provider's clinical judgment as to the determination of whether a condition was/was not present on admission. The provider should be queried regarding**

issues related to the linking of signs/symptoms, timing of test results, and the timing of findings.

General Reporting Requirements

All claims involving inpatient admissions to general acute care hospitals or other facilities that are subject to a law or regulation mandating collection of present on admission information.

Present on admission is defined as present at the time the order for inpatient admission occurs – conditions that develop during an outpatient encounter, including emergency department, observation, or outpatient surgery, are considered as present on admission.

POA indicator is assigned to principal and secondary diagnoses (as defined in Section II of the Official Guidelines for Coding and Reporting) and the external cause of injury codes.

Issues related to inconsistent, missing, conflicting or unclear documentation must still be resolved by the provider.

If a condition would not be coded and reported based on UHDDS definitions and current official coding guidelines, then the POA indicator would not be reported.

Reporting Options
Y – Yes
N – No
U – Unknown
W – Clinically undetermined
Unreported/Not used **(or "1" for Medicare usage)** – (Exempt from POA reporting)

For more specific instructions on Medicare POA indicator reporting options, refer to http://www.cms.hhs.gov/HospitalAcqCond/02_Statute_Regulations_Program_Instructions.asp#TopOfPage

Reporting Definitions
Y = present at the time of inpatient admission N = not present at the time of inpatient admission U = documentation is insufficient to determine if condition is present on admission W = provider is unable to clinically determine whether condition was present on admission or not

Timeframe for POA Identification and Documentation

There is no required timeframe as to when a provider (per the definition of "provider" used in these guidelines) must identify or document a condition to be present on admission. In some clinical situations, it may not be possible for a provider to make a definitive diagnosis (or a condition may not be recognized or reported by the patient) for a period of time after admission. In some cases it may be several days before the provider arrives at a definitive diagnosis. This does not mean that the condition was not present on admission. Determination of whether the condition was present on admission or not will be based on the applicable POA guideline as identified in this document, or on the provider's best clinical judgment.

If at the time of code assignment the documentation is unclear as to whether a condition was present on admission or not, it is appropriate to query the provider for clarification.

Assigning the POA Indicator

Condition is on the "Exempt from Reporting" List

Leave the "present on admission" field blank if the condition is on the list of ICD-9-CM codes for which this field is not applicable. This is the only circumstance in which the field may be left blank.

POA Explicitly Documented

Assign Y for any condition the provider explicitly documents as being present on admission.

Assign N for any condition the provider explicitly documents as not present at the time of admission.

Conditions Diagnosed Prior to Inpatient Admission

Assign "Y" for conditions that were diagnosed prior to admission (example: hypertension, diabetes mellitus, asthma)

Conditions Diagnosed During the Admission but Clearly Present Before Admission

Assign "Y" for conditions diagnosed during the admission that were clearly present but not diagnosed until after admission occurred.

Diagnoses subsequently confirmed after admission are considered present on admission if at the time of admission they are documented as suspected, possible, rule out, differential diagnosis, or constitute an underlying cause of a symptom that is present at the time of admission.

Condition Develops During Outpatient Encounter Prior to Inpatient Admission

Assign Y for any condition that develops during an outpatient encounter prior to a written order for inpatient admission.

Documentation does not Indicate Whether Condition was Present on Admission

Assign "U" when the medical record documentation is unclear as to whether the condition was present on admission. "U" should not be routinely assigned and used only in very limited circumstances. Coders are encouraged to query the providers when the documentation is unclear.

Documentation States That It Cannot be Determined Whether the Condition Was or Was Not Present on Admission

Assign "W" when the medical record documentation indicates that it cannot be clinically determined whether or not the condition was present on admission.

Chronic Condition with Acute Exacerbation During the Admission

If the code is a combination code that identifies both the chronic condition and the acute exacerbation, see POA guidelines pertaining to combination codes.

If the combination code only identifies the chronic condition and not the acute exacerbation (e.g., acute exacerbation of CHF), assign "Y."

Conditions Documented as Possible, Probable, Suspected, or Rule out At the Time of Discharge

If the final diagnosis contains a possible, probable, suspected, or rule out diagnosis, and this diagnosis was suspected at the time of inpatient admission, assign "Y."

If the final diagnosis contains a possible, probable, suspected, or rule out diagnosis, and this diagnosis was based on symptoms or clinical findings that were not present on admission, assign "N".

Conditions Documented as Impending or Threatened at the Time of Discharge

If the final diagnosis contains an impending or threatened diagnosis, and this diagnosis is based on symptoms or clinical findings that were present on admission, assign "Y".

If the final diagnosis contains an impending or threatened diagnosis, and this diagnosis is based on symptoms or clinical findings that were **not** present on admission, assign "N".

Acute and Chronic Conditions

Assign "Y" for acute conditions that are present at time of admission and N for acute conditions that are not present at time of admission.

Assign "Y" for chronic conditions, even though the condition may not be diagnosed until after admission.

If a single code identifies both an acute and chronic condition, see the POA guidelines for combination codes.

Combination Codes

Assign "N" if any part of the combination code was not present on admission (e.g., obstructive chronic bronchitis with acute exacerbation and the exacerbation was not present on admission; gastric ulcer that does not start bleeding until after admission; asthma patient develops status asthmaticus after admission)

Assign "Y" if all parts of the combination code were present on admission (e.g., patient with diabetic nephropathy is admitted with uncontrolled diabetes)

If the final diagnosis includes comparative or contrasting diagnoses, and both were present, or suspected, at the time of admission, assign "Y".

For infection codes that include the causal organism, assign "Y" if the infection (or signs of the infection) was present on admission, even though the culture results may not be known until after admission (e.g., patient is admitted with pneumonia and the provider documents pseudomonas as the causal organism a few days later).

Same Diagnosis Code for Two or More Conditions

When the same ICD-9-CM diagnosis code applies to two or more conditions during the same encounter (e.g. bilateral condition, or two separate conditions classified to the same ICD-9-CM diagnosis code):

Assign "Y" if all conditions represented by the single ICD-9-CM code were present on admission (e.g. bilateral fracture of the same bone, same site, and both fractures were present on admission)

Assign "N" if any of the conditions represented by the single ICD-9-CM code was not present on admission (e.g. dehydration with hyponatremia is assigned to code 276.1, but only one of these conditions was present on admission).

Obstetrical Conditions

Whether or not the patient delivers during the current hospitalization does not affect assignment of the POA indicator. The determining factor for POA assignment is whether the pregnancy complication or obstetrical condition described by the code was present at the time of admission or not.

If the pregnancy complication or obstetrical condition was present on admission (e.g., patient admitted in preterm labor), assign "Y".

If the pregnancy complication or obstetrical condition was not present on admission (e.g., 2nd degree laceration during delivery, postpartum hemorrhage that occurred during current hospitalization, fetal distress develops after admission), assign "N".

If the obstetrical code includes more than one diagnosis and any of the diagnoses identified by the code were not present on admission assign "N".

(e.g., Code 642.7, Pre-eclampsia or eclampsia superimposed on pre-existing hypertension).

If the obstetrical code includes information that is not a diagnosis, do not consider that information in the POA determination.

(e.g. Code 652.1x, Breech or other malpresentation successfully converted to cephalic presentation should be reported as present on admission if the fetus was breech on admission but was converted to cephalic presentation after admission (since the conversion to cephalic presentation does not represent a diagnosis, the fact that the conversion occurred after admission has no bearing on the POA determination).

Perinatal Conditions

Newborns are not considered to be admitted until after birth. Therefore, any condition present at birth or that developed in utero is considered present at admission and should be assigned "Y". This includes conditions that occur during delivery (e.g., injury during delivery, meconium aspiration, exposure to streptococcus B in the vaginal canal).

Congenital Conditions and Anomalies

Assign "Y" for congenital conditions and anomalies. Congenital conditions are always considered present on admission.

External Cause of Injury Codes

Assign "Y" for any E code representing an external cause of injury or poisoning that occurred prior to inpatient admission (e.g., patient fell out of bed at home, patient fell out of bed in emergency room prior to admission)

Assign "N" for any E code representing an external cause of injury or poisoning that occurred during inpatient hospitalization (e.g., patient fell out of hospital bed during hospital stay, patient experienced an adverse reaction to a medication administered after inpatient admission)

CATEGORIES AND CODES EXEMPT FROM DIAGNOSIS PRESENT ON ADMISSION REQUIREMENT

Effective Date: October 1, 2008

Note: "Diagnosis present on admission" for these code categories are exempt because they represent circumstances regarding the healthcare encounter or factors influencing health status that do not represent a current disease or injury or are always present on admission

137-139, Late effects of infectious and parasitic diseases

268.1, Rickets, late effect

326, Late effects of intracranial abscess or pyogenic infection

412, Old myocardial infarction

438, Late effects of cerebrovascular disease

650, Normal delivery

660.7, Failed forceps or vacuum extractor, unspecified

677, Late effect of complication of pregnancy, childbirth, and the puerperium

905-909, Late effects of injuries, poisonings, toxic effects, and other external causes

V02, Carrier or suspected carrier of infectious diseases

V03, Need for prophylactic vaccination and inoculation against bacterial diseases

V04, Need for prophylactic vaccination and inoculation against certain viral diseases

V05, Need for other prophylactic vaccination and inoculation against single diseases

V06, Need for prophylactic vaccination and inoculation against combinations of diseases

V07, Need for isolation and other prophylactic measures

V10, Personal history of malignant neoplasm

V11, Personal history of mental disorder

V12, Personal history of certain other diseases

V13, Personal history of other diseases

V14, Personal history of allergy to medicinal agents

V15.01-V15.09, Other personal history, Allergy, other than to medicinal agents

V15.1, Other personal history, Surgery to heart and great vessels

V15.2, Other personal history, Surgery to other major organs

V15.3, Other personal history, Irradiation

V15.4, Other personal history, Psychological trauma

V15.5, Other personal history, Injury

V15.6, Other personal history, Poisoning

V15.7, Other personal history, Contraception

V15.81, Other personal history, Noncompliance with medical treatment

V15.82, Other personal history, History of tobacco use

V15.88, Other personal history, History of fall

V15.89, Other personal history, Other

V15.9 Unspecified personal history presenting hazards to health

V16, Family history of malignant neoplasm

V17, Family history of certain chronic disabling diseases

V18, Family history of certain other specific conditions

V19, Family history of other conditions

V20, Health supervision of infant or child

V21, Constitutional states in development

V22, Normal pregnancy

V23, Supervision of high-risk pregnancy

V24, Postpartum care and examination

V25, Encounter for contraceptive management

V26, Procreative management

V27, Outcome of delivery

V28, Antenatal screening

V29, Observation and evaluation of newborns for suspected condition not found

V30-V39, Liveborn infants according to type of birth

V42, Organ or tissue replaced by transplant

V43, Organ or tissue replaced by other means

V44, Artificial opening status

V45, Other postprocedural states

V46, Other dependence on machines

V49.60-V49.77, Upper and lower limb amputation status

V49.81-V49.84, Other specified conditions influencing health status

V50, Elective surgery for purposes other than remedying health states

V51, Aftercare involving the use of plastic surgery

V52, Fitting and adjustment of prosthetic device and implant

V53, Fitting and adjustment of other device

V54, Other orthopedic aftercare

V55, Attention to artificial openings

V56, Encounter for dialysis and dialysis catheter care

V57, Care involving use of rehabilitation procedures

V58, Encounter for other and unspecified procedures and aftercare

V59, Donors

V60, Housing, household, and economic circumstances

V61, Other family circumstances

V62, Other psychosocial circumstances

V64, Persons encountering health services for specific procedures, not carried out

V65, Other persons seeking consultation

V66, Convalescence and palliative care

V67, Follow-up examination

V68, Encounters for administrative purposes

V69, Problems related to lifestyle

V70, General medical examination

V71, Observation and evaluation for suspected condition not found

V72, Special investigations and examinations

V73, Special screening examination for viral and chlamydial diseases

V74, Special screening examination for bacterial and spirochetal diseases

V75, Special screening examination for other infectious diseases

V76, Special screening for malignant neoplasms

V77, Special screening for endocrine, nutritional, metabolic, and immunity disorders

V78, Special screening for disorders of blood and blood-forming organs

V79, Special screening for mental disorders and developmental handicaps

V80, Special screening for neurological, eye, and ear diseases

V81, Special screening for cardiovascular, respiratory, and genitourinary diseases

V82, Special screening for other conditions

V83, Genetic carrier status

V84, Genetic susceptibility to disease

V85, Body Mass Index

V86, Estrogen receptor status

V87.4, Personal history of drug therapy

V88, Acquired absence of cervix and uterus

V89, Suspected maternal and fetal conditions not found

E800-E807, Railway accidents

E810-E819, Motor vehicle traffic accidents

E820-E825, Motor vehicle nontraffic accidents

E826-E829, Other road vehicle accidents

E830-E838, Water transport accidents

E840-E845, Air and space transport accidents

E846-E848, Vehicle accidents not elsewhere classifiable

E849.0-E849.6, Place of occurrence

E849.8-E849.9, Place of occurrence

E883.1, Accidental fall into well

E883.2, Accidental fall into storm drain or manhole

E884.0, Fall from playground equipment

E884.1, Fall from cliff

E885.0, Fall from (nonmotorized) scooter

E885.1, Fall from roller skates

E885.2, Fall from skateboard

E885.3, Fall from skis

E885.4, Fall from snowboard

E886.0, Fall on same level from collision, pushing, or shoving, by or with other person, In sports

E890.0-E89.9, Conflagration in private dwelling

E893.0, Accident caused by ignition of clothing, from controlled fire in private dwelling

E893.2, Accident caused by ignition of clothing, from controlled fire not in building or structure

E894, Ignition of highly inflammable material

E895, Accident caused by controlled fire in private dwelling

E897, Accident caused by controlled fire not in building or structure

E898.0-E898.1, Accident caused by other specified fire and flames

E917.0, Striking against or struck accidentally by objects or persons, in sports without subsequent fall

E917.1, Striking against or struck accidentally by objects or persons, caused by a crowd, by collective fear or panic without subsequent fall

E917.2, Striking against or struck accidentally by objects or persons, in running water without subsequent fall

E917.5, Striking against or struck accidentally by objects or persons, object in sports with subsequent fall

E917.6, Striking against or struck accidentally by objects or persons, caused by a crowd, by collective fear or panic with subsequent fall

E919.0-E919.1, Accidents caused by machinery

E919.3-E919.9, Accidents caused by machinery

E921.0-E921.9, Accident caused by explosion of pressure vessel

E922.0-E922.9, Accident caused by firearm and air gun missile

E924.1, Caustic and corrosive substances

E926.2, Visible and ultraviolet light sources

E927, Overexertion and strenuous movements

E928.0-E928.8, Other and unspecified environmental and accidental causes

E929.0-E929.9, Late effects of accidental injury

E959, Late effects of self-inflicted injury

E970-E978, Legal intervention

E979, Terrorism

E981.0-E981.8, Poisoning by gases in domestic use, undetermined whether accidentally or purposely inflicted

E982.0-E982.9, Poisoning by other gases, undetermined whether accidentally or purposely inflicted

E985.0-E985.7, Injury by firearms, air guns and explosives, undetermined whether accidentally or purposely inflicted

E987.0, Falling from high place, undetermined whether accidentally or purposely inflicted, residential premises

E987.2, Falling from high place, undetermined whether accidentally or purposely inflicted, natural sites

E989, Late effects of injury, undetermined whether accidentally or purposely inflicted

E990-E999, Injury resulting from operations of war

POA EXAMPLES

General Medical Surgical

1. Patient is admitted for diagnostic work-up for cachexia. The final diagnosis is malignant neoplasm of lung with metastasis.

   Assign "Y" on the POA field for the malignant neoplasm. The malignant neoplasm was clearly present on admission, although it was not diagnosed until after the admission occurred.

2. A patient undergoes outpatient surgery. During the recovery period, the patient develops atrial fibrillation and the patient is subsequently admitted to the hospital as an inpatient.

   Assign "Y" on the POA field for the atrial fibrillation since it developed prior to a written order for inpatient admission.

3. A patient is treated in observation and while in Observation, the patient falls out of bed and breaks a hip. The patient is subsequently admitted as an inpatient to treat the hip fracture.

   Assign "Y" on the POA field for the hip fracture since it developed prior to a written order for inpatient admission.

4. A patient with known congestive heart failure is admitted to the hospital after he develops decompensated congestive heart failure.

   Assign "Y" on the POA field for the congestive heart failure. The ICD-9-CM code identifies the chronic condition and does not specify the acute exacerbation.

5. A patient undergoes inpatient surgery. After surgery, the patient develops fever and is treated aggressively. The physician's final diagnosis documents "possible postoperative infection following surgery."

   Assign "N" on the POA field for the postoperative infection since final diagnoses that contain the terms "possible", "probable", "suspected" or "rule out" and that are based on symptoms or clinical findings that were not present on admission should be reported as "N".

6. A patient with severe cough and difficulty breathing was diagnosed during his hospitalization to have lung cancer.

   Assign "Y" on the POA field for the lung cancer. Even though the cancer was not diagnosed until after admission, it is a chronic condition that was clearly present before the patient's admission.

7. A patient is admitted to the hospital for a coronary artery bypass surgery. Postoperatively he developed a pulmonary embolism.

   Assign "N" on the POA field for the pulmonary embolism. This is an acute condition that was not present on admission.

8. A patient is admitted with a known history of coronary atherosclerosis, status post myocardial infarction five years ago is now admitted for treatment of impending myocardial infarction. The final diagnosis is documented as "impending myocardial infarction."

   Assign "Y" to the impending myocardial infarction because the condition is present on admission.

9. A patient with diabetes mellitus developed uncontrolled diabetes on day 3 of the hospitalization.

   Assign "N" to the diabetes code because the "uncontrolled" component of the code was not present on admission.

10. A patient is admitted with high fever and pneumonia. The patient rapidly deteriorates and becomes septic. The discharge diagnosis lists sepsis and pneumonia. The documentation is unclear as to whether the sepsis was present on admission or developed shortly after admission.

    Query the physician as to whether the sepsis was present on admission, developed shortly after admission, or it cannot be clinically determined as to whether it was present on admission or not.

11. A patient is admitted for repair of an abdominal aneurysm. However, the aneurysm ruptures after hospital admission.

    Assign "N" for the ruptured abdominal aneurysm. Although the aneurysm was present on admission, the "ruptured" component of the code description did not occur until after admission.

12. A patient with viral hepatitis B progresses to hepatic coma after admission.

    Assign "N" for the viral hepatitis B with hepatic coma because part of the code description did not develop until after admission.

13. A patient with a history of varicose veins and ulceration of the left lower extremity strikes the area against the side of his hospital bed during an inpatient hospitalization. It bleeds profusely. The final diagnosis lists varicose veins with ulcer and hemorrhage.

    Assign "Y" for the varicose veins with ulcer. Although the hemorrhage occurred after admission, the code description for varicose veins with ulcer does not mention hemorrhage.

14. The nursing initial assessment upon admission documents the presence of a decubitus ulcer. There is no mention of the decubitus ulcer in the physician documentation until several days after admission.

    Query the physician as to whether the decubitus ulcer was present on admission, or developed after admission. Both diagnosis code assignment and determination of whether a condition was present on admission must be based on provider documentation in the medical record (per the definition of "provider" found at the beginning of these POA guidelines and in the introductory section of the ICD-9-CM Official Guidelines for Coding and Reporting). If it cannot be determined from the provider documentation whether or not a condition was present on admission, the provider should be queried.

15. **A urine culture is obtained on admission. The provider documents urinary tract infection when the culture results become available a few days later.**

    Assign "Y" to the urinary tract infection since the diagnosis is based on test results from a specimen obtained on admission. It may not be possible for a provider to make a definitive diagnosis for a period of time after admission. There is no required timeframe as to when a provider must identify or document a condition to be present on admission.

16. **A patient tested positive for Methicillin resistant Staphylococcus (MRSA) on routine nasal culture on admission to the hospital. During the hospitalization, he underwent insertion of a central venous catheter and later developed an infection and was diagnosed with MRSA sepsis due to central venous catheter infection.**

    Assign "Y" to the positive MRSA colonization. Assign "N" for the MRSA sepsis due to central venous catheter infection since the patient did not have a MRSA infection at the time of admission.

Obstetrics

1. A female patient was admitted to the hospital and underwent a normal delivery.

Leave the "present on admission" (POA) field blank. Code 650, Normal delivery, is on the "exempt from reporting" list.

2. Patient admitted in late pregnancy due to excessive vomiting and dehydration. During admission patient goes into premature labor

   Assign "Y" for the excessive vomiting and the dehydration.

   Assign "N" for the premature labor

3. Patient admitted in active labor. During the stay, a breast abscess is noted when mother attempted to breast feed. Provider is unable to determine whether the abscess was present on admission

   Assign "W" for the breast abscess.

4. Patient admitted in active labor. After 12 hours of labor it is noted that the infant is in fetal distress and a Cesarean section is performed

   Assign "N" for the fetal distress.

5. **Pregnant female was admitted in labor and fetal nuchal cord entanglement was diagnosed. Physician is queried, but is unable to determine whether the cord entanglement was present on admission or not.**

   Assign "W" for the fetal nuchal cord entanglement.

Newborn

1. A single liveborn infant was delivered in the hospital via Cesarean section. The physician documented fetal bradycardia during labor in the final diagnosis in the newborn record.

   Assign " Y" because the bradycardia developed prior to the newborn admission (birth).

2. A newborn developed diarrhea which was believed to be due to the hospital baby formula.

   Assign " N" because the diarrhea developed after admission.

3. **A newborn born in the hospital, birth complicated by nuchal cord entanglement.**

   Assign "Y" for the nuchal cord entanglement on the baby's record. Any condition that is present at birth or that developed in utero is considered present at admission, including conditions that occur during delivery.

Medical Terminology

ablation	removal or destruction by cutting, chemicals, or electrocautery
abortion	termination of pregnancy
absence	without
actinotherapy	treatment of acne using ultraviolet rays
adenoidectomy	removal of adenoids
adipose	fatty
adrenals	glands, located at the top of the kidneys, that produce steroid hormones
albinism	lack of color pigment
allograft	homograft, same species graft
alopecia	condition in which hair falls out
amniocentesis	percutaneous aspiration of amniotic fluid
amniotic sac	sac containing the fetus and amniotic fluid
A-mode	one-dimensional ultrasonic display reflecting the time it takes a sound wave to reach a structure and reflect back; maps the structure's outline
anastomosis	surgical connection of two tubular structures, such as two pieces of the intestine
aneurysm	abnormal dilation of vessels, usually an artery
angina	sudden pain
angiography	radiography of the blood vessels
angioplasty	procedure in a vessel to dilate the vessel opening
anhidrosis	deficiency of sweat
anomaloscope	instrument used to test color vision
anoscopy	procedure that uses a scope to examine the anus
antepartum	before childbirth
anterior (ventral)	in front of
anterior segment	those parts of the eye in the front of and including the lens, orbit, extraocular muscles, and eyelid

anteroposterior	from front to back
antigen	a substance that produces a specific response
aortography	radiographic recording of the aorta
apex cardiography	recording of the movement of the chest wall
aphakia	absence of the lens of the eye
apicectomy	excision of a portion of the temporal bone
apnea	cessation of breathing
arthrocentesis	injection and/or aspiration of joint
arthrodesis	surgical immobilization of joint
arthrography	radiography of joint
arthroplasty	reshaping or reconstruction of joint
arthroscopy	use of scope to view inside joint
arthrotomy	incision into a joint
articular	pertains to joint
asphyxia	lack of oxygen
aspiration	use of a needle and a syringe to withdraw fluid
assignment	Medicare's payment for the service, which participating physicians agree to accept as payment in full
asthma	shortage of breath caused by contraction of bronchi
astigmatism	condition in which the refractive surfaces of the eye are unequal
atelectasis	incomplete expansion of lung, collapse
atherectomy	removal of plaque by percutaneous method
atrophy	wasting away
audiometry	hearing test
aural atresia	congenital absence of the external auditory canal
auscultation	listening to sounds within the body
autograft	from patient's own body
avulsion	ripping or tearing away of part either surgically or accidentally
axillary nodes	lymph nodes located in the armpit
bacilli	plural of bacillus, a rod-shaped bacterium
barium enema	radiographic contrast medium
beneficiary	person who benefits from health or life insurance
bifocal	two focuses in eyeglasses, one usually for close work and the other for improvement of distance vision
bilaminate skin	skin substitute usually made of silicone-covered nylon mesh
bilateral	occurring on two sides
biliary	refers to gallbladder, bile, or bile duct
bilobectomy	surgical removal of two lobes of a lung
biofeedback	process of giving a person self-information

biometry	application of a statistical measure to a biologic fact
biopsy	removal of a small piece of living tissue for diagnostic purposes
block	frozen piece of a sample
brachytherapy	therapy using radioactive sources that are placed inside the body
bronchiole	smaller division of bronchial tree
bronchography	radiographic recording of the lungs
bronchoplasty	surgical repair of the bronchi
bronchoscopy	inspection of the bronchial tree using a bronchoscope
B-scan	two-dimensional display of tissues and organs
bulbocavernosus	muscle that constricts the vagina in a female and the urethra in a male
bulbourethral	gland with duct leading to the urethra
bundle of His	muscular cardiac fibers that provide the heart rhythm to the ventricles; blockage of this rhythm produces heart block
bundled codes	one code that represents a package of services
bunion	hallux valgus, abnormal increase in size of metatarsal head that results in displacement of the great toe
burr	drill used to create an entry into the cranium
bursa	fluid-filled sac that absorbs friction
bursitis	inflammation of bursa (joint sac)
bypass	to go around
calcaneal	pertaining to the heel bone
calculus	concretion of mineral salts, also called a stone
calycoplasty	surgical reconstruction of a recess of the renal pelvis
calyx	recess of the renal pelvis
cancellous	lattice-type structure, usually of bone
cardiopulmonary	refers to the heart and lungs
cardiopulmonary bypass	blood bypasses the heart through a heart-lung machine
cardioversion	electrical shock to the heart to restore normal rhythm
cardioverter-defibrillator	surgically placed device that directs an electrical shock to the heart to restore rhythm
carotid body	located on each side of the common carotid artery, often a site of tumor
cartilage	connective tissue
cataract	opaque covering on or in the lens
catheter	tube placed into the body to put fluid in or take fluid out
caudal	same as inferior; away from the head, or the lower part of the body

causalgia	burning pain
cauterization	destruction of tissue by the use of cautery
cavernosa	connection between the cavity of the penis and a vein
cavernosography	radiographic recording of a cavity, e.g., the pulmonary cavity or the main part of the penis
cavernosometry	measurement of the pressure in a cavity, e.g., the penis
central nervous system	brain and spinal cord
cervical	pertaining to the neck or to the cervix of the uterus
cervix uteri	rounded, cone-shaped neck of the uterus
cesarean	surgical opening through abdominal wall for delivery
cholangiography	radiographic recording of the bile ducts
cholangiopancreatography	ERCP, radiographic recording of the biliary system or pancreas
cholecystectomy	surgical removal of the gallbladder
cholecystoenterostomy	creation of a connection between the gallbladder and intestine
cholecystography	radiographic recording of the gallbladder
cholesteatoma	tumor that forms in middle ear
chondral	referring to the cartilage
chordee	condition resulting in the penis being bent downward
chorionic villus sampling	CVS, biopsy of the outermost part of the placenta
circumflex	a coronary artery that circles the heart
Cloquet's node	also called a gland; it is the highest of the deep groin lymph nodes
closed fracture repair	not surgically opened with/without manipulation and with/without traction
closed treatment	fracture site that is not surgically opened and visualized
coccyx	caudal extremity of vertebral column
collagen	protein substance of skin
Colles' fracture	fracture at lower end of radius that displaces the bone posteriorly
colonoscopy	fiberscopic examination of the entire colon that may include part of the terminal ileum
colostomy	artificial opening between the colon and the abdominal wall
component	part
computed axial tomography	CAT or CT, procedure by which selected planes of tissue are pinpointed through computer enhancement, and images may be reconstructed by analysis of variance in absorption of the tissue
conjunctiva	the lining of the eyelids and the covering of the sclera
contraction	drawn together

contralateral	opposite side
cordectomy	surgical removal of the vocal cord(s)
cordocentesis	procedure to obtain a fetal blood sample; also called a percutaneous umbilical blood sampling
corneosclera	cornea and sclera of the eye
corpectomy	removal of vertebrae
corpora cavernosa	the two cavities of the penis
corpus uteri	uterus
crackle	abnormal sound when breathing (heard on auscultation)
craniectomy	permanent, partial removal of skull
craniotomy	opening of the skull
cranium	that part of the skeleton that encloses the brain
curettage	scraping of a cavity using a spoon-shaped instrument
curette	spoon-shaped instrument used to scrape a cavity
cutdown	incision into a vessel for placement of a catheter
cyanosis	bluish discoloration
cystocele	herniation of the bladder into the vagina
cystography	radiographic recording of the urinary bladder
cystolithectomy	removal of a calculus (stone) from the urinary bladder
cystolithotomy	cystolithectomy
cystometrogram	CMG, measurement of the pressures and capacity of the urinary bladder
cystoplasty	surgical reconstruction of the bladder
cystorrhaphy	suture of the bladder
cystoscopy	use of a scope to view the bladder
cystostomy	surgical creation of an opening into the bladder
cystotomy	incision into the bladder
cystourethroplasty	surgical reconstruction of the bladder and urethra
cystourethroscopy	use of a scope to view the bladder and urethra
dacryocystography	radiographic recording of the lacrimal sac or tear duct sac
dacryostenosis	narrowing of the lacrimal duct
debridement	cleansing of or removal of dead tissue from a wound
deductible	amount the patient is liable for before the payer begins to pay for covered services
delayed flap	pedicle of skin with blood supply that is separated from origin over time
delivery	childbirth
dermabrasion	planing of the skin by means of sander, brush, or sandpaper

dermatologist	physician who treats conditions of the skin
dermatoplasty	surgical repair of skin
dialysis	filtration of blood
dilation	expansion
diskectomy	removal of a vertebral disk
diskography	radiographic recording of an intervertebral joint
dislocation	placement in a location other than the original location
distal	farther from the point of attachment or origin
diverticulum	protrusion in the wall of an organ
Doppler	ultrasonic measure of blood movement
dosimetry	scientific calculation of radiation emitted from various radioactive sources
drainage	free flow or withdrawal of fluids from a wound or cavity
duodenography	radiographic recording of the duodenum or first part of the small intestine
dysphagia	difficulty swallowing
dysphonia	speech impairment
dyspnea	shortness of breath, difficult breathing
dysuria	painful urination
echocardiography	radiographic recording of the heart or heart walls or surrounding tissues
echoencephalography	ultrasound of the brain
echography	ultrasound procedure in which sound waves are bounced off an internal organ and the resulting image is recorded
ectopic	pregnancy outside the uterus (i.e., in the fallopian tube)
edema	swelling due to abnormal fluid collection in the tissue spaces
elective surgery	nonemergency procedure
electrocardiogram	ECG, written record of the electrical action of the heart
electrocautery	cauterization by means of heated instrument
electrocochleography	test to measure the eighth cranial nerve (hearing test)
electrode	lead attached to a generator that carries the electrical current from the generator to the atria or ventricles
electroencephalogram	EEG, written record of the electrical action of the brain
electromyogram	EMG, written record of the electrical activity of the skeletal muscles
electronic claim submission	claims prepared and submitted via a computer
electronic signature	identification system of a computer
electro-oculogram	EOG, written record of the electrical activity of the eye

electrophysiology	study of the electrical system of the heart, including the study of arrhythmias
embolectomy	removal of blockage (embolism) from vessel
emphysema	air accumulated in organ or tissue
encephalography	radiographic recording of the subarachnoid space and ventricles of the brain
endarterectomy	incision into an artery to remove the inner lining so as to eliminate disease or blockage
endomyocardial	pertaining to the inner and middle layers of the heart
endopyelotomy	procedure involving the bladder and ureters, including the insertion of a stent into the renal pelvis
endoscopy	inspection of body organs or cavities using a lighted scope that may be inserted through an existing opening or through a small incision
enterolysis	releasing of adhesions of intestine
enucleation	removal of an organ or organs from a body cavity
epicardial	over the heart
epidermolysis	loosening of the epidermis
epidermomycosis	superficial fungal infection
epididymectomy	surgical removal of the epididymis
epididymis	tube located at the top of the testes that stores sperm
epididymography	radiographic recording of the epididymis
epididymovasostomy	creation of a new connection between the vas deferens and epididymis
epiglottidectomy	excision of the covering of the larynx
episclera	connective covering of sclera
epistaxis	nose bleed
epithelium	surface covering of internal and external organs of the body
erythema	redness of skin
escharotomy	surgical incision into necrotic (dead) tissue
eventration	protrusion of the bowel through an opening in the abdomen
evisceration	pulling the viscera outside of the body through an incision
evocative	tests that are administered to evoke a predetermined response
exenteration	removal of an organ all in one piece
exophthalmos	protrusion of the eyeball
exostosis	bony growth
exstrophy	condition in which an organ is turned inside out
extracorporeal	occurring outside of the body
false aneurysm	sac of clotted blood that has completely destroyed the vessel and is being contained by the tissue that surrounds the vessel

fasciectomy	removal of a band of fibrous tissue
Federal Register	official publication of all "Presidential Documents," "Rules and Regulations," "Proposed Rules," and "Notices"; government-instituted national changes are published in the *Federal Register*
fee schedule	services and payment allowed for each service
femoral	pertaining to the bone from the pelvis to knee
fenestration	creation of a new opening in the inner wall of the middle ear
fissure	cleft or groove
fistula	abnormal opening from one area to another area or to the outside of the body
fluoroscopy	procedure for viewing the interior of the body using x-rays and projecting the image onto a television screen
fracture	break in a bone
free full-thickness graft	graft of epidermis and dermis that is completely removed from donor area
fulguration	use of electrical current to destroy tissue
fundoplasty	repair of the bottom of the bladder
furuncle	nodule in the skin caused by *Staphylococci* entering through hair follicle
ganglion	knot
gastrointestinal	pertaining to the stomach and intestine
gastroplasty	operation on the stomach for repair or reconfiguration
gastrostomy	artificial opening between the stomach and the abdominal wall
gatekeeper	a physician who manages a patient's access to health care
glaucoma	eye diseases that are characterized by an increase of intraocular pressure
globe	eyeball
glottis	true vocal cords
gonioscopy	use of a scope to examine the angles of the eye
Group Practice Model	an organization of physicians who contract with a Health Maintenance Organization to provide services to the enrollees of the HMO
grouper	computer used to input the principal diagnosis and other critical information about a patient and then provide the correct DRG code
Health Maintenance Organization	HMO, a healthcare delivery system in which an enrollee is assigned a primary care physician who manages all the healthcare needs of the enrollee
hematoma	mass of blood that forms outside the vessel
hemodialysis	cleansing of the blood outside of the body
hemolysis	breakdown of red blood cells

hemoptysis	bloody sputum
hepatography	radiographic recording of the liver
hernia	organ or tissue protruding through the wall or cavity that usually contains it
histology	study of structure of tissue and cells
homograft	allograft, same species graft
hormone	chemical substance produced by the body's endocrine glands
hydrocele	sac of fluid
hyperopia	farsightedness, eyeball is too short from front to back
hypogastric	lowest middle abdominal area
hyposensitization	decreased sensitivity
hypothermia	low body temperature; sometimes induced during surgical procedures
hypoxemia	low level of oxygen in the blood
hypoxia	low level of oxygen in the tissue
hysterectomy	surgical removal of the uterus
hysterorrhaphy	suturing of the uterus
hysterosalpingography	radiographic recording of the uterine cavity and fallopian tubes
hysteroscopy	visualization of the canal and cavity of the uterus using a scope placed through the vagina
ichthyosis	skin disorder characterized by scaling
ileostomy	artificial opening between the ileum and the abdominal wall
ilium	portion of hip
imbrication	overlapping
immunotherapy	therapy to increase immunity
incarcerated	regarding hernias, a constricted, irreducible hernia that may cause obstruction of an intestine
incise	to cut into
Individual Practice Association	IPA, an organization of physicians who provide services for a set fee; Health Maintenance Organizations often contract with the IPA for services to their enrollees
inferior	away from the head or the lower part of the body; also known as caudalingual
inguinofemoral	referring to the groin and thigh
inofemoral	referring to the groin and thigh
internal/external fixation	application of pins, wires, and/or screws placed externally or internally to immobilize a body part
intracardiac	inside the heart

intramural	within the organ wall
intramuscular	into a muscle
intrauterine	inside the uterus
intravenous	into a vein
intravenous pyelography	IVP, radiographic recording of the urinary system
introitus	opening or entrance to the vagina from the uterus
intubation	insertion of a tube
intussusception	slipping of one part of the intestine into another part
invasive	entering the body, breaking skin
iontophoresis	introduction of ions into the body
ischemia	deficient blood supply due to obstruction of the circulatory system
island pedicle flap	contains a single artery and vein that remains attached to origin temporarily or permanently
isthmus	connection of two regions or structures
isthmus, thyroid	tissue connection between right and left thyroid lobes
isthmusectomy	surgical removal of the isthmus
jejunostomy	artificial opening between the jejunum and the abdominal wall
jugular nodes	lymph nodes located next to the large vein in the neck
keratomalacia	softening of the cornea associated with a deficiency of vitamin A
keratoplasty	surgical repair of the cornea
Kock pouch	surgical creation of a urinary bladder from a segment of the ileum
kyphosis	humpback
labyrinth	inner connecting cavities, such as the internal ear
labyrinthitis	inner ear inflammation
lacrimal	related to tears
lamina	flat plate
laminectomy	surgical excision of the lamina
laparoscopy	exploration of the abdomen and pelvic cavities using a scope placed through a small incision in the abdominal wall
laryngeal web	congenital abnormality of connective tissue between the vocal cords
laryngectomy	surgical removal of the larynx
laryngography	radiographic recording of the larynx
laryngoplasty	surgical repair of the larynx
laryngoscope	fiberoptic scope used to view the inside of the larynx

laryngoscopy	direct visualization and examination of the interior of larynx with a laryngoscope
laryngotomy	incision into the larynx
lateral	away from the midline of the body (to the side)
lavage	washing out
leukoderma	depigmentation of skin
leukoplakia	white patch on mucous membrane
ligament	fibrous band of tissue that connects cartilage or bone
ligation	binding or tying off, as in constricting the blood flow of a vessel or binding fallopian tubes for sterilization
lipocyte	fat cell
lipoma	fatty tumor
lithotomy	incision into an organ or a duct for the purpose of removing a stone
lithotripsy	crushing of a stone by sound waves or force
lobectomy	surgical excision of lobe of the lung
lordosis	anterior curve of spine
lumbodynia	pain in the lumbar area
lunate	one of the wrist (carpal) bones
lymph node	station along the lymphatic system
lymphadenectomy	excision of a lymph node or nodes
lymphadenitis	inflammation of a lymph node
lymphangiography	radiographic recording of the lymphatic vessels and nodes
lymphangiotomy	incision into a lymphatic vessel
lysis	releasing
magnetic resonance imaging	MRI, procedure that uses nonionizing radiation to view the body in a cross-sectional view
Major Diagnostic Categories	MDC, the division of all principal diagnoses into 25 mutually exclusive principal diagnosis areas within the DRG system
mammography	radiographic recording of the breasts
Managed Care Organization	MCO, a group that is responsible for the health care services offered to an enrolled group of persons
manipulation	movement by hand
manipulation or reduction	alignment of a fracture or joint dislocation to its normal position
mastoidectomy	removal of the mastoid bone
Maximum Actual Allowable Charge	MAAC, limitation on the total amount that can be charged by physicians who are not participants in Medicare
meatotomy	surgical enlargement of the opening of the urinary meatus

medial	toward the midline of the body
Medical Volume Performance Standards	MVPS, government's estimate of how much growth is appropriate for nationwide physician expenditures paid by the Part B Medicare program
Medicare Economic Index	MEI, government mandated index that ties increases in the Medicare prevailing charges to economic indicators
Medicare Fee Schedule	MFS, schedule that listed the allowable charges for Medicare services; was replaced by the Medicare reasonable charge payment system
Medicare Risk HMO	a Medicare-funded alternative to the standard Medicare supplemental coverage
melanin	dark pigment of skin
melanoma	tumor of epidermis, malignant and black in color
Ménière's disease	condition that causes dizziness, ringing in the ears, and deafness
M-mode	one-dimensional display of movement of structures
modality	treatment method
Mohs' surgery or Mohs' micrographic surgery	removal of skin cancer in layers by a surgeon who also acts as pathologist during surgery
monofocal	eyeglasses with one vision correction
multipara	more than one pregnancy
muscle	organ of contraction for movement
muscle flap	transfer of muscle from origin to recipient site
myasthenia gravis	syndrome characterized by muscle weakness
myelography	radiographic recording of the subarachnoid space of the spine
myopia	nearsightedness, eyeball too long from front to back
myringotomy	incision into tympanic membrane
nasal button	synthetic circular disk used to cover a hole in the nasal septum
nasopharyngoscopy	use of a scope to visualize the nose and pharynx
National Provider Identifier	NPI, a 10-digit number assigned to a physician by Medicare
nephrectomy, paraperitoneal	kidney transplant
nephrocutaneous fistula	a channel from the kidney to the skin
nephrolithotomy	removal of a kidney stone through an incision made into the kidney
nephrorrhaphy	suturing of the kidney
nephrostolithotomy	creation of an artificial channel to the kidney
nephrostolithotomy, percutaneous	procedure to establish an artificial channel between the skin and the kidney
nephrostomy	creation of a channel into the renal pelvis of the kidney
nephrostomy, percutaneous	creation of a channel from the skin to the renal pelvis

nephrotomy	incision into the kidney
neurovascular flap	contains artery, vein, and nerve
noninvasive	not entering the body, not breaking skin
nuclear cardiology	diagnostic specialty that uses radiologic procedures to aid in diagnosis of cardiologic conditions
nystagmus	rapid involuntary eye movements
ocular adnexa	orbit, extraocular muscles, and eyelid
olecranon	elbow bone
Omnibus Budget Reconciliation Act of 1989	OBRA, act that established new rules for Medicare reimbursement
oophorectomy	surgical removal of the ovary(ies)
opacification	area that has become opaque (milky)
open fracture repair	surgical opening (incision) over or remote opening as access to a fracture site
open treatment	fracture site that is surgically opened and visualized
ophthalmodynamometry	test of the blood pressure of the eye
ophthalmology	body of knowledge regarding the eyes
ophthalmoscopy	examination of the interior of the eye by means of a scope, also known as funduscopy
optokinetic	movement of the eyes to objects moving in the visual field
orchiectomy	castration, removal of the testes
orchiopexy	surgical procedure to release undescended testes and fixate them within the scrotum
order	shows subordination of one thing to another; family or class
orthopnea	difficulty in breathing, needing to be in erect position to breathe
orthoptic	corrective; in the correct place
osteoarthritis	degenerative condition of articular cartilage
osteoclast	absorbs or removes bone
osteotomy	cutting into bone
otitis media	noninfectious inflammation of the middle ear; serous otitis media produces liquid drainage (not purulent) and suppurative otitis media produces purulent (pus) matter
otoscope	instrument used to examine the internal and external ear
oviduct	fallopian tube
papilledema	swelling of the optic disk (papilla)
paraesophageal hiatus hernia	hernia that is near the esophagus
parathyroid	produces a hormone to mobilize calcium from the bones to the blood
paronychia	infection around nail

Part A	Medicare's Hospital Insurance; covers hospital/facility care
Part B	Medicare's Supplemental Medical Insurance; covers physician services and durable medical equipment that are not paid for under Part A
participating provider program	Medicare providers who have agreed in advance to accept assignment on all Medicare claims, now termed Quality Improvement Organizations (QIO)
patella	knee cap
pedicle	growth attached with a stem
Peer Review Organizations	PROs, groups established to review hospital admission and care
pelviolithotomy	pyeloplasty
penoscrotal	referring to the penis and scrotum
percussion	tapping with sharp blows as a diagnostic technique
percutaneous	through the skin
percutaneous fracture repair	repair of a fracture by means of pins and wires inserted through the fracture site
percutaneous skeletal fixation	considered neither open nor closed; the fracture is not visualized, but fixation is placed across the fracture site under x-ray imaging
pericardiocentesis	procedure in which a surgeon withdraws fluid from the pericardial space by means of a needle inserted percutaneously
pericardium	membranous sac enclosing heart and ends of great vessels
perineum	area between the vulva and anus; also known as the pelvic floor
peripheral nerves	12 pairs of cranial nerves, 31 pairs of spinal nerves, and autonomic nervous system; connects peripheral receptors to the brain and spinal cord
peritoneal	within the lining of the abdominal cavity
peritoneoscopy	visualization of the abdominal cavity using one scope placed through a small incision in the abdominal wall and another scope placed in the vagina
pharyngolaryngectomy	surgical removal of the pharynx and larynx
phlebotomy	cutting into a vein
phonocardiogram	recording of heart sounds
photochemotherapy	treatment by means of drugs that react to ultraviolet radiation or sunlight
physics	scientific study of energy
pilosebaceous	pertains to hair follicles and sebaceous glands
placenta	a structure that connects the fetus and mother during pregnancy
plethysmography	determining the changes in volume of an organ part or body
pleura	covers the lungs and lines the thoracic cavity
pleurectomy	surgical excision of the pleura

pleuritis	inflammation of the pleura
pneumonocentesis	surgical puncturing of a lung to withdraw fluid
pneumonolysis	surgical separation of the lung from the chest wall to allow the lung to collapse
pneumonostomy	surgical procedure in which the chest cavity is exposed and the lung is incised
pneumonotomy	incision of the lung
pneumoplethysmography	determining the changes in the volume of the lung
posterior (dorsal)	in back of
posterior segment	those parts of the eye behind the lens
posteroanterior	from back to front
postpartum	after childbirth
Preferred Provider Organization	PPO, a group of providers who form a network and who have agreed to provide services to enrollees at a discounted rate
priapism	painful condition in which the penis is constantly erect
primary care physician	PCP, physician who oversees a patient's care within a managed care organization
primary diagnosis	chief complaint of a patient in outpatient setting
primipara	first pregnancy
prior approval	also known as a prior authorization, the payer's approval of care
proctosigmoidoscopy	fiberscopic examination of the sigmoid colon and rectum
Professional Standards Review Organization	PSRO, voluntary physicians' organization designed to monitor the necessity of hospital admissions, treatment costs, and medical records of hospitals
prognosis	probable outcome of an illness
prostatotomy	incision into the prostate
Provider Identification Number	PIN, assigned to physicians by payers for use in claims submission
pyelography	radiographic recording of the kidneys, renal pelvis, ureters, and bladder
qualitative	measuring the presence or absence of
Quality Improvement Organizations	QIO, consists of a national network of 53 entities that work with consumers, physicians, hospitals, and caregivers to refine care delivery systems
quantitative	measuring the presence or absence of and the amount of
rad	radiation-absorbed dose, the energy deposited in patient's tissues
radiation oncology	branch of medicine concerned with the application of radiation to a tumor site for treatment (destruction) of cancerous tumors
radiograph	film on which an image is produced through exposure to x-radiation

radiologist	physician who specializes in the use of radioactive materials in the diagnosis and treatment of disease and illness
radiology	branch of medicine concerned with the use of radioactive substances for diagnosis and therapy
rales	coarse sound on inspiration, also known as crackle (heard on auscultation)
real time	two-dimensional display of both the structures and the motion of tissues and organs, with the length of time also recorded as part of the study
reduction	replacement to normal position
Relative Value Unit	RVU, unit value that has been assigned for each service
Resource-Based Relative Value Scale	RBRVS, scale designed to decrease Medicare expenditures, redistribute physician payment, and ensure quality health care at reasonable rates
resource intensity	refers to the relative volume and type of diagnostic, therapeutic, and bed services used in the management of a particular illness
retrograde	moving backward or against the usual direction of flow
rhinoplasty	surgical repair of nose
rhinorrhea	nasal mucous discharge
salpingectomy	surgical removal of the uterine tube
salpingostomy	creation of a fistula into the uterine tube
scan	mapping of emissions of radioactive substances after they have been introduced into the body; the density can determine normal or abnormal conditions
sclera	outer covering of the eye
scoliosis	lateral curve of the spine
sebaceous gland	secretes sebum
seborrhea	excess sebum secretion
sebum	oily substance
section	slice of a frozen block
segmentectomy	surgical removal of a portion of a lung
septoplasty	surgical repair of the nasal septum
serum	blood from which the fibrinogen has been removed
severity of illness	refers to the levels of loss of function and mortality that may be experienced by patients with a particular disease
shunt	an artificial passage
sialography	radiographic recording of the salivary duct and branches
sialolithotomy	surgical removal of a stone of the salivary gland or duct
sinography	radiographic recording of the sinus or sinus tract
sinusotomy	surgical incision into a sinus

skeletal traction	application of pressure to the bone by means of pins and/or wires inserted into the bone
skin traction	application of pressure to the bone by means of tape applied to the skin
skull	entire skeletal framework of the head
somatic nerve	sensory or motor nerve
specimen	sample of tissue or fluid
spirometry	measurement of breathing capacity
splenectomy	excision of the spleen
splenography	radiographic recording of the spleen
splenoportography	radiographic procedure to allow visualization of the splenic and portal veins of the spleen
split-thickness graft	all epidermis and some of dermis
spondylitis	inflammation of vertebrae
Staff Model	a Health Maintenance Organization that directly employs the physicians who provide services to enrollees
steatoma	fat mass in sebaceous gland
stem cell	immature blood cell
stereotaxis	method of identifying a specific area or point in the brain
strabismus	extraocular muscle deviation resulting in unequal visual axes
stratified	layered
stratum (strata)	layer
subcutaneous	tissue below the dermis, primarily fat cells that insulate the body
subluxation	partial dislocation
subungual	beneath the nail
superior	toward the head or the upper part of the body; also known as cephalic
supination	supine position
supine	lying on the back
Swan-Ganz catheter	a catheter that measures pressure in the heart
sympathetic nerve	part of the peripheral nervous system that controls automatic body function and sympathetic nerves activated under stress
symphysis	natural junction
synchondrosis	union between two bones (connected by cartilage)
tachypnea	quick, shallow breathing
tarsorrhaphy	suturing together of the eyelids
Tax Equity and Fiscal Responsibility Act	TEFRA, act that contains language to reward cost-conscious healthcare providers

tendon	attaches a muscle to a bone
tenodesis	suturing of a tendon to a bone
tenorrhaphy	suture repair of tendon
thermogram	written record of temperature variation
third-party payer	insurance company or entity that is liable for another's health care services
thoracentesis	surgical puncture of the thoracic cavity, usually using a needle, to remove fluids
thoracic duct	collection and distribution point for lymph, and the largest lymph vessel located in the chest
thoracoplasty	surgical procedure that removes rib(s) and thereby allows the collapse of a lung
thoracoscopy	use of a lighted endoscope to view the pleural spaces and thoracic cavity or to perform surgical procedures
thoracostomy	incision into the chest wall and insertion of a chest tube
thoracotomy	surgical incision into the chest wall
thromboendarterectomy	procedure to remove plaque or clot formations from a vessel by percutaneous method
thymectomy	surgical removal of the thymus
thymus	gland that produces hormones important to the immune response
thyroglossal duct	connection between the thyroid and the tongue
thyroid	part of the endocrine system that produces hormones that regulate metabolism
thyroidectomy	surgical removal of the thyroid
tinnitus	ringing in the ears
titer	measure of a laboratory analysis
tocolysis	repression of uterine contractions
tomography	procedure that allows viewing of a single plane of the body by blurring out all but that particular level
tonography	recording of changes in intraocular pressure in response to sustained pressure on the eyeball
tonometry	measurement of pressure or tension
total pneumonectomy	surgical removal of an entire lung
tracheostomy	creation of an opening into trachea
tracheotomy	incision into trachea
traction	application of pressure to maintain normal alignment
transcutaneous	entering by way of the skin
transesophageal echocardiogram	TEE, echocardiogram performed by placing a probe down the esophagus and sending out sound waves to obtain images of the heart and its movement

transmastoid	creates an opening in the mastoid for drainage antrostomy
transplantation	grafting of tissue from one source to another
transseptal	through the septum
transtracheal	across the trachea
transureteroureterostomy	surgical connection of one ureter to the other ureter
transurethral resection, prostate	procedure performed through the urethra by means of a cystoscopy to remove part or all of the prostate
transvenous	through a vein
transvesical ureterolithotomy	removal of a ureter stone (calculus) through the bladder
trephination	surgical removal of a disk of bone
trocar needle	needle with a tube on the end; used to puncture and withdraw fluid from a cavity
tubercle	lesion caused by infection of tuberculosis
tumescence	state of being swollen
tunica vaginalis	covering of the testes
tympanolysis	freeing of adhesions of the tympanic membrane
tympanometry	test of the inner ear using air pressure
tympanostomy	insertion of ventilation tube into tympanum
ultrasound	technique using sound waves to determine the density of the outline of tissue
unbundling	reporting with multiple codes that which can be reported with one code
unilateral	occurring on one side
uptake	absorption of a radioactive substance by body tissues; recorded for diagnostic purposes in conditions such as thyroid disease
ureterectomy	surgical removal of a ureter, either totally or partially
ureterocolon	pertaining to the ureter and colon
ureterocutaneous fistula	channel from the ureter to exterior skin
ureteroenterostomy	creation of a connection between the intestine and the ureter
ureterolithotomy	removal of a stone from the ureter
ureterolysis	freeing of adhesions of the ureter
ureteroneocystostomy	surgical connection of the ureter to a new site on the bladder
ureteropyelography	ureter and bladder radiography
ureterotomy	incision into the ureter
urethrocystography	radiography of the bladder and urethra
urethromeatoplasty	surgical repair of the urethra and meatus
urethropexy	fixation of the urethra by means of surgery
urethroplasty	surgical repair of the urethra

urethrorrhaphy	suturing of the urethra
urethroscopy	use of a scope to view the urethra
urography	same as pyelography; radiographic recording of the kidneys, renal pelvis, ureters, and bladder
uveal	vascular tissue of the choroid, ciliary body, and iris
varices	varicose veins
varicocele	swelling of a scrotal vein
vas deferens	tube that carries sperm from the epididymis to the urethra
vasectomy	removal of segment of vas deferens
vasogram	recording of the flow in the vas deferens
vasotomy	incision in the vas deferens
vasorrhaphy	suturing of the vas deferens
vasovasostomy	reversal of a vasectomy
vectorcardiogram	VCG, continuous recording of electrical direction and magnitude of the heart
venography	radiographic recording of the veins and tributaries
vertebrectomy	removal of vertebra
vertigo	dizziness
vesicostomy	surgical creation of a connection of the viscera of the bladder to the skin
vesicovaginal fistula	creation of a tube between the vagina and the bladder
vesiculectomy	excision of the seminal vesicle
vesiculography	radiographic recording of the seminal vesicles
vesiculotomy	incision into the seminal vesicle
viscera	an organ in one of the large cavities of the body
volvulus	twisted section of the intestine
vomer	flat bones of the nasal septum
xanthoma	tumor composed of cells containing lipid material, yellow in color
xenograft	different species graft
xeroderma	dry, discolored, scaly skin
xeroradiography	photoelectric process of radiographs

Combining Forms

abdomin/o	abdomen
acetabul/o	hip socket
acr/o	height/extremities
aden/o	in relationship to a gland
adenoid/o	adenoids
adip/o	fat
adren/o, adrenal/o	adrenal gland
albin/o	white
albumin/o	albumin
alveol/o	alveolus
ambly/o	dim
amni/o	amnion
an/o	anus
andr/o	male
andren/o	adrenal gland
andrenal/o	adrenal gland
angi/o	vessel
ankyl/o	bent, fused
aort/o	aorta
aponeur/o	tendon type
appendic/o	appendix
aque/o	water
arche/o	first
arter/o, arteri/o	artery
arthr/o	joint
atel/o	incomplete
ather/o	plaque
atri/o	atrium

audi/o	hearing
aut/o	self
axill/o	armpit
azot/o	urea
balan/o	glans penis
bi/o	life
bil/i	bile
bilirubin/o	bile pigment
blephar/o	eyelid
brachi/o	arm
bronch/o	bronchus
bronchi/o	bronchus
bronchiol/o	bronchiole
burs/o	fluid-filled sac in a joint
calc/o, calc/i	calcium
cardi/o	heart
carp/o	carpals (wrist bones)
cauter/o	burn
cec/o	cecum
celi/o	abdomen
cephal/o	head
cerebell/o	cerebellum
cerebr/o	cerebrum
cervic/o	neck/cervix
chol/e	gall/bile
cholangio/o	bile duct
cholecyst/o	gallbladder
choledoch/o	common bile duct
cholester/o	cholesterol
chondr/o	cartilage
chori/o	chorion
clavic/o, clavicul/o	clavicle (collar bone)
col/o	colon
colp/o	vagina
coni/o	dust
conjunctiv/o	conjunctiva

cor/o, core/o	pupil
corne/o	cornea
coron/o	heart
cortic/o	cortex
cost/o	rib
crani/o	cranium (skull)
crin/o	secrete
crypt/o	hidden
culd/o	cul-de-sac
cutane/o	skin
cyan/o	blue
cycl/o	ciliary body
cyst/o	bladder
dacry/o	tear
dacryocyst/o	prefix meaning pertaining to the lacrimal sac
dent/i	tooth
derm/o, dermat/o	skin
diaphragmat/o	diaphragm
dips/o	thirst
disk/o	intervertebral disk
diverticul/o	diverticulum
duoden/o	duodenum
dur/o	dura mater
encephal/o	brain
enter/o	small intestine
eosin/o	rosy
epididym/o	epididymis
epiglott/o	epiglottis
episi/o	vulva
erythr/o, erythem/o	red
esophag/o	esophagus
essi/o, esthesi/o	sensation
estr/o	female
femor/o	thighbone
fet/o	fetus
fibul/o	fibula

galact/o	milk
gangli/o	ganglion
ganglion/o	ganglion
gastr/o	stomach
gingiv/o	gum
glomerul/o	glomerulus
gloss/o	tongue
gluc/o	sugar
glyc/o	sugar
glycos/o	sugar
gonad/o	ovaries and testes
gyn/o	female
gynec/o	female
hepat/o	liver
herni/o	hernia
heter/o	different
hidr/o	sweat
home/o	same
hormon/o	hormone
humer/o	humerus (upper arm bone)
hydr/o	water
hymen/o	hymen
hyster/o	uterus
ichthy/o	dry/scaly
ile/o	ileus
ili/o	ilium (upper pelvic bone)
immun/o	immune
inguin/o	groin
ir/o	iris
irid/o	iris
ischi/o	ischium (posterior pelvic bone)
jaund/o	yellow
jejun/o	jejunum
kal/i	potassium
kerat/o	hard, cornea

kinesi/o	movement
kyph/o	hump
lacrim/o	tear
lact/o	milk
lamin/o	lamina
lapar/o	abdomen
laryng/o	larynx
lingu/o	tongue
lip/o	fat
lith/o	stone
lob/o	lobe
lord/o	curve
lumb/o	lower back
lute/o	yellow
lymph/o	lymph
lymphaden/o	lymph gland
mamm/o	breast
mandibul/o	mandible (lower jawbone)
mast/o	breast
maxill/o	maxilla (upper jawbone)
meat/o	meatus
melan/o	black
men/o	menstruation, month
mening/o, meningi/o	meninges
menisc/o, menisci/o	meniscus
ment/o	mind
metacarp/o	metacarpals (hand)
metatars/o	metatarsals (foot)
metr/o	uterus, measure
metr/i	uterus
mon/o	one
muc/o	mucus
my/o, muscul/o	muscle
myc/o	fungus

myel/o	bone marrow, spinal cord
myring/o	ear drum
myx/o	mucus
nas/o	nose
nat/a, nat/i	birth
natr/o	sodium
necr/o	death
nephr/o	kidney
neur/o	nerve
noct/i	night
ocul/o	eye
olecran/o	olecranon (elbow)
olig/o	scant, few
onych/o	nail
oo/o	egg
oophor/o	ovary
ophthalm/o	eye
opt/o	eye, vision
optic/o	eye
or/o	mouth
orch/i, orch/o, orchi/o, orchid/o	testicle
orth/o	straight
oste/o	bone
ot/o	ear
ov/o	egg
ovari/o	ovary
ovul/o	ovulation
ox/i, ox/o	oxygen
oxy/o	oxygen
pachy/o	thick
palat/o	palate
palpebr/o	eyelid
pancreat/o	pancreas

papill/o	optic nerve
patell/o	patella (kneecap)
pelv/i	pelvis (hip)
pericardi/o	pericardium
perine/o	perineum
peritone/o	peritoneum
petr/o	stone
phac/o	eye lens
phak/o	eye lens
phalang/o	phalanges (finger or toe)
pharyng/o	pharynx
phas/o	speech
phleb/o	vein
phren/o	mind, diaphragm
phys/o	growing
pil/o	hair
pituitar/o	pituitary gland
pleur/o	pleura
pneumat/o	lung/air
pneumon/o	lung/air
poli/o	gray matter
polyp/o	polyp
pont/o	pons
proct/o	rectum
prostat/o	prostate gland
psych/o	mind
pub/o	pubis
pulmon/o	lung
pupill/o	pupil
py/o	pus
pyel/o	renal pelvis
pylor/o	pylorus
quadr/i	four
rachi/o	spine
radi/o	radius (lower arm)
radic/o, radicul/o	nerve root
rect/o	rectum

ren/o	kidney
retin/o	retina
rhin/o	nose
rhiz/o	nerve root
rhytid/o	wrinkle
rube/o	red
sacr/o	sacrum
salping/o	uterine tube, Fallopian tube
scapul/o	scapula (shoulder)
scler/o	sclera
scoli/o	bent
seb/o	sebum/oil
semin/i	semen
sept/o	septum
sial/o	saliva
sigmoid/o	sigmoid colon
sinus/o	sinus
somat/o	body
son/o	sound
sperm/o, spermat/o	sperm
sphygm/o	pulse
spir/o	breath
splen/o	spleen
spondyl/o	vertebra
staped/o	middle ear, stapes
staphyl/o	clusters
steat/o	fat
ster/o, stere/o	solid, having three dimensions
stern/o	sternum (breast bone)
steth/o	chest
stomat/o	mouth
strept/o	twisted chain
synovi/o	synovial joint membrane
tars/o	tarsal (ankle)
ten/o	tendon

tend/o, tendin/o	tendon (connective tissue)
test/o	testicle
thorac/o	thorax
thromb/o	clot
thym/o	thymus gland
thyr/o, thyroid/o	thyroid gland
tibi/o	shin bone
toc/o	childbirth
tonsill/o	tonsil
top/o	place
tox/o, toxic/o	poison
trache/o	trachea
trich/o	hair
tympan/o	ear drum
uln/o	ulna (lower arm bone)
ungu/o	nail
ur/o	urine
ureter/o	ureter
urethr/o	urethra
urin/o	urine
uter/o	uterus
uve/o	uvea
uvul/o	uvula
vagin/o	vagina
valv/o, valvul/o	valve
vas/o, vascul/o	vessel
ven/o	vein
ventricul/o	ventricle
vertebr/o	vertebra
vesic/o	bladder
vesicul/o	seminal vesicles
vitre/o	glass/glassy
vulv/o	vulva
xanth/o	yellow
xer/o	dry

Prefixes

a-	not
an-	not
ante-	before
audi-	hearing
bi-	two
brady-	slow
de-	lack of
dys-	difficult, painful
ecto-	outside
endo-	in
epi-	on/upon
eso-	inward
eu-	good/normal
exo-	outward
extra-	outside
hemi-	half
hyper-	excess, over
hypo-	under
in-	into
inter-	between
intra-	within
meta-	change, after
multi-	many
neo-	new
nulli-, nulti-	none
oxy-	sharp, oxygen
pan-	all
para-	beside

per-	through
peri-	surrounding
poly-	many
post-	after
primi-	first
pseudo-	false
quadri-	four
retro-	behind
sub-	under
supra-	above
sym-	together
syn-	together
tachy-	fast
tetra-	four
tri-	three
tropin-	act upon
uni-	one

Suffixes

-agon	assemble
-algesia	pain sensation
-algia	pain
-ar	pertaining to
-arche	beginning
-ary	pertaining to
-asthenia	weakness
-blast	embryonic
-capnia	carbon dioxide
-cele	hernia
-centesis	puncture to remove (drain)
-chezia	defecation
-clast, -clasia, -clasis	break
-coccus	spherical bacterium
-cyesis	pregnancy
-desis	fusion
-dilation	widening, expanding
-drome	run
-dynia	pain
-eal	pertaining to
-ectasis	stretching
-ectomy	removal
-edema	swelling
-emia	blood
-esthesis	feeling
-gram	record
-graph	recording instrument
-graphy	recording process

-gravida	pregnancy
-ia	condition
-iatrist	physician specialist
-iatry	medical treatment
-ical	pertaining to
-ictal	pertaining to
-in	a substance
-ine	a substance
-itis	inflammation
-listhesis	slipping
-lithiasis	condition of stones
-lysis	separation
-malacia	softening
-megaly	enlargement
-meta	change
-meter	measurement; instrument that measures
-metry	measurement of
-oid	resembling
-oma	tumor
-omia	smell
-one	hormone
-opia	vision
-opsy	view of
-orrhexis	rupture
-osis	condition
-oxia	oxygen
-para	woman who has given birth
-paresis	incomplete paralysis
-parous	to bear
-penia	deficient
-pexy	fixation
-phagia	eating
-phonia	sound
-phylaxis	protection
-physis	to grow
-plasty	repair
-plegia	paralysis

-pnea	breathing
-poiesis	production
-poly	many
-porosis	passage
-retro	behind
-rrhagia	bursting of blood
-rrhaphy	suture
-rrhea	discharge
-schisis	split
-sclerosis	hardening
-scopy	to examine
-spasm	contraction of muscle
-steat/o	fat
-stenosis	blockage, narrowing
-stomy	opening
-thorax	chest
-tocia	labor
-tom/o	to cut
-tome	an instrument that cuts
-tomy	cutting, incision
-tripsy	crush
-tropia	to turn
-tropin	act upon
-uria	urine
-version	turning

Abbreviations

ABG	arterial blood gas
ABN	Advanced Beneficiary Notice used by CMS to notify beneficiary of payment of provider services
ACL	anterior cruciate ligament
AD	right ear
AFB	acid-fast bacillus
AFI	amniotic fluid index
AGA	appropriate for gestational age
AGCUS	atypical glandular cells of undetermined significance
AKA	above-knee amputation
ANS	autonomic nervous system
APCs	Ambulatory Payment Classifications, patient classification that provides a payment system for outpatients
ARDS	adult respiratory distress syndrome
ARF	acute renal failure
ARM	artificial rupture of membrane
AS	left ear
ASCUS	atypical squamous cells of undetermined significance
ASCVD	arteriosclerotic cardiovascular disease
ASD	atrial septal defect
ASHD	arteriosclerotic heart disease
AU	both ears
AV	atrioventricular
BCC	benign cellular changes
BiPAP	bi-level positive airway pressure
BKA	below-knee amputation
BP	blood pressure
BPD	biparietal diameter

BPH	benign prostatic hypertrophy
BPP	biophysical profile
BUN	blood urea nitrogen
BV	bacterial vaginosis
bx	biopsy
C1-C7	cervical vertebrae
ca	cancer
CABG	coronary artery bypass graft
CBC	complete blood (cell) count
CF	conversion factor, national dollar amount that is applied to all services paid on the Medicare Fee Schedule basis
CHF	congestive heart failure
CHL	crown-to-heel length
CK	creatine kinase
CMS	Centers for Medicare and Medicaid Services, formerly HCFA, Health Care Financing Administration
CNM	certified nurse midwife
CNS	central nervous system
COB	coordination of benefits, management of payment between two or more third-party payers for a service
COPD	chronic obstructive pulmonary disease
CPAP	continuous positive airway pressure
CPD	cephalopelvic disproportion
CPK	creatine phosphokinase
CPP	chronic pelvic pain
CSF	cerebrospinal fluid
CTS	carpal tunnel syndrome
CVA	stroke/cerebrovascular accident
CVI	cerebrovascular insufficiency
D&C	dilation and curettage
D&E	dilation and evacuation
derm	dermatology
DHHS	Department of Health and Human Services
DLCO	diffuse capacity of lungs for carbon monoxide
DRGs	Diagnosis Related Groups, disease classification system that relates the type of inpatients a hospital treats (case mix) to the costs incurred by the hospital
DSE	dobutamine stress echocardiography

DUB	dysfunctional uterine bleeding
ECC	endocervical curettage
EDC	estimated date of confinement
EDD	estimated date of delivery
EDI	electronic data interchange, exchange of data between multiple computer terminals
EEG	electroencephalogram
EFM	electronic fetal monitoring
EFW	estimated fetal weight
EGA	estimated gestational age
EGD	esophagogastroduodenoscopy
EGJ	esophagogastric junction
EMC	endometrial curettage
EOB	explanation of benefits, remittance advice
EPO	Exclusive Provider Organization, similar to a Health Maintenance Organization except that the providers of the services are not prepaid, but rather are paid on a fee-for-service basis
EPSDT	Early and Periodic Screening, Diagnosis, and Treatment
ERCP	endoscopic retrograde cholangiopancreatography
ERT	estrogen replacement therapy
ESRD	end-stage renal disease
FAS	fetal alcohol syndrome
FEF	forced expiratory flow
FEV_1	forced expiratory volume in 1 second
$FEV_1 : FVC$	maximum amount of forced expiratory volume in 1 second
FHR	fetal heart rate
FI	fiscal intermediary, financial agent acting on behalf of a third-party payer
FRC	functional residual capacity
FSH	follicle-stimulating hormone
FVC	forced vital capacity
fx	fracture
GERD	gastroesophageal reflux disease
GI	gastrointestinal
H or E	hemorrhage or exudate
HCFA	Health Care Financing Administration, now known as Centers for Medicare and Medicaid Services (CMS)
HCVD	hypertensive cardiovascular disease
HD	hemodialysis

HDL	high-density lipoprotein
HEA	hemorrhage, exudate, aneurysm
HHN	hand-held nebulizer
HJR	hepatojugular reflux
H&P	history and physical
HPV	human papillomavirus
HSG	hysterosalpingogram
HSV	herpes simplex virus
I&D	incision and drainage
IO	intraocular
IOL	intraocular lens
IPAP	inspiratory positive airway pressure
IRDS	infant respiratory distress syndrome
IVF	in vitro fertilization
IVP	intravenous pyelogram
JBP	jugular blood pressure
KUB	kidneys, ureter, bladder
L1-L5	lumbar vertebrae
LBBB	left bundle branch block
LEEP	loop electrosurgical excision procedure
LGA	large for gestational age
LLQ	left lower quadrant
LP	lumbar puncture
LUQ	left upper quadrant
LVH	left ventricular hypertrophy
MAT	multifocal atrial tachycardia
MDI	metered dose inhaler
MI	myocardial infarction
MRI	magnetic resonance imaging
MSLT	multiple sleep latency testing
MVV	maximum voluntary ventilation
NCPAP	nasal continuous positive airway pressure
NSR	normal sinus rhythm
OA	osteoarthritis
OD	right eye
OS	left eye
OU	each eye

PAC	premature atrial contraction
PAT	paroxysmal atrial tachycardia
PAWP	pulmonary artery wedge pressure
PCWP	pulmonary capillary wedge pressure
PEAP	positive end-airway pressure
PEEP	positive end-expiratory pressure
PEG	percutaneous endoscopic gastrostomy
PERL	pupils equal and reactive to light
PERRL	pupils equal, round, and reactive to light
PERRLA	pupils equal, round, and reactive to light and accommodation
PFT	pulmonary function test
pH	symbol for acid/base level
PICC	peripherally inserted central catheter
PID	pelvic inflammatory disease
PND	paroxysmal nocturnal dyspnea
PNS	peripheral nervous system
PROM	premature rupture of membranes
PSA	prostate-specific antigen
PST	paroxysmal supraventricular tachycardia
PSVT	paroxysmal supraventricular tachycardia
PT	prothrombin time
PTCA	percutaneous transluminal coronary angioplasty
PTT	partial thromboplastin time
PVC	premature ventricular contraction
RA	remittance advice, explanation of services
RA	rheumatoid arthritis
RBBB	right bundle branch block
RDS	respiratory distress syndrome
REM	rapid eye movement
RLQ	right lower quadrant
RSR	regular sinus rhythm
RUQ	right upper quadrant
RV	respiratory volume
RVG	*Relative Value Guide*
RVH	right ventricular hypertrophy
RVS	relative value studies, list of procedures with unit values assigned to each
RV:TLC	ratio of respiratory volume to total lung capacity

SHG	sonohysterogram
sp gr	specific gravity
SROM	spontaneous rupture of membranes
subcu, subq, SC, SQ	subcutaneous
SUI	stress urinary incontinence
SVT	supraventricular tachycardia
T1-T12	thoracic vertebrae
TAH	total abdominal hysterectomy
TEE	transesophageal echocardiography
TENS	transcutaneous electrical nerve stimulation
TIA	transient ischemic attack
TLC	total lung capacity
TLV	total lung volume
TM	tympanic membrane
TMJ	temporomandibular joint
TPA	tissue plasminogen activator
TSH	thyroid-stimulating hormone
TST	treadmill stress test
TURBT	transurethral resection of bladder tumor
TURP	transurethral resection of prostate
UA	urinalysis
UCR	usual, customary, and reasonable—third-party payers' assessment of the reimbursement for health care services: usual, that which would ordinarily be charged for the service; customary, the cost of that service in that locale; and reasonable, as assessed by the payer
UPJ	ureteropelvic junction
URI	upper respiratory infection
UTI	urinary tract infection
V/Q	ventilation/perfusion scan
VBAC	vaginal birth after cesarean
WBC	white blood (cell) count

Further Text Resources

ANATOMY AND PHYSIOLOGY

Book Title	Author	Imprint	Copyright Date	ISBN
The Anatomy and Physiology Learning System, 3rd Edition	Applegate	Saunders	2006	978-1-4160-2586-3
Gray's Anatomy for Students, 2nd Edition	Drake, Vogl, Mitchell	Churchill Livingstone	2009	978-0-443-06952-9
Anthony's Textbook of Anatomy and Physiology, 19th Edition	Thibodeau, Patton	Mosby	2010	978-0-323-05539-0

CODING

Book Title	Author	Imprint	Copyright Date	ISBN
Step-by-Step Medical Coding, 2009 Edition	Buck	Saunders	2009	978-1-4160-4566-3
2009 ICD-9-CM, Volumes 1 & 2 (Professional Edition)	Buck	Saunders	2009	978-1-4160-4448-2
2009 ICD-9-CM, Volumes 1, 2, & 3 (Professional Edition)	Buck	Saunders	2009	978-1-4160-4450-5
2009 HCPCS Level II (Professional Edition)	Buck	Saunders	2009	978-1-4160-5203-6
The Next Step, Advanced Medical Coding, 2009 Edition	Buck	Saunders	2009	978-1-4160-5679-9
The Extra Step: Facility-Based Coding Practice	Buck	Saunders	2006	978-1-4160-3450-6
The Extra Step: Physician-Based Coding Practice	Buck	Saunders	2009	978-1-4160-6162-5
CPC Coding Exam Review 2009: The Certification Step	Buck	Saunders	2009	978-1-4160-3713-2
The Evaluation and Management Step: An Auditing Tool, 2009 Edition	Buck	Saunders	2009	978-1-4160-6724-5
ICD-9-CM Coding: Theory and Practice, 2009 Edition	Lovaasen, Schwerdtfeger	Saunders	2009	978-1-4160-5881-6

PATHOPHYSIOLOGY

Book Title	Author	Imprint	Copyright Date	ISBN-13
Pathology for the Health Professions, 3rd Edition	Damjanov	Saunders	2006	978-1-4160-0031-0
Essentials of Human Diseases and Conditions, 4th Edition	Frazier, Drzymkowski	Saunders	2008	978-1-4160-4714-8
Pathophysiology for the Health Related Professions, 3rd Edition	Gould	Saunders	2006	978-1-4160-0210-9
The Human Body in Health and Illness, 3rd Edition	Herlihy	Saunders	2007	978-1-4160-2885-7
The Human Body in Health and Disease, 5th Edition	Thibodeau, Patton	Mosby	2010	978-0-323-05492-8

MEDICAL TERMINOLOGY

Book Title	Author	Imprint	Copyright Date	ISBN-13
The Language of Medicine, 8th Edition	Chabner	Saunders	2007	978-1-4160-3492-6
Jablonski's Dictionary of Medical Acronyms & Abbreviations, 6th edition	Jablonski	Saunders	2009	978-1-4160-5899-1
Exploring Medical Language, 7th Edition	LaFleur, Brooks	Mosby	2008	978-0-323-04950-4
Building a Medical Vocabulary (with Spanish Translations), 7th Edition	Leonard	Saunders	2009	978-1-4160-5627-0
Quick & Easy Medical Terminology, 5th Edition	Leonard	Saunders	2007	978-1-4160-2494-1
Mastering Healthcare Terminology, 3rd Edition	Shiland	Mosby	2010	978-0-323-05506-2
Dorland's Illustrated Medical Dictionary, 31st Edition		Saunders	2007	978-1-4160-2364-7

INTRODUCTION TO COMPUTER

Book Title	Author	Imprint	Copyright Date	ISBN-13
Computerized Medical Office Procedures: A Worktext, 2nd Edition	Larsen	Saunders	2008	978-1-4160-4834-3

BASICS OF WRITING/MEDICAL TRANSCRIPTION

Book Title	Author	Imprint	Copyright Date	ISBN-13
Medical Transcription Guide: Do's and Don'ts, 3rd Edition	Diehl	Saunders	2005	978-0-7216-0684-2
Diehl & Fordney's Medical Transcribing: Techniques and Procedures, 6th Edition	Diehl	Saunders	2007	978-1-4160-2347-0

COMPREHENSION BUILDING/STUDY SKILLS

Book Title	Author	Imprint	Copyright Date	ISBN-13
Career Development for Health Professionals: Success in School and on the Job, 2nd Edition	Haroun	Saunders	2006	978-0-7216-0609-5

BASIC MATH

Book Title	Author	Imprint	Copyright Date	ISBN-13
Basic Mathematics for the Health-Related Professions	Doucette	Saunders	2000	978-0-7216-7938-9
Using Maths in Health Sciences	Gunn	Churchill Livingstone	2001	978-0-443-07074-7

MEDICAL BILLING/INSURANCE

Book Title	Author	Imprint	Copyright Date	ISBN-13
Health Insurance Today: A Practical Approach, 2nd Edition	Beik	Saunders	2009	978-1-4160-5320-0
Medical Insurance Made Easy: Understanding the Claim Cycle, 2nd Edition	Brown	Saunders	2006	978-0-7216-0556-2
Insurance Handbook for the Medical Office, 10th Edition	Fordney	Saunders	2008	978-1-4160-3666-1

Pharmacology Review

Generic Name	Registered Brand or Trade Name	Therapeutic Use/Medication Action
ANTI-ATTENTION DEFICIT HYPERACTIVITY DISORDER		
atomoxetine	Strattera	Attention Deficit Hyperactivity Disorder (ADHD) therapy
AMNESIC		
diazepam	Valium	amnesic, antianxiety, anticonvulsant, antipain, anti-tremor agent, sedative-hypnotic, skeletal muscle relaxant adjunct
lorazepam	Ativan	amnesic, antianxiety, anticonvulsant, antiemetic, antipanic, anti-tremor, sedative-hypnotic, skeletal muscle relaxant
ANALGESIC		
acetaminophen-codeine	Phenaphen with Codeine	analgesic
acetaminophen-codeine	Tylenol with Codeine	analgesic
celecoxib	Celebrex	analgesic, antirheumatic NSAID
fentanyl	Duragesic	analgesic
fentanyl	Actiq	analgesic, anesthetic adjunct
fentanyl	Sublimaze	analgesic, anesthetic adjunct
hydrocodone	Hycodan	analgesic
hydrocodone-acetaminophen	Lortab	analgesic
hydrocodone-acetaminophen	Vicodin	analgesic
ibuprofen	Advil	analgesic
ibuprofen	Motrin	analgesic
naproxen	Aleve	analgesic, nonsteroid anti-inflammatory, antidysmenorreal, antigout, antipyretic, antirheumatic, vascular headache prophylactic and suppressant
naproxen	Naprosyn	analgesic, nonsteroid anti-inflammatory, antidysmenorreal, antigout, antipyretic, antirheumatic, vascular headache prophylactic and suppressant
oxycodone	OxyContin	analgesic
oxycodone-acetaminophen	Endocet	analgesic
oxycodone-acetaminophen	Percocet	analgesic
oxycodone-acetaminophen	Tylox	analgesic
propoxyphene-acetaminophen	Darvocet-N 100	analgesic

Generic Name	Registered Brand or Trade Name	Therapeutic Use/Medication Action
ANALGESIC—cont'd		
tramadol	Ultram	analgesic
tramadol-acetaminophen	Ultracet	analgesic
ANTI HIV AIDS		
efavirenz	Sustiva	anti HIV AIDS
emtricitabine	Emtriva	anti HIV AIDS
tenofovir	Viread	anti HIV AIDS
ANTI-IMPOTENCE		
sildenafil	Viagra	impotence, anti-erectile dysfunction
ANTI-PARKINSONISM		
cabergoline	Dostinex	anti-parkinsonism, anti-migraine headache
ANTIPROSTATIC HYPERTROPHY		
finasteride	Propecia	benign prostatic hyperplasia therapy, hair growth stimulant
finasteride	Proscar	benign prostatic hyperplasia therapy, hair growth stimulant
tamsulosin HCL	Flomax	benign prostatic hyperplasia therapy
ANTIACNE		
ethinyl estradiol-norethindrone	Estrostep Fe	antiacne, antiendometriotic, systemic contraceptive, estrogen-progestin, gonadotropin inhibitor
ethinyl estradiol-norethindrone	Femhrt	antiacne, antiendometriotic, systemic contraceptive, estrogen-progestin, gonadotropin inhibitor
ethinyl estradiol-norethindrone	Loestrin Fe	antiacne, antiendometriotic, systemic contraceptive, estrogen-progestin, gonadotropin inhibitor
ethinyl estradiol-norethindrone	Ovcon	antiacne, antiendometriotic, systemic contraceptive, estrogen-progestin, gonadotropin inhibitor
ethinyl estrodiol-norgestinmate	Ortho Tri-Cyclen	antiacne, antiendometriotic, systemic contraceptive, estrogen-progestin, gonadotropin inhibitor
ANTIADRENERGIC		
metoprolol	Lopressor	antiadrenergic, antianginal, antianxiety, antiarrhythmic, antihypertensive, anti-tremor, hypertrophic cardiomyopathy, MI therapy
metoprolol succinate	Toprol XL	antiadrenergic, antianginal, antianxiety, antiarrhythmic, antihypertensive, anti-tremor, hypertrophic cardiomyopathy, MI therapy
propranolol	Inderal	antiadrenergic, antianginal, antianxiety, antiarrhythmic, antihypertensive, anti-tremor, hypertrophic cardiomyopathy, MI prophylactic, MI therapy, neuroleptic-induced akathisia therapy
timolol	Blocadren	antiadrenergic, antianginal, antianxiety, antiarrhythmic, systemic antiglaucoma, antihypertensive, anti-tremor, hypertrophic cardiomyopathy, MI prophylactic

Generic Name	Registered Brand or Trade Name	Therapeutic Use/Medication Action
ANTIANGINAL		
diltiazem	Cardizem	antianginal, antiarrhythmic, antihypertensive
diltiazem	Dilacor	antianginal, antiarrhythmic, antihypertensive
felodipine	Plendil	antianginal, antihypertensive
isosorbide mononitrate	Imdur	antianginal
isosorbide mononitrate	Ismo	antianginal
nifedipine	Procardia	antianginal, antihypertensive
nitroglycerin	Nitrolingual	antianginal, CHS, vasodilator
nitroglycerin	Nitrostat	antianginal, CHS, vasodilator
nitroglycerin	Minitran	antianginal, congestive heart failure (CHF), vasodilator
verapamil	Isoptin	antianginal, antiarrhymic, antihypertensive, hypertrophic cardiomyopathy therapy vascular headache prophylactic
verapamil	Verelan	antianginal, antiarrhymic, antihypertensive, hypertrophic cardiomyopathy therapy vascular headache prophylactic
verapamil	Calan	antianginal, antiarrhythmic, antihypertensive, hypertrophic cardiomyopathy therapy, vascular headache prophylactic
verapamil	Covera HS	antianginal, antiarrhythmic, antihypertensive, hypertrophic cardiomyopathy therapy, vascular headache prophylactic
ANTIANXIETY		
alprazolam	Xanax	antianxiety
buspirone	BuSpar	antianxiety
escitalopram oxalate	Lexapro	antianxiety, antidepressant
paroxetine HCL	Paxil	antianxiety, antidepressant, antiobsessional, antipanic, posttraumatic stress disorder, social anxiety disorder agent
sertraline	Zoloft	antianxiety, antidepressant, antiobsessional, antipanic, posttraumatic stress disorder, premenstrual dysphoric disorder therapy
ANTIARRHYTHMIC		
digoxin	Digitek	antiarrhythmic, cardiotonic
digoxin	Lanoxicaps	antiarrhythmic, cardiotonic
digoxin	Lanoxin	antiarrhythmic, cardiotonic
phenytoin	Dilantin	antiarrhythmic, anticonvulsant, trigeminal neuralgic antineuralgic, skeletal muscle relaxant
ANTIASTHMATIC		
budesonide	Pulmicort	antiasthmatic
fluticasone-salmeterol	Advair Diskus	antiasthmatic, inhalation anti-inflammatory, bronchodilator
ipratropium bromide	Atrovent	antiasthmatic bronchodilator
lipatropium-albuterol	Combivent	antiasthmatic-bronchodilator
montelukast sodium	Singular	antiasthmatic, leukotriene receptor antagonist

Generic Name	Registered Brand or Trade Name	Therapeutic Use/Medication Action
ANTIASTHMATIC—cont'd		
salmeterol maleate	Serevent	antiasthmatic
zafirlukast	Accolate	antiasthmatic
ANTIBACTERIAL		
amoxicillin	Trimax	systemic antibacterial
amoxicillin-clavulanate	Augmentin	systemic antibacterial
azithromycin	Zithromax	systemic antibacterial
cefadroxil	Duricef	systemic antibacterial
cefdinir	Omnicef	systemic antibacterial
cefluroximine axetil	Ceflin	systemic antibacterial
cefprozil	Cefzil	systemic antibacterial
cephalexin	Keflex	systemic antibacterial
ciprofloxacin	Ciloxan	ophthalmic antibacterial
ciprofloxacin	Cipro	systemic antibacterial
clarithromycin	Biaxin	systemic antibacterial, antimycobacterial
clindamycin	Cleocin	systemic antibacterial
doxycycline	Vibramycin	systemic antibacterial, antiprotozoal
levofloxacin	Levaquin	systemic antibacterial
metronidazole	Flagyl	systemic antibacterial
minocycline	Minocin	systemic antibacterial
moxifloxacin	Vigamox	ophthalmic antibacterial
moxifloxacin	Avelox	systemic antibacterial
mupirocin	Bactroban	topical antibacterial
nitrofurantoin	Macrodantin	systemic antibacterial
nitrofurantoin monohydrate	Macrobid	systemic antibacterial
ofloxacin	Floxin	systemic antibacterial
penicillin V	Veetids	systemic antibacterial
sulfamethoxazole-trimethoprim	Bactrim	systemic antibacterial, antiprotozoal
sulfamethoxazole-trimethoprim	Cotrim	systemic antibacterial, antiprotozoal
sulfamethoxazole-trimethoprim	Septra DS	systemic antibacterial, antiprotozoal
trimethoprim	Bactrim	systemic antibacterial
ANTICOAGULANT		
dipyridamole/ASA	Aggrenox	anticoagulant
warfarin	Coumadin	anticoagulant

Generic Name	Registered Brand or Trade Name	Therapeutic Use/Medication Action
ANTICONVULSANT		
clonazepam	Klonopin	anticonvulsant
divalproex sodium	Depakote	anticonvulsant, antimanic, migraine headache prophylactic
gabapentin	Neurontin	anticonvulsant, antineuralgic
lamotrigine	Lamictal	anticonvulsant
levetiracetam	Keppra	anticonvulsant
oxcarbazepine	Trileptal	anticonvulsant
tiagabine	Gabitril	anticonvulsant
topiramate	Topamax	anticonvulsant, antimigraine headache
zonisamide	Zonegran	anticonvulsant
ANTIDEMENTIA		
donepezil	Aricept	anti dementia
galantamine HBr	Reminyl	antidementia-mild/moderate Alzheimer's
rivastigmine tartrate	Exelon	antidementia of Parkinson's
ANTIDEPRESSANT		
amitriptyline	Elavil	antidepressant
bupropion	Zyban	antidepressant, smoking cessation
bupropion HCL	Wellbutrin	antidepressant, smoking cessation
citalopram hydrobromide	Celexa	antidepressant
doxepin	Sinequan	antidepressant
fluoxetine	Prozac	antidepressant, antiobsessional agent
fluoxetine	Sarafem	antidepressant, antiobsessional, antibulimic agent
mirtazapine	Remeron	antidepressant
trazodone	Desyrel	antidepressant, antineuralgic
venlafaxine HLC	Effexor	antidepressant, antianxiety agent
ANTIDIABETIC		
doxazosin mesylate	Diabinese	antidiabetic
glimepiride	Amaryl	antidiabetic
glipizide	Glucotrol	antidiabetic
glyburide	DiaBeta	antidiabetic
glyburide	Glynase	antidiabetic
glyburide	Micronase	antidiabetic
glyburide-metformin	Glucovance	antidiabetic
insulin	Nolog	antidiabetic
insulin	Novolin	antidiabetic
insulin glargine	Lantus	antidiabetic

Generic Name	Registered Brand or Trade Name	Therapeutic Use/Medication Action
ANTIDIABETIC—cont'd		
insulin lispro	Humalog	antidiabetic
metformin HCL	Glucophage	antihyperglycemic
miglitol	Glyset	antidiabetic
NPH isophane insulin	Humulin N	antidiabetic
NPH regular insulin	Humulin 70/30	antidiabetic
pioglitazone	Actos	antidiabetic
repaglinide	Prandin	antidiabetic
rosiglitazone	Avandia	antidiabetic
ANTIEMETIC		
meclizine	Antivert	antiemetic, antivertigo
promethazine	Phenergan	antiemetic, antihistaminic, H1 receptor, antivertigo, sedative-hypnotic
ANTIENDOMETRIOTIC		
ethinyl estradiol-desogestrel	Cyclessa	antiendometriotic, systemic contraceptive, gonadotropin inhibitor
ethinyl estradiol-desogestrel	Desogen	antiendometriotic, systemic contraceptive, gonadotropin inhibitor
ethinyl estradiol-desogestrel	Kariva	antiendometriotic, systemic contraceptive, gonadotropin inhibitor
ethinyl estradiol-desogestrel	Mircette	antiendometriotic, systemic contraceptive, gonadotropin inhibitor
ethinyl estradiol-desogestrel	Ortho-Cept	antiendometriotic, systemic contraceptive, gonadotropin inhibitor
ethinyl estradiol-levonorgestrel	Levlen	antiendometriotic, systemic postcoital contraceptive, systemic contraceptive, estrogen progestin, gonadotropin inhibitor
ethinyl estradiol-levonorgestrel	Nordette	antiendometriotic, systemic postcoital contraceptive, systemic contraceptive, estrogen-progestin, gonadotropin inhibitor
ethinyl estradiol-levonorgestrel	Seasonale	antiendometriotic, systemic postcoital contraceptive, systemic contraceptive, estrogen-progestin, gonadotropin inhibitor
ethinyl estradiol-levonorgestrel	Tri-Levlen	antiendometriotic, systemic postcoital contraceptive, systemic contraceptive, estrogen-progestin, gonadotropin inhibitor
ethinyl estradiol-levonorgestrel	Triphasil	antiendometriotic, systemic postcoital contraceptive, systemic contraceptive, estrogen-progestin, gonadotropin inhibitor
ethinyl estradiol-levonorgestrel	Trivora-28	antiendometriotic, systemic postcoital contraceptive, systemic contraceptive, estrogen-progestin, gonadotropin inhibitor
ethinyl estradiol-norgestrel	Lo/Ovral	antiendometriotic, systemic postcoital contraceptive, systemic contraceptive, estrogen-progestin, gonadotropin inhibitor
ethinyl estradiol-norgestrel	Low-Ogestrel	antiendometriotic, systemic postcoital contraceptive, systemic contraceptive, estrogen-progestin, gonadotropin inhibitor
ethinyl estradiol-norgestrel	Ovral	antiendometriotic, systemic postcoital contraceptive, systemic contraceptive, estrogen-progestin, gonadotropin inhibitor

Generic Name	Registered Brand or Trade Name	Therapeutic Use/Medication Action
ANTIFUNGAL		
clotrimazole	Mycelex Cream	antifungal
clotrimazole-betamethasone	Lotrisone	antifungal, corticosteroid
econazole	Sporanox	antifungal
econazole	Spectazole Cream	antifungal
fluconazole	Diflucan	systemic antifungal
griseofulvin	Grifulvin	antifungal
itraconazole	Sporanox	antifungal
ketoconazole	Nizoral	antifungal
miconazole	Monistat Derm	cream antifungal
terbinafine	Lamisil	antifungal
terconazole	Terazol	vaginal antifungal cream, suppositories
ANTIGLAUCOMA		
bimatoprost	Lumigan Ophthalmic	antiglaucoma solution
brimonidine	Alphagan P	antiglaucoma solution
dorzolamide/timolol maleate	Cosopt	decreases ocular hypertension
latanoprost	Xalatan	antiglaucoma
latanoprost	Xalatan Ophthalmic	antiglaucoma, ocular antihypertensive
timolol	Timoptic	ophthalmic antiglaucoma
ANTIGOUT		
allopurinol	Zyloprim	antigout agent
ANTIHISTAMINE		
cetirizine	Zyrtec	antihistaminic, H1 receptor
cetirizine-pseudoephedrine	Zyrtec-D	antihistaminic, H1 receptor-decongestant
desloratadine	Clarinex	antihistamine, H1 receptor
fexofenadine	Allegra	antihistamine, H1 receptor
fexofenadine-pseudoephedrine	Allegra D	antihistamine, H1 receptor-decongestant
hydrocodone-chlorpheniramine	Tussionex	antihistaminic, H1 receptor antitussive
hydroxyzine	Vistaril	antihistamine
loratadine	Claritin	antihistamine
olopatadine	Patanol	ophthalmic antihistamine, H1 receptor, mask cell stabilizer, antiallergic
promethazine-codeine	Prometh with Codeine	antihistamine, H1 receptor-antitussive
ANTIHYPERCALCEMIC		
furosemide	Lasix	antihypercalcemic, antihypertensive, renal disease diagnostic aid, diuretic

Generic Name	Registered Brand or Trade Name	Therapeutic Use/Medication Action
ANTIHYPERLIPIDEMIC		
atorvastatin	Lipitor	antilipidemic, statin
colesevelam	WelChol	antihyperlipidemic
ezetimibe	Zetia	antihyperlipidemic
fenofibrate	TriCor	antihyperlipidemic
fluvastatin sodium	Lescol	antihyperlipidemic
gemfibrozil	Lopid	antihyperlipidemic
lovastatin	Mevacor	antihyperlipidemic
pravastatin sodium	Pravachol	antihyperlipidemic, HMG-CoA reductase inhibitor
simvastatin	Zocor	antihyperlipidemic, HMG-CoA reductase inhibitor
ANTIHYPERTENSIVE		
amlodipine/atorvastatin	Caduet	antihypertensive, calcium channel blocker
amlodipine-benazepril HCL	Lotrel	antihypertensive, calcium channel blocker
amlodipine-besylate	Norvasc	antihypertensive, calcium channel blocker
atenolol	Tenormin	antihypertensive
benazepril	Lotensin	antihypertensive, ACE Inhibitor
bepridil	Vascor	antihypertensive, calcium channel blocker
candesartan	Atacand	antihypertensive
captopril	Capoten	antihypertensive, ACE Inhibitor
carvedilol	Coreg	antihypertensive
clonidine	Duraclon	antihypertensive
clonidine HCL	Catapres	antihypertensive
doxazosin	Cardura	antihypertensive, Alpha blocker
enalapril	Vasotec	antihypertensive, vasodilator, ACE Inhibitor
fosinopril sodium	Monopril	antihypertensive, vasodilator, ACE Inhibitor
hydrochlorothiazide	Esidrix	antihypertensive, diuretic, antiurolithic
irbesartan	Avapro	antihypertensive
irbesartan-hydrochlorothiazide	Avalide	antihypertensive
lisinopril	Prinivil	antihypertensive, vasodilator
lisinopril	Zestril	antihypertensive, vasodilator, ACE Inhibitor
losartan potassium	Cozaar	antihypertensive, angiotensin II-receptor antagonist
losartan-hydrochlorothiazide	Hyzaar	antihypertensive
perindopril	Coversyl	antihypertensive, vasodilator, ACE Inhibitor
prazosin	Minipress	antihypertensive, Alpha blocker
prazosin/polythiazide	Minizide	antihypertensive, Alpha blocker
quinapril	Accupril	antihypertensive, vasodilator, ACE Inhibitor
ramipril	Altace	antihypertensive, vasodilator, ACE Inhibitor

Generic Name	Registered Brand or Trade Name	Therapeutic Use/Medication Action
ANTIHYPERTENSIVE—cont'd		
spironolactone	Aldactone	antihypertensive, antihypokalemic, hyperaldosteronism diagnostic aid, diuretic, aldosterone antagonist
terazosin	Hytrin	antihypertensive, benign prostatic hyperplasia
trandolapril	Mavik	antihypertensive, vasodilator, ACE inhibitor
travoprost	Travatan	antihypertensive reducing intraocular pressure
triamterene-hydrochlorothiazide	Dyazide	antihypertensive, antihypokalemia, diuretic
triamterene-hydrochlorothiazide	Maxzide	antihypertensive, antihypokalemia, diuretic
valsartan	Diovan	antihypertensive
valsartan-hydrochlorothiazide	Diovan HCT	antihypertensive
verapamil/trandolapril	Tarka	antihypertensive, calcium channel blocker
ANTIHYPOKALEMIC		
potassium chloride	Klor-Con	antihypokalemic, electrolyte replenisher
ANTI-INFLAMMATORY (nonsteroid)		
diclofenac	Arthrotec	anti-inflammatory, analgesic
hydroxychloroquine	Plaquenil	systemic antiinflammatory
hydroxychloroquine	Plaquenil	systemic antiinflammatory
mesalamine	Asacol	antiinflammatory in colon/rectum
piroxicam	Feldene	anti-inflammatory, analgesic
tolmetin	Tolectin	anti-inflammatory, analgesic
triamcinolone	Azmacort	inhalation anti-inflammatory, antiasthmatic
valdecoxib	Bextra	nonsteroidal anti-inflammatory antirheumatic antidysmenorrheal
ANTIMETASTATIC		
bicalutamide	Casodex	antimetastatic—used with LHRH-A to treat advanced prostate cancer
ANTIMIGRAINE		
eletriptan HBr	Relpax	antimigraine
sumatriptan	Imitrex	antimigraine
ANTINEOPLASTIC		
conjugated estrogen	Enjuvia	antineoplastic, systemic estrogen, osteoporosis prophylactic, ovarian hormone therapy agent
conjugated estrogen	Premarin	antineoplastic, systemic estrogen, osteoporosis prophylactic, ovarian hormone therapy agent
levothyroxine sodium	Synthroid	antineoplastic, thyroid function diagnostic aid, thyroid hormone
levothyroxine T4	Levothroid	antineoplastic, thyroid function diagnostic aid, thyroid hormone

Generic Name	Registered Brand or Trade Name	Therapeutic Use/Medication Action
ANTIPSYCHOTIC		
olanzapine	Zyprexa	antipsychotic
quetiapine	Seroquel	antipsychotic
risperidone	Risperdal	antipsychotic
thiothixene	Navane	antipsychotic
ziprasidone	Geodon	antipsychotic
ziprasidone	Geodon	antipsychotic
ANTIRHEUMATIC		
meloxicam	Mobic	antirheumatic (NSAID)
ANTISEIZURE		
ethosuximide	Zarontin	antiseizure
ANTISPASMOTIC		
oxybutynin chloride	Ditropan XL	urinary tract antispasmodic
tolterodine tartrate	Detrol	urinary bladder antispasmodic
ANTITHROMBOTIC		
clopidogrel bisulfate	Plavix	antithrombotic, platelet aggregation inhibitor
ANTIULCER		
esomeprazole magnesium	Nexium	gastric acid pump inhibitor, antiulcer
lansoprazole SR	Prevacid	gastric acid pump inhibitor, antiulcer
misoprostol	Cytotec	gastric acid pump inhibitor, antiulcer
omeprazole SA	Prilosec	gastric acid pump inhibitor, antiulcer
pantoprazole	Protonix	gastric acid pump inhibitor, antiulcer
rabeprazole	AcipHex	gastric acid pump inhibitor, antiulcer
ranitidine	Zantac	histamine H2-receptor antagonist, antiulcer, gastric acid secretion inhibitor
ANTIVIRAL		
acyclovir	Zovirax	systemic antiviral
ribavirin	Rebetol	antiviral
ribavirin	Copegus	antiviral
valacyclovir	Valtrex	systemic antiviral
ANTIWRINKLE (topical)		
tretinoin	Retin-A	antiwrinkle cream

Generic Name	Registered Brand or Trade Name	Therapeutic Use/Medication Action
BRONCHODILATOR		
albuterol	Proventil	bronchodilator
albuterol	Ventolin	bronchodilator
BONE RESORPTION INHIBITOR		
alendronate sodium	Fosamax	bone resorption inhibitor
calcitonin-salmon	Miacalcin	bone resorption inhibitor
raloxifene sodium	Evista	selective estrogen receptor modulator, osteoporosis prophylactic
risedronate sodium	Actonel	bone resorption inhibitor
CATHARTIC		
polyethylene glycol	MiraLax	hyperosmotic laxative
CENTRAL NERVOUS SYSTEM STIMULANT		
dextroamphetamine-amphetamine	Adderall	CNS stimulant, ADHD therapy
methylphenidate	Concerta	CNS stimulant, ADHD therapy
methylphenidate	Metadate	CNS stimulant, ADHD therapy
methylphenidate	Ritalin	CNS stimulant, ADHD therapy
CONTRACEPTIVE		
ethinyl estradiol-drospirenone	Yasmin	systemic contraceptive
ethinyl estradiol-norelgestromin	Ortho Evra	systemic contraceptive
ethinyl estradiol-norelgestromin	Ortho Evra	systemic contraceptive
ENZYME		
pancrelipase	Pancrease	pancreatic enzyme replacement
HEMOPOIETIC		
erythropoietin	Epogen	hematopoietic
erythropoietin	Procrit	hematopoietic
HORMONE		
conjugated estrogen-medroxyprogesterone	Premphase	estrogen-progestin, osteoporosis prophylactic, ovarian hormone therapy
conjugated estrogen-medroxyprogesterone	Prempro	estrogen-progestin, osteoporosis prophylactic, ovarian hormone therapy
estrogen conjugated	Premarin	hormone replacement—estrogen
IMMUNE ENHANCER		
pimecrolimus	Elidel	immunomodulator

Generic Name	Registered Brand or Trade Name	Therapeutic Use/Medication Action
NEOPLASTIC		
anastrozole	Arimidex	chemotherapeutic-hormone receptor-positive
SEDATIVE		
temazepam	Restoril	sedative-hypnotic
zolpidem tartrate	Ambien	sedative-hypnotic
SKELETAL MUSCLE RELAXANT		
carisoprodol	Soma	skeletal muscle relaxant
chlorzoxazone	Parafon Forte DSC	skeletal muscle relaxant
cyclobenzaprine	Flexeril	skeletal muscle relaxant
metaxalone	Skelaxin	skeletal muscle relaxant
STEROIDS		
fluticasone	Flonase	steroidal nasal anti-inflammatory, nasal corticosteroid
fluticasone	Flovent	steroidal nasal anti-inflammatory, nasal corticosteroid
methylprednisolone	Medrol	steroidal anti-inflammatory, corticoid, steroid, immunosuppressant
mometasone furoate	Nasonex	nasal steroid anti-inflammatory, nasal corticosteroid
prednisone	Deltasone	systemic steroidal anti-inflammatory, cancer chemotherapy antiemetic, corticosteroid immunosuppressant
tobramycin-dexamethasone	TobraDex	ophthalmic corticosteroid, steroidal anti-inflammatory, antibacterial
triamcinolone	Nasacort AQ	nasal steroid anti-inflammatory, nasal corticosteroid
VITAMIN		
niacin	Niacor	nutritional supplement, vitamin

Index

Note: *page numbers followed by f refer to figures.*

"3-day window", 306
72-hour Rule, 306

A

Abdominal pain, 178, 202
ABG. *See* Arterial blood gas
ABN. *See* Advance Beneficiary Notice
Abnormal menstruation types, 108
Abortion, A-35
  with liveborn fetus, A-36
  methods, 119
  services, 370
  types, 118
Above-knee amputation (AKA), 2, 43
Abruptio placentae, 117
Absorption atelectasis, 66
Abuse, 312
  medicare fraud and, 310
Accessory organs, 98, 123, 164. *See also* Digestive system
Accessory sinuses, 55, 351
Accounts receivable (AR), 306
Acetabulum, 34
Acetaminophen-codeine, trade name and use of, A-127
Achilles tendon, 40
Acid-fast bacillus (AFB), 59
Acidosis, respiratory, 66
ACL. *See* Anterior cruciate ligament
Acne vulgaris, 18
Acquired immunodeficiency syndrome (AIDS), 25
Acromegaly, 220
Actinic keratosis, 24
Acuity sheet, in emergency department, 415
Acute bronchitis, with COPD, A-30
Acute fractures vs. Aftercare, A-36, A-41
Acute infection, of B cells, 203
Acute lymphocytic leukemia, treatment, 205
Acute myelogenous leukemia (AML), 204
Acute myocardial infarction (AMI), A-29
Acute necrotizing fasciitis, 21
Acute organ dysfunction, A-16
Acute pericarditis, 92
Acute poststreptococcal glomerulonephritis (APSGN), 153–154
Acute pyelonephritis, 151f, 152
Acute renal failure (ARF), 144, 149
Acute respiratory failure, 65, A-30
Acute superficial gastritis, 174
Acyclovir, trade name and use of, A-136
AD. *See* Ear, right

Addison's disease
  cause, 224
  symptoms, 224
  treatment, 225
Adenomyosis, 112
Adrenal glands, 212
  disorders, 224
Adrenal insufficiency, primary, 224
Adrenal medulla, 255
Adult respiratory distress syndrome (ARDS), 59, 66, 186
Advance Beneficiary Notice (ABN)
  reimbursement terminology, 316
Adverse effect, A-43
AFB. *See* Acid-fast bacillus
AFI. *See* Amniotic fluid index
Aftercare, A-50
  acute fractures vs., A-36, A-41
AGA. *See* Appropriate for gestational age
AIDS, 237
Air-conducting structure, 55
AKA. *See* Above-knee amputation
Albuterol, trade name and use of, A-137
Alcohol, 175
Aldosterone, 212
Alendronate sodium, trade name and use of, A-137
Allergic contact dermatitis
  diagnosis and treatment, 14
  manifestations, 14
  potential causes, 13
Allopurinol, trade name and use of, A-133
Alphabetic index and tabular list, use of, A-9
Alprazolam, trade name and use of, A-129
Alveolar ducts, 56
Alzheimer's disease, 237
Amblyopia, 263
Ambulance modifiers, 376
Ambulatory Payment Classifications (APCS), 285
Amenorrhea, 107
American Health Information Management Association (AHIMA), A-1
American Hospital Association (AHA), A-1
Amitriptyline, trade name and use of, A-131
AML. *See* Acute myelogenous leukemia
Amlodipine/atorvastatin, trade name and use of, A-134
Amlodipine-benazepril HCL, trade name and use of, A-134
Amniotic fluid index (AFI), 101
Amoxicillin, trade name and use of, A-130
Amoxicillin-clavulanate, trade name and use of, A-130

Index

Amphiarthrosis, 36
Amyotrophic lateral sclerosis (ALS), 238
Analgesia, 333
Anastrozole, trade name and use of, A-138
Ancillary Service, reimbursement terminology, 316
"And" codes, A-9
Androgen, 212, 226
Anemia
    aplastic, 201
    with chemotherapy, immunotherapy and radiation
        therapy, A-19
    of chronic disease, A-22
    in kidney disease, A-22
    with malignancy, A-19
    in neoplastic disease, A-22
Anesthesia, uses of, 333
Aneurysm
    cerebral, 244
    false, 87
    symptoms, 245
    treatment, 245
    true, 87
Angioma, 249
Angioplasty, 358
Angiotensin-converting enzyme inhibitors, 156
Ankylosing spondylitis (AS), treatment, 50
Anorexia, 176
ANS. See Autonomic nervous system
Antacids, 176
Anterior cruciate ligament (ACL), 43
Anti HIV aids, A-128
Antiacne, A-128
Antiadrenergic, A-128
Antianginal, A-129
Antianxiety, A-129
Antiarrhythmic, A-129
Antibacterial, A-130
Antibiotic therapy, 24
Antibiotics, 133, 151, 176
Anticoagulant, A-130
Anticonvulsant, A-131
Antidementia, A-131
Antidepressant, A-131
Antiemetic, trade name and use of, A-132
Antifungal, A-133
Antiglaucoma, A-133
Antigout, A-133
Antihistamine, A-133
Antihypercalcemic, A-133
Antihyperlipidemic, A-134
Antihypokalemic, A-135
Anti-impotence, A-128
Anti-inflammatory (nonsteroid), trade name and use of,
    A-135
Anti-inflammatory medications, 181
Antimetastatic, A-135
Antimicrobial therapy, for acute necrotizing fasciitis, 21
Antimigraine, A-135
Antimotility agents, 181
Antineoplastic, A-135
Anti-Parkinsonism, A-128
Antipsychotic, A-136
Antirheumatic, A-136
Antiseizure, A-136
Antispasmotic, A-136
Antithrombotic, A-136

Antiulcer, trade name and use of, A-136
Antiviral, A-136
Antiwrinkle (topical), A-136
Aorta, 76
Aortic regurgitation (AR), 92
Aortic valve disease, 91
Aortic valve stenosis, 92
APC (ambulatory patient classification)
    payment rate, and co-insurance amount, 289f
    reimbursement terminology, 316
    structure, 286
Aplastic anemia, 201
Appendicitis, 178
Appendicular skeleton, 34
Appropriate for gestational age (AGA), 101
ARDS. See Adult respiratory distress syndrome
ARF. See Acute renal failure
ARM. See Artificial rupture of membrane
Arterial blood gas (ABG), 59
Arterial grafting, for coronary artery bypass, 356
Arterial-venous grafting, combined, 356
Arteries and veins, 356
Arteriosclerotic cardiovascular disease (ASCVD), 79
Arteriosclerotic heart disease (ASHD), 79
Arteriovenous fistula, repair, 358
Arthralgia, 202
Arthritis, infectious and septic, 50
Articulations, 36
Artificial rupture of membrane (ARM), 101
AS. See Ear, left
ASC modifiers, 325
ASCVD. See Arteriosclerotic cardiovascular disease
ASD. See Atrial septal defect
ASHD. See Arteriosclerotic heart disease
Aspirin, 175
Assignment, reimbursement terminology, 316
Asthma, COPD and, A-29
Astigmatism, 263
Astrocytoma, 249
Atenolol, trade name and use of, A-134
Atherectomy, transluminal, 358
Athlete's foot, 23
Atomoxetine, trade name and use of, A-127
Atopic dermatitis, 13
Atorvastatin, trade name and use of, A-134
Atrial fibrillation, 90, 222
Atrial septal defect (ASD), 79
Atrioventricular, 79
Atrioventricular node (AVN), 77
Atrophy
    illustration, 10f
    lesions, pathophysiology, 11
Attending Physician, reimbursement terminology, 316
AU. See Ears, both
Auditory system, subsection, 374
Autogenous grafts, 346
Autonomic nervous system (ANS), 232, 233
AV. See Atrioventricular
Avian influenza virus, A-31
Axial skeleton, 30
Axon. See also Myelinated axon
Azithromycin, trade name and use of, A-130

B

B cells, acute infection of, 203
B vitamins, 238

Bacterial impetigo, 19
Bacterial sepsis and septicemia, A-16
Bacterial vaginosis, 101
Balanitis, 133
Balloon, 357
Basal cell carcinoma, 25
Basophilia, 203
Below-knee amputation, 43
Benazepril, trade name and use of, A-134
Beneficiary, reimbursement terminology, 316
Benign lesions, 111, 336
Benign prostatic hyperplasia (BPH)
    screening, 135
    symptoms, 135
    treatment, 135
Benign prostatic hypertrophy (BPH), 124
Benign tumors, 24
Bepridil, trade name and use of, A-134
Beta blockers, 156
Bicalutamide, trade name and use of, A-135
Bicuspid, 76
Bi-level positive airway pressure (BiPAP), 59
Bimatoprost, trade name and use of, A-133
Biophysical profile (BPP), 101
Biopsy, 5, 335
    codes, 365
BiPAP. See Bi-level positive airway pressure
Biparietal diameter (BPD), 101
Birthday Rule, reimbursement terminology,
    316
BKA. See Below-knee amputation
Bladder carcinoma, 155, 364
Blood, 73
Blood accumulation, 247
Blood cultures, negative or inconclusive, A-17
Blood pressure (BP)
    classification of, 86f
    elevated, A-28
    readouts, 77
Blood urea nitrogen (BUN), 144
Blood vessels, 76, 249
Boils, 20
Bone marrow, 361
Bone resorption inhibitor, A-137
Bone tumors, origin of, 51
Bones
    cancellous, 29
    classification of, 29
    compact, 29
    cortical, 29
    disorders, 48
    long, 29
    structure of, 30f
Bowen's disease, 134
BP. See Blood pressure
BPD. See Biparietal diameter
BPH. See Benign prostatic hypertrophy
BPP. See Biophysical profile
Bradycardia, 90
Brain, 230
    and spinal cord, 230f
    tumors of, 249
Brain abscess, 246
Brainstem, 231
BRCA-1, 112, 114
BRCA-2, 112

Breast, 98
    carcinoma of, 112
    procedures, 342
    structure of, 98f
Breech presentation, 119
Brimonidine, trade name and use of, A-133
Bronchial tree, branches of, 56
Bronchiectasis, 66
Bronchioles, 56
Bronchiolitis, 66
Bronchitis, COPD and, A-30
Bronchodilator, A-137
Budesonide, trade name and use of, A-129
Buerger's disease, 89
Bulla
    illustration, 10f
    lesions, pathophysiology, 9
BUN. See Blood urea nitrogen
Bundle of His, 77
Bupropion, trade name and use of, A-131
Bupropion HCL, trade name and use of, A-131
Burkitt's lymphoma, 207
Burns treatment, 340

C
C. trachomatis, 132
CA modifier, 289
Cabergoline, trade name and use of, A-128
CABG. See Coronary artery bypass graft
Calcitonin-salmon, trade name and use of,
    A-137
Cancellous bones, 29
Cancer, of scrotum, 5
    endometrial, 113
    of esophagus, 173
    of liver, 182
    of oral cavity, 172
    of penis, 134–135
    of prostate
        stages, 137
        symptoms, 136
        treatment, 137
    symptoms, 132
    of testes, 131
    treatment, 132
Candesartan, trade name and use of, A-134
Candida albicans, 23, 133
Candidiasis, 23, 171
    treatment for, 109
Canker sore, 171
Capillaries, 74
Carcinoma. See also Basal cell carcinoma; Squamous cell
        carcinoma
    of breast, 112
    of cervix, 113
    of fallopian tubes, 115
    of ovary, 114
    of uterus, 113
    of vagina, 116
    of vulva, 116
Cardiac muscle, 37
Cardiac valves, 355
Cardiology, nuclear, 354
Cardiology coding terminology, 353
Cardiomegaly. See Heart
Cardiomyopathy, 93

Cardiovascular system
  anatomy and terminology, 73–77
  combining forms, 77
  pathophysiology, 85
  prefixes, 78
  subsection, 353
  suffixes, 79
  in surgery section, 354
Cardioverter-defibrillators
  pacemakers and, 354
Carisoprodol, trade name and use of, A-138
Carotid body, 371
Carvedilol, trade name and use of, A-134
Case mix, analyzing, 302
Casting, and strapping, 348
Cataracts, 265–266
Cathartic, A-137
Cefadroxil, trade name and use of, A-130
Cefdinir, trade name and use of, A-130
Cefluroximine axetil, trade name and use of, A-130
Cefprozil, trade name and use of, A-130
Celecoxib, trade name and use of, A-127
Celiac disease, 177
Cellular structures, 73
Cellulitis, 20
Centers for Medicare and Medicaid Services (CMS), A-1
Central nervous system (CNS), 233
  disorders, 243
  divisions of, 230
  stimulant, A-137
Central venous access (CVA), procedures, 359
Cephalexin, trade name and use of, A-130
Cephalopelvic disproportion (CPD), 101
Cerebellum, 231
Cerebral cortex, 254
Cerebral infarction, A-28
Cerebrospinal fluid (CSF), shunt category, 233, 372
Cerebrovascular accident (CVA), 233, A-28
  causes, 244
  postoperative, A-28
  symptoms, 244
  treatment, 244
Cerebrovascular disease
  hypertensive, A-27
  late effects of, A-28
Cerebrovascular insufficiency (CVI), 79
Cerebrum, 231
Certified nurse midwife (CNM), 101
Certified Registered Nurse Anesthetist, reimbursement
    terminology, 316
Cervical vertebrae (CV), 43
Cervix, 97
  carcinoma of, 113
  symptoms, 114
  treatment, 114
Cetirizine, trade name and use of, A-133
Cetirizine-pseudoephedrine, trade name and use of,
    A-133
Chambers, of the heart
  lower, 74
  upper, 74
  walls, 75
Chapter-specific coding guidelines, A-12
Charge Description Master
  example of, 310
  reimbursement terminology, 316

Chemotherapy, 112, 155, A-19
  Kaposi's sarcoma and, 25
CHF. See Congestive heart failure
Child and adult abuse guideline, A-65
CHL. See Crown-to-heel length
Chlamydia, 110
Chlorzoxazone, trade name and use of, A-138
Cholangitis, 185
Cholecystitis, 185
Cholelithiasis, 185–186
Chondroblastoma, 51
Chondrosarcoma, 52
Chorea, 238
Choroid, 254
Chronic atrophic gastritis, 174–175
Chronic bronchitis, 69
Chronic diseases, A-22, A-72
Chronic glaucoma, 266
Chronic kidney disease (CKD)
  anemia in, A-22
  hypertensive, A-26
  and kidney transplant, A-31
  stages of, A-31
Chronic lymphocytic leukemia (CLL), 205
Chronic myelogenous leukemia (CML)
  symptoms, 205
  treatment, 205
Chronic obstructive pulmonary disease (COPD), 68
  acute bronchitis with, A-30
  and asthma, A-29
  and bronchitis, A-30
Chronic pain, A-25
Chronic pelvic pain (CPP), 101
Chronic pyelonephritis
  symptoms, 152
  treatment, 152
Chronic renal failure
  cause, 150
  stages, 149
  symptoms, 150
  treatment, 150
Cicatrix, pathophysiology, 13
Ciprofloxacin, trade name and use of, A-130
Circulatory system, 73
  arteries of, 74f
  veins of, 75f
Cirrhosis, 184–185
Citalopram hydrobromide, trade name and use of, A-131
CK. See Creatine kinase
Cleft lip, and cleft palate, 171
Cleft palate, 171f
  cleft lip and, 171
Clonazepam, trade name and use of, A-131
Clonidine, trade name and use of, A-134
Clopidogrel bisulfate, trade name and use of, A-136
Clot, 247
Clotrimazole, trade name and use of, A-133
Clotrimazole-betamethasone, trade name and use of, A-133
CMS. See Centers for Medicare and Medicaid Services
CMS-1450/UB-04, 301f
  blocks 66–81 of, 377
CMS-1500 health insurance claim form, 282f
CNM. See Certified nurse midwife
CNS. See Central nervous system
Coal tar, 16
Coarctation of aorta (CoA), 93

COB. *See* Coordination of benefits
Coding challenge
  examination, 410
    final examination, 411
      grading of examination, 411–413
      guidelines, 410
      pre-examination and post-examination, 410–411
Coding guidelines, general, A-9
Coding of burns, A-41
Co-insurance, reimbursement terminology, 316
Colesevelam, trade name and use of, A-134
Colorectal cancer, 181
Combination code, A-11
Compact bones, 29
Compliance Plan, reimbursement terminology, 316
Conchae, 55
Concurrent Care, reimbursement terminology, 316
Concussion, 247
Conduction system, 76
Congenital anomalies, A-37
Congenital disorders, 156
Congenital heart defects, 93
Congenital neurologic disorders, 241
Congestive heart failure (CHF), 79, 89
Conjugated estrogen, trade name and use of, A-135
Conjugated estrogen-medroxyprogesterone, trade name
  and use of, A-137
Conjunctiva, 254
Conjunctivitis, 264
Constrictive pericarditis, 93
Contraceptive, A-137
Contusion, 247
Coordination of benefits (COB), reimbursement
  terminology, 316
Co-payment, reimbursement terminology, 316
COPD. *See* Chronic obstructive pulmonary disease
Cor pulmonale, 67
Cornea, 253–254
Coronary artery bypass graft (CABG), 79, 355
Coronary artery disease (CAD), 85
Corpus uteri, 368
Correct Coding Initiative, reimbursement terminology, 316
Cortical bones, 29
Cortisol, 212
Cough, 65
Counseling, A-52
CPD. *See* Cephalopelvic disproportion
CPK. *See* Creatine phosphokinase
CPP. *See* Chronic pelvic pain
CPT manual, parenthetical information in, 334f
CPT/HCPCS level I modifiers, 325
Cranial, 30
Cranial nerve tumors, 250
Craniectomy, 371
Creatine kinase (CK), 79
Creatine phosphokinase (CPK), 79
Crohn's disease, 177–178
Crown-to-heel length (CHL), 101
Crust, of the skin
  illustration, 10f
  lesions, pathophysiology, 11
Cryotherapy, squamous cell carcinoma and, 25
Cryptorchidism, 129
CSF. *See* Cerebrospinal fluid
CTS. *See* Carpal tunnel syndrome
Cuboidal bones, 29

Curvatures, spinal, 49
Cushing syndrome, 224
CVA. *See* Cerebrovascular accident
CVI. *See* Cerebrovascular insufficiency
Cyclobenzaprine, trade name and use of, A-138
Cyclosporin, 16
Cystitis
  bacterial, 150–151
  nonbacterial, 151

D
Data quality, 309
  reimbursement issues and, 277–321
Decubitis ulcer, 11, 340
Deductible, reimbursement terminology, 316
Dehydration, management of, due to malignancy, A-19
Dementias, classified by causative factor, 237
Denial, reimbursement terminology, 316
Department of Health and Human Services (DHHS), 283,
  A-1
Depression, 243
Dermatitis
  allergic contact, 13
  irritant contact, 14
  seborrheic, 15
Dermatology, 5
Dermis, 2
Desloratadine, trade name and use of, A-133
Destruction, 341
Developed Ambulatory Patient Groups, 285
DHHS. *See* Department of Health and Human Services
Diabetes codes, A-21
Diabetes insipidus, 221
Diabetes mellitus, 219, A-20
  acute complications, 219
  chronic complications, 219
  gestational, 220
  and insulin, A-21
  in pregnancy, A-33
  in pregnancy and gestational diabetes, A-22
  symptoms, 219
  types of, 219
Diabetic ketoacidosis, 219
Diabetic macular edema, A-21
Diabetic retinopathy, A-21
Diagnosis codes, ICD-9-CM, 324
Diagnosis Related Groups (DRGs), 307, 315
  categories of, 294f
  reimbursement terminology, 316
Diaper dermatitis
  causes of, 18
  treatment for, 19
Diaphragm
  anatomy and terminology, 191
  mediastinum and, 191f
Diaphragmatic hernia, 173
Diaphysis, 29
Diarthrosis, types, 36
Diazepam, trade name and use of, A-127
Diclofenac, trade name and use of, A-135
Diencephalon, 231
Diffuse capacity of lungs for carbon monoxide (DLCO), 59
Digestive system, 163f
  accessory organs, 164
  anatomy and terminology, 161–165
  combining forms, 165

Index

Digestive system *(Continued)*
  diseases of, A-31
  function, 161
  pathophysiology, 171
  suffixes, 166–167
Digital rectal examination (DRE), 135
Digoxin, trade name and use of, A-129
Dilation, 145
Dilation and curettage, 101
Dilation and evacuation, 101
Diltiazem, trade name and use of, A-129
Diplopia, 263
Dipyridamole/ASA, trade name and use of, A-130
Dislocation, 48, 344
Disorders
  joint, 49
  of pancreas, 186
  papulosquamous, 15
  of prostate gland, 135
Divalproex sodium, trade name and use of, A-131
Diverticulitis, 180
Diverticulosis, 180
DJD, degenerative joint disease, 49
DLCO. *See* Diffuse capacity of lungs for carbon monoxide
Dobutamine stress echocardiography (DSE), 79
Documentation, reimbursement terminology, 316
Donepezil, trade name and use of, A-131
Donor, A-52
Dorzolamide/timolol, trade name and use of, A-133
Doxazosin, trade name and use of, A-134
Doxazosin mesylate, trade name and use of, A-131
Doxepin, trade name and use of, A-131
DRGs. *See* Diagnosis Related Groups
Drugs
  and chemicals, table of, 381
  overdose of, A-44
DSE. *See* Dobutamine stress echocardiography
Duodenal ulcers, 178
Duodenum, 164
  disorders of the, 174
Durable Medical equipment, reimbursement terminology, 316
Dwarfism, 220
Dysfunctional uterine bleeding, 108
Dysmenorrhea, 107–108
  primary, 107
  secondary, 107
Dyspnea, 65, 222

E

E codes, 382
  coding guidelines, A-63
E. coli, 130, 152
Ear(s)
  bones, middle, 30
  both, 257
  divisions of, 31f, 255
  infections, 267
  left, 257
  right, 257
  structure of, 31f
Eburnation, sclerosis of bone, 49
ECC. *See* Endocervical curettage
Eclampsia, 117
Econazole, trade name and use of, A-133
Ectopic pregnancy, 118

ED acuity sheet, example of, 330f
EDC. *See* Estimated date of confinement
EDD. *See* Estimated date of delivery
Edema. 80, 153. *See also* Diabetic macular edema; Pulmonary edema
EDI. *See* Electronic data interchange
Efavirenz, trade name and use of, A-128
EFM. *See* Electronic fetal monitoring
EFW. *See* Estimated fetal weight
EGJ. *See* Esophagogastric junction
Electroencephalogram (EEG), 233
Electronic data interchange (EDI), 315
  reimbursement terminology, 316
Electronic fetal monitoring (EFM), 101
Electrophysiologic operative procedures, 355
Electrophysiology (EPS), 353
Eletriptan HBr, trade name and use of, A-135
Embolectomy, and thrombectomy, 357
Embolism, 67, 88
Embolus, 357
EMC. *See* Endometrial curettage
Emergency department (ED)
  acuity sheet, 415
  services, 330
Emphysema, 69
Employer Identification Number, reimbursement terminology, 316
Empyema, 67
Emtricitabine, trade name and use of, A-128
Enalapril, trade name and use of, A-134
Encephalitis, 245
Encounter Form, reimbursement terminology, 317
Endocarditis, infective, 90
Endocardium, 75
Endocervical curettage (ECC), 101
Endocrine glands, 211
Endocrine system
  anatomy and terminology, 211–213
  combining forms, 213
  illustration, 211f
  pathophysiology, 219
  prefixes, 214
  subsection, 370
  suffixes, 214
Endometrial cancer, 113
Endometrial curettage (EMC), 102
Endometriosis
  causes, 108
  risks, 109
  treatment, 109
Endometrium, 97
  repair, 98
Endoscopic retrograde cholangiopancreatography (ERCP), 166
Endoscopy, 349
  laparoscopy and, 348, 362
Endosteum, 29
Endovascular repair, of descending thoracic aorta, 356
End-stage renal disease (ESRD), 144, 315
Enzyme, A-137
EOB. *See* Explanation of benefits
Eosinophilia, 202–203
Ependymoma, 249
Epicardium, 75
Epidermis, 2
Epididymis, disorders of, 129

Epididymitis
  symptoms, 130
  treatment, 130
  types, 129
Epilepsies
  causes, 246
  treatment, 247
  types, 246
Epiphyseal line, 29
Epiphysis, 29
Epispadias, 132
Epithelial tumors, 115
Eponychium, 2
ERCP. *See* Endoscopic retrograde cholangiopancreatography
Erosion
  illustration, 10f
  lesions, pathophysiology, 11
ERT. *See* Estrogen replacement therapy
Erysipelas
  cause, 20
  lesions, 21
Erythrocytes, 73
Erythropoietin, trade name and use of, A-137
Escitalopram oxalate, trade name and use of, A-129
Esomeprazole magnesium, trade name and use of, A-136
Esophageal disorders, 172
Esophagitis
  acute, 172
  chronic, 173
Esophagogastric junction (EGJ), 166
Esophagogastroduodenoscopy (EGD), 166
Esophagus, 163
ESRD. *See* End–stage renal disease
Estimated date of confinement (EDC), 101
Estimated date of delivery (EDD), 101
Estimated fetal weight (EFW), 101
Estimated gestational age (EGA), 102
Estrogen conjugated, trade name and use of, A-137
Estrogen hypersecretion, 226
Estrogen replacement therapy (ERT), 102
Estropia, 264
Ethinyl estradiol-desogestrel, trade name and use of, A-132
Ethinyl estradiol-drospirenone, trade name and use of, A-137
Ethinyl estradiol-levonorgestrel, trade name and use of, A-132
Ethinyl estradiol-norelgestromin, trade name and use of, A-137
Ethinyl estradiol-norethindrone, trade name and use of, A-128
Ethinyl estradiol-norgestrel, trade name and use of, A-132
Ethosuximide, trade name and use of, A-136
Evaluation and management (E/M) section, 329–333
Exotropia, 264
Explanation of Benefits (EOB), reimbursement terminology, 315, 317
Extrauterine, 118
Extremities, 39
  lower, 34, 40
  upper, 34
Eye
  layers of, 253
  left, 258
  and ocular adnexa, 253
  right, 258
Ezetimibe, trade name and use of, A-134

F

Fallopian tubes, 97
  carcinoma, of, 115
  ectopic pregnancy in, 118
  primary, 115
  symptoms, 115
  treatment, 116
FAS. *See* Fetal alcohol syndrome
Federal Register, example of page from, 284
Fee schedule, reimbursement terminology, 317
FEF. *See* Forced expiratory flow
Female genital system
  anatomy and terminology, 97–99
  pathophysiology, 107
  subsection, 366
Female reproductive system, 97f
  combining forms, 99
  prefixes, 100
  suffixes, 101
Femur, 34
Fenofibrate, trade name and use of, A-134
Fentanyl, trade name and use of, A-127
Fetal alcohol syndrome (FAS), 102
Fetal conditions, affecting management of mother, A-33
Fetal heart rate, 102
FEV_1. *See* Forced expiratory volume in 1 second
Fever, rheumatic, 91
Fexofenadine, trade name and use of, A-133
Fexofenadine-pseudoephedrine, trade name and use of, A-133
Fibrillation, 90
Fibroid, 111
Fibroma, 111
Fibromyalgia syndrome, primary, 51
Fibromyoma, 111
Fibrous lesions, encase heart, 93
Final examination, 437
Fissure
  illustration, 10f
  lesions, pathophysiology, 11
Fistulectomy codes, 363
Fixation
  external, 346
  spinal instrumentation and, 347
Fixator, as joint stabilizer, 38
Fluconazole, trade name and use of, A-133
Fluid replacement, for acute necrotizing fasciitis, 21
Fluids, 254
Fluoxetine, trade name and use of, A-131
Fluticasone, trade name and use of, A-138
Flutter, treatment, 90
Fluvastatin sodium, trade name and use of, A-134
Follicle-stimulating hormone (FSH), 102
Folliculitis, 20
Follow-Up Days, reimbursement terminology, 317
Forced expiratory flow (FEF), 59
Forced expiratory volume in 1 second (FEV_1), 59
Forced vital capacity (FVC), 59
Fosinopril sodium, trade name and use of, A-134
Fractures, 43–44
  classification of, 47
  treatment, 47, 344
Fraud
  abuse, complaints of, 312
  examples, 311
FRC. *See* Functional residual capacity

FSH. *See* Follicle-stimulating hormone
Functional residual capacity (FRC), 59
Fundus, 97
Fungal, 23
Furosemide, trade name and use of, A-133
Furuncles, 20
FVC. *See* Forced vital capacity

G

Gabapentin, trade name and use of, A-131
Galantamine HBr, trade name and use of, A-131
Gallbladder
    containing gallstones, 185f
    disorders of, 182, 185
Gamma globulin, 183
Gastric cancer, 176
Gastritis
    causes, 174
    symptoms, 174
    treatment, 174
Gastrocnemius, 40
Gastroesophageal reflux disease (GERD), 166, 174
Gemfibrozil, trade name and use of, A-134
Genital herpes, 110
Genital warts, 110
Genitalia, external, 123
Genitourinary system, diseases of, A-31
GERD. *See* Gastroesophageal reflux disease
Germ cell tumors, 114, 249
Gestation, 99, 370
Gestational diabetes mellitus, 220, A-34
GI. *See* Gastrointestinal
Gigantism, 220, 221f
Glands, 2
Glaucoma, 266
Glia, 229
Glimepiride, trade name and use of, A-131
Glioblastoma, 249
Glipizide, trade name and use of, A-131
Glomerular disorders, 152
Glomerulonephritis
    cause, 152
    treatment, 153
Glucagons, 212
Glyburide, trade name and use of, A-131
Glyburide-metformin, trade name and use of, A-131
Goiter, 222f
    cause for, 221
Gonadal stromal tumors, 115
Gonads, 123
Gonorrhea, 110, 133
Gout, 50
Gouty arthritis, 50
Grafts, 339, 346
Granulocytosis, 202
Griseofulvin, trade name and use of, A-133
Group A beta-hemolytic streptococcus, 19
Group Practice Group Provider Number, reimbursement
    terminology, 317
Guillain-Barré syndrome, 241

H

Hand-held nebulizer (HHN), 59
HCPCS codes, APC grouping of, 286f, 315, 375
HCPCS National Level II index, 376
HCVD. *See* Hypertensive cardiovascular disease

Head injury, 247
Health care, managed, 312
Health Insurance Portability and Accountability Act
    (HIPAA), A-1
Health maintenance organization (HMO), 313
Hearing, 255
Hearing loss
    conductive, 267
    ototoxic, 268
Heart, 74, 354
    and chronic kidney disease, hypertensive, A-27
    electrical system of, 77f
    internal view of, 76f
Heart block, bradycardia and, 90
Heart disease, 91
Heart disorders, 89
Heart muscle, 37
Heart rhythms, abnormal, 90
Heart wall, disorders, 92
Heartbeat, 77
Hemangioblastoma, 249
Hematoma, 247
Hematopoietic organ, 195
Hemic system
    anatomy and terminology, 195
    combining forms, 195
    and lymphatic system, 195
    pathophysiology, 201
    prefixes, 197
    subsection, 361
    suffixes, 197
Hemodialysis, 144
Hemolytic anemia, treatment, 202
Hemopoietic, A-137
Hemorrhoidectomy codes, 363
Hepatitis, 184
Hepatitis A (HAV), 182
Hepatitis B (HBV), 183
Hepatitis C (HCV), 183
Hepatitis D (HDV), 183
Hepatitis E (HEV), 183
Hepatitis G, 183
Hepatojugular reflux (HJR), 166
Hernia
    sliding and paraesophageal, 173
Hernia codes, 363
Herpes simplex virus (HSV), 25, 102
    type 1 (HSV-1), 21, 172
    type 2 (HSV-2), 21
Herpes zoster, 22
HHN. *See* Hand-held nebulizer
Hiatal hernia, 173
HIV codes, selection and sequencing of, A-12
HIV infection, in pregnancy, childbirth and puerperium,
    A-13, A-33
Hodgkin's disease, 206
Home health prospective payment system (HHPPS),
    307
Hordeolum, 264
Hormonal disorders, 107
Hormone, A-137
Hospital Outpatient, reimbursement terminology, 317
Hospital Payment Monitoring System, reimbursement
    terminology, 317
HPV. *See* Human papillomavirus
HSG. *See* Hysterosalpingogram

HSV. *See* Herpes simplex virus

Human chorionic gonadotropin (HCG), 99

Human immunodeficiency virus (HIV), 25
  asymptomatic, A-13
  infections, A-12

Human papillomavirus (HPV), 22, 102

Huntington's disease, 238

Hydatidiform mole, 118

Hydrocele, 130, 130f

Hydrocephalus, 241

Hydrochlorothiazide, trade name and use of, A-134

Hydrocodone, trade name and use of, A-127

Hydrocodone-acetaminophen, trade name and use of, A-127

Hydrocodone-chlorpheniramine, trade name and use of, A-133

Hydronephrosis, 155–156

Hydroxychloroquine, trade name and use of, A-135

Hydroxyzine, trade name and use of, A-133

Hyperaldosteronism, 225

Hyperbilirubinemia, 182

Hypercapnia, 65

Hypercholesterolemia, 153

Hypercoagulability, 153

Hypercortisolism, 224

Hyperopia, 263

Hyperparathyroidism, 223

Hyperpituitarism, 220

Hypertension (HTN), A-26
  controlled, A-27
  essential, or NOS, A-26
  with heart disease, A-26
  secondary, A-27
  transient, A-27
  treatment for, 86
  uncontrolled, A-28

Hypertensive cardiovascular disease (HCVD), 79

Hypertensive retinopathy, A-27

Hyperthyroidism, 221–222

Hypertropia, 264

Hyperventilation, 65

Hypoalbuminemia, 153

Hypodermis, 2

Hypomenorrhea, 108

Hypoparathyroidism
  symptoms, 223
  treatment, 224

Hypophysis glands, 211

Hypopituitarism, 220

Hypospadias, 132

Hypotension, 87

Hypothalamus, 213

Hypothyroidism
  treatment, 223
  types, 222

Hypotropia, 264

Hypoventilation, 65

Hysterosalpingogram, 102

I

Ibuprofen, trade name and use of, A-127

ICD-9-CM
  with 3, 4, or 5 digits, A-71
  conventions, 378, A-7
  format of, 378
  on insurance forms, 377

ICD-9-CM (Continued)
  overview of, 376
  uses of, 377, 383

ICD-9-CM official guidelines for coding and reporting, A-1

Immune enhancer, A-137

Immunotherapy, A-19

Improper union, 48

In vitro fertilization, 102, 369

Incision and drainage, 5

Individual Practice Infant respiratory distress syndrome, 59

Infections, 109, 171, 264
  causes, 172
  ear, 267
  treatment, 172

Infectious arthritis, 50

Infectious disease, 68, A-12

Infectious mononucleosis, 203

Infectious pleural effusion, 67

Inferior vena cava, 76

Inflammation, 109
  thrombophlebitis caused by, 88

Inflammatory bowel disease (IBD), 177

Inflammatory disorders, pathophysiology, 13

Injury, in musculoskeletal systems, 47

Inpatient, reimbursement terminology, 317

Inpatient psychiatric facility (IPF), prospective payment system, 308

Inpatient rehabilitation facility (IRF), prospective payment system, 308

Inspiratory positive airway pressure (IPAP), 59

Insulin, 212, A-22

Insulin, trade name and use of, A-131

Insulin glargine, trade name and use of, A-131

Insulin pump malfunction, A-22

Insulin-dependent diabetes mellitus, 219

Integumentary system, 3f
  anatomy and terminology, 2
  combining forms, 3
  pathophysiology, 9
  prefixes, 4
  subsection, 335
  suffixes, 5

Interleukin-2 inhibitors, 16

Intestinal disorders, 177

Intestine
  large, 164, 180
  small, 164

Intraocular, 258

Intraocular lens (IOL), 258

Intravenous pyelogram (IVP), 144

Introitus, 366

Invalid Claim, reimbursement terminology, 317

IOL. *See* Intraocular lens

IPAP. *See* Inspiratory positive airway pressure

Irbesartan, trade name and use of, A-134

IRDS. *See* Infant respiratory distress syndrome

Iron deficiency anemia, 201

Irreversible ischemia, 85

Irritant contact dermatitis, 14–15

Ischemia, 85

Ischemic heart disease (IHD), 85

Ischium, 34

Isosorbide mononitrate, trade name and use of, A-129

Itching, 19

Itraconazole, trade name and use of, A-133

IVP. *See* Intravenous pyelogram

J

Jaundice, 182
Joints, 36
    disorders of, 49

K

Kaposi's sarcoma, 25, 172
Keloids, pathophysiology, 12
Keratin plates, 2
Keratitis, 264
Keratoacanthoma, 24
Keratosis, 24
Ketoacidosis, 219
Ketoconazole, trade name and use of, A-133
Kickbacks, 312
Kidney, 141
    disease, chronic, A-31
    illustration, 142f
    stones
        symptoms, 154
        treatment, 155
    structure, 142
    subheading, 364
    transplant, complications, A-45
    ureter, bladder (KUB), 144
Kyphosis, 49

L

Laboratory pathological revenue code, chart of, 309
Labyrinth, 255
Lactase deficiency
    symptoms, 177
    treatment, 177
Lamotrigine, trade name and use of, A-131
Lansoprazole SR, trade name and use of, A-136
Laparoscopy, and endoscopy, 362
Large for gestational age (LGA), 102
Large intestine, 164
Laryngoscopic procedures, 352
Larynx, 55, 351
Laser therapy, 132
Latanoprost, trade name and use of, A-133
LEEP. *See* Loop electrosurgical excision procedure
Left bundle branch block, 79
Left lower quadrant (LLQ), 167
Left upper quadrant (LUQ), 167
Left ventricular hypertrophy (LVH), 79
Leiomyomas, 111
Lens, 254
Lesion
    calculating size of, 336
    in integumentary system, 9
    removal of, 343
    shaving of, 336
    of skin, 10
Leukemia, 204
Leukocytopenia, cause, 203
Leukocytosis, cause, 203
Levetiracetam, trade name and use of, A-131
Levothyroxine sodium, trade name and use of, A-135
Levothyroxine T4, trade name and use of, A-135
LGA. *See* Large for gestational age
Lichen planus
    lesions, 17
    treatment for, 18

Ligament disorders, 51
Lisinopril, trade name and use of, A-134
Liveborn fetus, abortion with, A-36
Liver, disorders of, 182
LLQ. *See* Left lower quadrant
Loop electrosurgical excision procedure (LEEP), 102
Loratadine, trade name and use of, A-133
Lorazepam, trade name and use of, A-127
Lordosis, 49
Losartan potassium, trade name and use of, A-134
Losartan-hydrochlorothiazide, trade name and use of,
    A-134
Lovastatin, trade name and use of, A-134
Lower respiratory infection (LRI), 68
Lower respiratory tract, 55
Lumbar puncture, 233
Lumbar vertebrae, 43
Lund-Browder chart, for estimating burns on children, 342
Lungs, 57
    and pleura, 352
LUQ. *See* Left upper quadrant
LVH. *See* Left ventricular hypertrophy
Lymph, 195
Lymph node, 132
    and lymphatic channels, 361
Lymph organs, 195
Lymph vessels, 195
Lymphadenitis, 205
Lymphadenopathy, 205
Lymphangitis, 205
Lymphatic channels, lymph nodes and, 361
Lymphatic system, 196f
    anatomy and terminology, 195
    combining forms, 195
    pathophysiology, 201
    prefixes, 197
    subsection, 361
    suffixes, 197
Lymphocytic leukemia, acute, 204

M

Macular degeneration, 265
Macule
    illustration, 10f
    lesions, pathophysiology, 9
Major diagnostic category, DRG structure for, 299
Malabsorption, 48
Male genital system
    anatomy and terminology, 123–124
    combining forms, 124
    disorders of, 129
    pathophysiology, 129
    subsection, 365
    suffixes, 124
Malignant lesions, 112, 336
Malignant lymphoma, 206
Malignant melanoma, 25
Malignant tumor, 24, 155, 176
Malposition, of fetus, types of, 118–119
Malpresentation, of fetus, types of, 118
Managed Care Organization, 313
Manipulation, 344
Mastectomy, 112
Master glands, 211
MAT. *See* Multifocal atrial tachycardia
Maternity care & delivery, subsection, 369

MDI. *See* Metered dose inhaler
Mechanoreceptors, 256
Meckel's diverticulum, 178
Mediastinum
  anatomy and terminology, 191
  and diaphragm, 191f, 193
Medical coding, introduction to, 324
Medical Record, reimbursement terminology, 317
Medical Volume Performance Medicare, 278
  funding for, 283
Medicare Administrative Contractors, reimbursement
    terminology, 317
Medicare Economic Medicare Fee Medicare fraud, and
    abuse, 310
Medicare Severity Diagnosis Related Groups
  classification, 297
  reimbursement terminology, 293, 295–296, 296f,
      317
  structure of, 293
Medulloblastoma, 250
Meloxicam, trade name and use of, A-136
Ménière's disease, 259, 268
Meningioma, 250
Meningocele, 242f
Menometrorrhagia, 108
Menorrhagia, 108
Menorrhea, 108
Menstrual, disorders, 107
Menstruation
  abnormal, 108
  and pregnancy, 98
Mental disorders, 241, A-23
Mesalamine, trade name and use of, A-135
Metaphysis, 29
Metaxalone, trade name and use of, A-138
Metered dose inhaler, 60
Metformin HCL, trade name and use of, A-132
Methylphenidate, trade name and use of, A-137
Methylprednisolone, trade name and use of, A-138
Metoprolol succinate, trade name and use of, A-128
Metrorrhagia, 108
Miconazole, trade name and use of, A-133
Miglitol, trade name and use of, A-132
Minocycline, trade name and use of, A-130
Mirtazapine, trade name and use of, A-131
Misoprostol, trade name and use of, A-136
Mitral regurgitation (MR), 92
Mitral valve stenosis, 92
Modifier functions, 325
Mohs' microscope surgery, 342
Moles (nevi), 24
Mometasone furoate, trade name and use of,
    A-138
Monocytosis, 203
Mononucleosis, infectious, 203
Motor neuron disease (MND), 238
Mouth, 161
  anatomic structures of, 161f
Movements, terms of, 39
Moxifloxacin, trade name and use of, A-130
MS-DRG payment, calculating, 300
MS-DRG reimbursement, monitoring, 306
Multifocal atrial tachycardia (MAT), 79
Multiple fractures, A-41
Multiple myeloma, 52
Multiple sclerosis (MS), 239

Muscle
  action, 38
  capabilities, 38
  disorders, 51
  movement, 38
  names of, 39
Muscle tissue, types of, 36
Muscle tumors, 52
Muscular dystrophy, familial disorder, 51
Muscular system
  anterior view, 38f
  functions, 36
  posterior view of, 37f
Musculoskeletal system
  anatomy and terminology, 29–42
    bone classification, 29
    skeletal system, 29
    structure, 29
  combining forms, 40
  prefixes, 42
  subsection, 343
  suffixes, 42
Musculoskeletal systems, pathophysiology, 47
Myasthenia gravis (MG)
  symptoms, 239
  treatment, 240
Myelomeningocele, 242f
Myocardial infarction, 79, 85, A-77
Myocardial ischemia, 85
Myocardium, 75, 93
Myoma, 111
Myometrium, 97

N

Nails, 2, 337
Naproxen, trade name and use of, A-127
Nasal turbinates, superior, inferior, and middle, 56
National Center for Health Statistics (NCHS), A-1
National Correct Coding Initiative (NCCI), 285
National Provider Identifier (NPI), 282f
  reimbursement terminology, 317
Nausea and vomiting, 184
Neoplasms, general guidelines, A-18
Neoplastic, A-138
Nephroblastoma, 157
Nephrolithiasis, 154
Nephron loss, stages of, 150
Nephrosclerosis, 156
Nephrosis, 153
Nephrotic syndrome, 153
Nervous system
  anatomy and terminology, 229
  cells of, 229
  combining forms, 232
  pathophysiology, 237
  prefixes, 232
  primary cells of, 229
  and sense organs, diseases of, A-23
  subsection, 371
  suffixes, 233
Neurons, 229
Neuropathy, 220f
Neutrophils, 202
Newborn, A-37
  congenital anomalies in, A-39
  infant and child, A-53

Niacin, trade name and use of, 238, A-138
Nifedipine, trade name and use of, A-129
Nitrofurantoin, trade name and use of, A-130
Nitroglycerin, trade name and use of, A-129
Nociceptors, 256
Nodule
   illustration, 10f
   lesions, pathophysiology, 9
Nonbacterial, 136
Noncoronary bypass grafts, 358
Noncovered Services, reimbursement terminology, 317
Non-healing burns, A-42
Non-Hodgkin lymphoma, 109, 206–207
Non-infectious process, SIRS due to, A-45
Non-insulin-dependent diabetes mellitus, 219
Noninvasive, 88
Nonprescribed drug, A-44
Nonviral hepatitis, 184
Normal delivery, A-34
Normal sinus rhythm (NSR), 79
Nose, 55
NPH isophane insulin, trade name and use of, A-132
NPH regular insulin, trade name and use of, A-132
NSR. *See* Normal sinus rhythm
Nuclear cardiology, 354
Nursing services, 279
Nutritional degenerative disease, 238
Nystagmus, 263

O

OA. *See* Osteoarthritis
Obstetric cases, general rules for, A-32
Obstruction, 179
Obstructs vessel, 88
Ocular adnexa
   eye and, 253
OD. *See* Eye, right
Olanzapine, trade name and use of, A-136
Olfactory sense receptors, 255
Oligodendrocytoma, 249
Oligomenorrhea, 108
Olopatadine, trade name and use of, A-133
Omeprazole SA, trade name and use of, A-136
Onychomycosis, 23
Opiates, 19
Optic chiasm, 254
Optic nerve fibers, 254
Oral cavity, disorders of, 171
Orchitis, 129
Organs, 141
   accessory, 123
   essential, in male genital system, 123
Orofacial cleft, 171
OS. *See* Eye, left
Ossicles, 255
Osteitis deformans, 49
Osteoarthritis (OA), 43–44, 49
Osteoma, 51
Osteomalacia, and rickets, 49
Osteomyelitis, 48
Osteoporosis, 48
Osteosarcoma, 57
Otitis externa, 267
Outpatient code edit (OCE), 292
Ovary, 97, 213, 369
   carcinoma of, 114

Oviduct, 97, 369
Ovulation, 98
Oxcarbazepine, trade name and use of, A-131
Oxybutynin chloride, trade name and use of, A-136
Oxycodone, trade name and use of, A-127
Oxycodone-acetaminophen, trade name and use of, A-127

P

PAC. *See* Premature atrial contraction
Pacemakers, and cardioverter-defibrillators, 354
Paget's disease, 49
Pain
   category, A-23
   chronic, A-25
   devices, implants and grafts, A-24
   neoplasm related, A-25
   postoperative, A-24–A-25
Pain control, admission/encounter for, A-20
Pain syndrome, chronic, A-25
Pancreas, 212
   disorders of, 182
Pancreatic cancer, 187
Pancreatic cells, 164
Pancreatitis, 186
Pancrelipase, trade name and use of, A-137
Pantoprazole, trade name and use of, A-136
Pantothenic acid, 238
Papule
   illustration, 10f
   lesions, pathophysiology, 9
Papulosquamous disorders
   conditions associated with, 15
   types of, 16
Paranasal sinuses, 55
Paraphimosis
   phimosis and, 133
   symptom, 134
   treatment, 134
Parathyroid disorders, 223
Parathyroid glands, 212
Parathyroid hormone (PTH), 223
Paring/cutting, 335
Parkinsonism, 238
Parkinson's disease, 239
Paronychium, 2
Paroxetine HCL, trade name and use of, A-129
Paroxysmal atrial tachycardia, 79
Paroxysmal nocturnal dyspnea (PND), 60
   and PSVT, 79
Patent ductus arteriosus (PDA), 93
Patient-activated event recorder, 355
Patient-controlled analgesia (PCA), 333
PAWP. *See* Pulmonary artery wedge pressure
PCWP. *See* Pulmonary capillary wedge pressure
PEAP. *See* Positive end-airway pressure
PEEP. *See* Positive end-expiratory pressure
Pelvic inflammatory disease (PID), 102, 109
Pelvis, 34
Penicillin V, trade name and use of, A-130
Penis, disorders of, 133
Peptic ulcers
   symptoms, 175
   treatment, 176
Percutaneous endoscopic gastrostomy, 167
Percutaneous transluminal coronary angioplasty (PTCA),
   79

Pericardial cavity, 76
Pericardial effusion, 93
Pericarditis
    acute, 92
    constrictive, 93
    restrictive, 93
    types of, 91
Pericardium, 76, 354
Perimetrium, 97
Perinatal morbidity, maternal causes of, A-39
Perindopril, trade name and use of, A-134
Perineum, 98, 366
Peripheral arterial disease, 89
Peripheral nervous system (PNS), 231, 233
Peritoneum, 164
Peritonitis, 178
    symptoms, 179
    treatment, 179
    types, 178
PERL. See Pupils equal and reactive to light
Pernicious anemia, 201–202
Pet modifiers, 376
Peyronie's disease, 134
PFT. See Pulmonary function test
Pharynx, 55, 163
Phimosis, 133–134
Phlebitis, 88
PID. See Pelvic inflammatory disease
Pimecrolimus, trade name and use of, A-137
Pineal region, 213, 249
Pineal tumors, 249
Pink eye, 264
Pioglitazone, trade name and use of, A-132
Piroxicam, trade name and use of, A-135
Pituitary glands, 211
    anterior, 220
    disorders, 220
    posterior, 221
Pituitary tumor, 250
Pityriasis rosea, 17
Placenta, 213
Placenta forms, within uterine wall, 99
Placenta previa, 116, 117f
Plaque
    illustration, 10f
    lesions, pathophysiology, 9
Pleura, lungs and, 352
Pleural effusion-fluid, in pleural space, 67
Pleural space, pleural effusion-fluid in, 67
Pleurisy, 67
Pleuritis, 67
PND. See Paroxysmal nocturnal dyspnea
Pneumoconiosis, 67
Pneumonia, 68
Pneumothorax, 67
PNS. See Peripheral nervous system
POA examples, A-81
Point of service (POS), 313
Poisoning, sequencing of, A-44
Poliomyelitis, 240
Polycystic kidney (PKD), 156
Polyethylene glycol, trade name and use of, A-137
Polymenorrhea, 108
Polymyositis, 51
Positive end-airway pressure (PEAP), 60
Positive end-expiratory pressure (PEEP), 60

Post acute transfer, 305
Posterior pituitary glands, 221
Post-examination, 417–435
Postpartum, and peripartum periods, A-34
Postpolio syndrome (PPS), 240
Potassium chloride, trade name and use of, A-135
Pravastatin sodium, trade name and use of, A-134
Prazosin
    polythiazide, trade name and use of, A-134
    trade name and use of, A-134
Prednisone, trade name and use of, A-138
Pre-examination, 417–435
Pregnancy, 99, 116
    anatomy and terminology, 97–99
    combining forms, 99
    current conditions complicating, A-33
    diabetes mellitus in, A-33
    ectopic, 118
    menstruation and, 98
    pathophysiology, 107
    prefixes, 100
    suffixes, 101
Premature atrial contraction (PAC), 79
Premature rupture of membranes (PROM), 102
Premature ventricular contraction (PVC), 79
Pre-MDC flow chart, 298f
Premenstrual syndrome (PMS), 108
Premenstrual tension (PMT), 108
Premenstruation, 98
Presbyopia, 263
Present on admission indicator (POA), 305
Pressure ulcers, 340
    locations, 11
    stage I, II, III, and IV of, 12
    staging or classification system, 11
Prior Authorization, reimbursement terminology, 317
Professional Standards Review Proliferation phase, 98
PROM. See Premature rupture of membranes
Promethazine-codeine, trade name and use of, A-133
Propoxyphene-acetaminophen, trade name and use of, A-127
Proprioceptors, 256
Prospective payment systems (PPS), 292
Prostate, vesical neck and, 365
Prostate gland, disorders of, 135
Prostate-specific antigen (PSA), 124, 135
Prostatitis
    acute, 136
    causes, 135
    chronic, 136
    symptoms, 136
    treatment, 136
Proteus, 152
Provider Identification Number, reimbursement terminology, 317
Pruritus, 19
PSA. See Prostate-specific antigen
Pseudomonas, 152
Psoralens and ultraviolet A (PUVA) light therapy, 16
Psoriasis, 16
Pseudoaneurysm, 87
PTCA. See Percutaneous transluminal coronary angioplasty
Pubis, 34
Pubis symphysis, 34
Pulmonale, cor, 67
Pulmonary artery stenosis, 76, 94

Index

Pulmonary artery wedge pressure (PAWP), 60
Pulmonary capillary wedge pressure (PCWP), 60
Pulmonary diseases, 65
Pulmonary disorders, signs and symptoms of, 65
Pulmonary edema, 66
Pulmonary embolism, 67
Pulmonary function test (PFT), 60
Pulmonary valve, 91
Pulmonary veins, 76
Pulmonic regurgitation (PR), 92
Pupils equal and reactive to light (PERL), 258
Purkinje fibers, 77
Pustule
    illustration, 10f
    lesions, pathophysiology, 9
PVC. See Premature ventricular contraction
Pyelonephritis, 151–152
Pyloric stenosis, 176–177

Q

Quality Improvement Quetiapine, trade name and use of, A-136
Quinapril, trade name and use of, A-134

R

RA. See Remittance advice; Rheumatoid arthritis
Rabeprazole, trade name and use of, A-136
Radiation, Kaposi's sarcoma and, 25
Radiation therapy, A-19
Radiotherapy, squamous cell carcinoma and, 25
Raloxifene sodium, trade name and use of, A-137
Ramipril, trade name and use of, A-134
Ranitidine, trade name and use of, A-136
Rapid eye movement (REM), 258
Raynaud's disease, 89
RBBB. See Right bundle branch block
RDS. See Respiratory distress syndrome
Red blood cells, 73
Regional enteritis, 177
Regular sinus rhythm (RSR), 79
Regurgitation, of the heart, 92
Reimbursement issues
    basic structure, 279
    and data quality, 277–321
    medicare, 278
        hospital and institutional care coverage, 279
        medicare advantage, 281
        prescription drug, improvement, and modernization act of 2003, 283
        supplemental, 281
    reimbursement terminology, 317
    responsibility, 278
Rejection, reimbursement terminology, 317
Relative Value Relative weights, hospital admissions with, 302f
REM. See Rapid eye movement
Remittance advice (RA), 43
Renal calculi, 154
Renal cancer, tumor staging for, 155
Renal failure, 149
Repaglinide, trade name and use of, A-132
Replantation, 346
Reproductive system, male, 123f
Resource utilization groups (RUGs), 307
Respiration, 40, 57, 66
Respiratory distress syndrome (RDS), 60

Respiratory system
    anatomy and terminology, 55–57
    combining forms, 57
    pathophysiology, 65
    prefixes, 58
    subsection, 348
    suffixes, 58
    upper and lower, 56f
Respiratory volume, 60
Restrictive pericarditis, 93
Retina, 254
Retina, detached, 265
Retinopathy, 219
Revenue codes, categories, 308
Reye's syndrome, 246
Rheumatic fever, 91
Rheumatic heart disease, 91
Rheumatoid arthritis (RA), 50
Ribavirin, trade name and use of, A-136
Rickets, osteomalacia and, 49
Right bundle branch block (RBBB), 79
Right lower quadrant (RLQ), 167, 178
Right upper quadrant (RUQ), 167, 186
Ringworm, 23
Risedronate sodium, trade name and use of, A-137
Risperidone, trade name and use of, A-136
Rivastigmine tartrate, trade name and use of, A-131
RLQ. See Right lower quadrant
Rosiglitazone, trade name and use of, A-132
RSR. See Regular sinus rhythm
Rule of Nines, to calculate burn area, 341
RUQ. See Right upper quadrant

S

Salivary glands, 161
    illustration, 162f
Scales
    illustration, 10f
    lesions, pathophysiology, 11
Scar
    illustration, 10f
    lesions, pathophysiology, 11
Schizophrenia, 241
    symptoms, 242
    treatment, 243
Sclera, 253
Scleroderma, 172
Scrotum, disorders of, 129
Sebaceous glands, 2, 6
Seborrheic dermatitis, 15
Seborrheic keratosis, 24
Secretory phase, 98
Sedation, moderate, 333
Sedative, A-138
"See Also" codes, A-9
"See" codes, A-9
Segmental bronchi, 55
Seizures, 246
Senses
    anatomy and terminology, 253
    combining forms, 256
    pathophysiology, 263
    prefixes, 257
    suffixes, 257
Sensorineural, 268
Sepsis, A-14

Sepsis and severe sepsis
with non-infectious process, A-17
as principal diagnosis, A-15
as secondary diagnosis, A-15
sequencing, A-15
and SIRS with localized infection, A-15
Septa, 75
Septic arthritis, 50
Septic shock, A-16
sepsis and, A-17
sequencing of, A-16
of severe sepsis, A-16
Septicemia, A-14
Service codes, levels of, 324
Sexually transmitted disease (STD), 109
SHG. See Sonohysterogram
Shingles, 22
Sickle cell anemia, 202
Sildenafil, trade name and use of, A-128
Simvastatin, trade name and use of, A-134
Sinuses, paranasal/ accessory, 55
SIRS, cause of injury codes with, A-17
Skeletal divisions, 30
Skeletal muscle, 36, A-138
Skeletal system, 29, 35f
Skeletal traction, 47f
Skeleton
appendicular, 34
axial, 30
Skin
epidermis and dermis, 2
lesions of, 10
tumors of, 24
Skin grafts, split-thickness and full-thickness, 339f
Skin infections, 19
Skin replacement surgery, 339
Skin substitutes, 339
Skin tag removal, 336
Skin traction, strapping in, 48f
Skull, 30
frontal view of, 32
lateral view of, 31f
meninges, and brain, subheading, 371
Skull base, surgery of, 372
Small intestine, 164, 177
Smell, 255
Smooth muscle, 37
Sonohysterogram, 102
Sores, cold, 21
Specific gravity, 144
Spina bifida, 49, 241
Spina bifida occulta, 242f
Spinal cord, 231
brain and, 230f
injury, 248
tumors of, 249, 250
Spinal curvatures, 49
Spinal instrumentation
and fixation, 347
types of, 348
Spine, 32
and spinal cord, subheading, 372
Spironolactone, trade name and use of, A-135
Spleen, 361
Squamous cell carcinoma, 24
Staphylococci, 130

Stasis dermatitis, 14
State License Number, reimbursement terminology, 318
Status indicators (SI), APC payment, 287, 288f
Stem cells, 361
Stenosis, 92
Sternum, 34f
Steroids, A-138
Stomach, 163
disorders, 174
malignant tumor of, 176
Strabismus, 264
Strains, sprains and, 48
Strapping, casting and, 348
Streptococcal sepsis, A-16
Streptococcal septicaemia, A-16
Streptococci, 130
Stress urinary incontinence (SUI), 102
Stroke, 244, A-28
Sudoriferous glands, 2
SUI. See Stress urinary incontinence
Sulfamethoxazole-trimethoprim, trade name and use of, A-130
Sumatriptan, trade name and use of, A-135
Supraventricular tachycardia, 80
Surgery section, 333–374
SVT. See Supraventricular tachycardia (SVT)
Synarthrosis, 36
Syphilis
cause, 110
symptoms, 110
treatment, 111
Systemic inflammatory response syndrome (SIRS), A-14, A-63

T

T. pallidum, 129
T. vaginalis, 129
T1-T12. See Thoracic vertebrae
Tachypnea, 65
Tamoxifen, 112
Tamsulosin HCL, trade name and use of, A-128
Taste, 256
Teeth, 161
Temazepam, trade name and use of, A-138
Temporomandibular joint (TMJ), 43
Tendons, 37
disorders of, 50
Tenofovir, trade name and use of, A-128
TENS. See Transcutaneous electrical nerve stimulation
Terazosin, trade name and use of, A-135
Terbinafine, trade name and use of, A-133
Terconazole, trade name and use of, A-133
Terminology, 97
Terrorism guidelines, A-66
Testes, 123, 213
disorders of, 129
Tetralogy of Fallot, 94
Text resources, further, A-124
Thermoreceptors, 256
Thighbone, 34
Thiothixene, trade name and use of, A-136
Thoracic aorta, endovascular repair of descending, 356
Thoracic cage, 34f
Thoracic vertebrae, 43
Thoracostomy, 81
Thorax, 33

Throat, 163

Thromboangiitis obliterans, 89

Thrombophlebitis, caused by inflammation, 88

Thrombus, 87, 357
 risks related to, 88
 treatment for, 88

Thymus, 213

Thyroid glands, 212, 371
 disorders, 221

Thyrotoxicosis, 221

TIA. *See* Transient ischemic attack

Tiagabine, trade name and use of, A-131

Tibialis anterior, 40

Timolol, trade name and use of, A-133

Tinea, 23

Tinea corporis, 23

Tinea pedis, 23

Tinea unguium, 23

Tissue, subcutaneous, 2

Tissue transfer, adjacent, 338

TLC. *See* Total lung capacity

TM. *See* Tympanic membrane

TMJ. *See* Temporomandibular joint

Tobramycin-dexamethasone, trade name and use of, A-138

Tolmetin, trade name and use of, A-135

Tolterodine tartrate, trade name and use of, A-136

Tongue, dorsum of, 162f

Topiramate, trade name and use of, A-131

Torsion of testes, 131

Total lung capacity (TLC), 60

Touch, 256

Tourette syndrome, 240

Toxic effects, A-44

Trachea
 and bronchi, 352
 opening to, 55

Traction, 344

Tramadol, trade name and use of, A-128

Tramadol-acetaminophen, trade name and use of, A-128

Trandolapril, trade name and use of, A-135

Transcatheter procedures, 360

Transcutaneous electrical nerve stimulation (TENS), 233

Transesophageal echocardiography, 80

Transfusion, 183

Transient ischemia, 85

Transient ischemic attack (TIA), 233, 243

Transmission, 182, 204

Transurethral resection of bladder tumor (TURBT), 124

Transurethral resection of prostate (TURP), 124, 125, 135

Trauma, 248

Traumatic brain injury (TBI), 247

Traumatic cataract, 266f

Travoprost, trade name and use of, A-135

Trazodone, trade name and use of, A-131

Treadmill stress test (TST), 80, 116, 207

Tretinoin, trade name and use of, A-136

Triamcinolone, trade name and use of, A-135, A-138

Triamterene-hydrochlorothiazide, trade name and use of, A-135

Trichomoniasis, 111, 133

Tricuspid, 76

Tricuspid regurgitation (TR), 92

Tricuspid valve, 91

Trimethoprim, trade name and use of, A-130

Trunk, 40

TST. *See* Treadmill stress test

Tuberculosis, 68

Tubular bones, 29

Tumors
 benign, 24
 of brain and spinal cord, 249
 categories, 114
 cranial nerve, 250
 epithelial, 115
 germ cell, 114
 gonadal stromal, 115
 illustration, 10f
 lesions, pathophysiology, 9
 of muscles, 52
 pituitary, 250
 spinal cord, 250

Turbinates, 55

TURBT. *See* Transurethral resection of bladder tumor

TURP. *See* Transurethral resection of prostate

Tympanic membrane (TM), 258

U

U. urealyticum, 132

UA. *See* Urinalysis

UB-04 field locators, 303

Ulcer
 decubitis, 11
 illustration, 10f
 lesions, pathophysiology, 11
 peptic, 175
 pressure, 11

Ulceration, 171

Ulcerative colitis, 180–181, 180f

Uniform hospital discharge data set (UHDDS), 294

"Unspecified" codes, A-8

UPJ. *See* Ureteropelvic junction

Upper respiratory infection (URI), 60, 68

Upper respiratory tract (URT), 55

Ureteropelvic junction (UPJ), 144

Ureters, 142, 364

Urethra, 143
 disorders of, 132

Urethritis, 132–133

URI. *See* Upper respiratory infection

Urinalysis (UA), 144

Urinary bladder, 142

Urinary system, 141
 anatomy and terminology, 141–143
 combining forms, 143
 illustration, 141f
 pathophysiology, 149
 prefixes, 144
 subsection, 363
 suffixes, 144

Urinary tract infection (UTI), 144, 150

Urinary tract obstructions, 154

Urodynamics, 365

Usual, Customary, and Reasonable, reimbursement terminology, 318

Uterine fibroids, 111

Uterine tubes, 97

Utero surgery, A-33

Uterus, 97

UTI. *See* Urinary tract infection

V

V codes, 387
  categories of, A-46
  miscellaneous, A-54
  nonspecific, A-55
  uses of, 387
V27.0, A-34
Vagina, carcinoma of 97, 367
Vaginal birth after cesarean (VBAC), 102
Vaginal delivery, 118
Valacyclovir, trade name and use of, A-136
Valdecoxib, trade name and use of, A-135
Valsartan, trade name and use of, A-135
Valsartan-hydrochlorothiazide, trade name and use of, A-135
Valves, 76
Valvular heart disease, 91
Valvular regurgitation, 92
Variable growth rate, 249
Varicella-zoster virus (VZV), 22
Varicocele, 130–131
Varicose veins, 89
Vas deferens, 123
Vascular dementia, 237
Vascular disorder, 85, 156, 243
Vascular injection procedures, 359
VBAC. *See* Vaginal birth after cesarean
Veins, 74
Venlafaxine HLC, trade name and use of, A-131
Venous reconstruction, 358
Ventilation/perfusion scan, 60
Ventricular fibrillation
  symptoms, 90
  treatment, 90
Ventricular hypertrophy, right, 80
Verapamil, trade name and use of, A-129, A-135
Verruca vulgaris, 22
Verrucae, 22
Vertebra injury, 248
Vertebral column, 231
  anterior view of, 33f
Vertex, 119

Vesical neck, and prostate, 365
Vesicle
  illustration, 10f
  lesions, pathophysiology, 9
Vessels, 73
  brachiocephalic vascular with, 357
  function, 73
  types of, 73
Viral hepatitis, 182
Viral herpes simplex, 21
Visceral muscle, 37
Visual disturbances, 263
Vitamin, A-138
Vitamin D analogs, 16
Voice box, 55
Vulva, carcinoma of 97, 366
Vulvectomy, 367

W

Warfarin, trade name and use of, A-130
Warts, 22–23
Wheal
  illustration, 10f
  lesions, pathophysiology, 9
White cells, 73
Whitmore-Jewett stages, 137
Wilms' tumor, 157
Windpipe, 55
"With" codes, A-9
Womb, 97
Wound exploration, 345
Wound repair
  codes, 338
  grouping of, 338
  repair factors in, 337
  types of, 337

Z

Ziprasidone, trade name and use of, A-136
Zolpidem tartrate, trade name and use of, A-138
Zonisamide, trade name and use of, A-131
Z-plasty, levels of service, 331

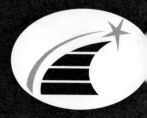

Trust Carol J. Buck and Elsevier for the
resources you need at *each step* of your coding career!

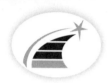
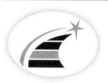
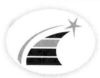

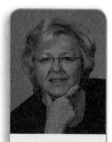